AN INTRODUCTION
TO NURSING RESEARCH

MARY ANNE SWEENEY, R.N., Ph.D.
BOSTON COLLEGE
BOSTON, MASSACHUSETTS

PETER OLIVIERI, Ph.D.
BOSTON COLLEGE
BOSTON, MASSACHUSETTS

AN INTRODUCTION TO NURSING RESEARCH

Research, Measurement, and Computers in Nursing

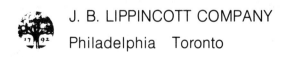
J. B. LIPPINCOTT COMPANY

Philadelphia   Toronto

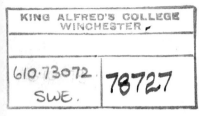
For information address J. B. Lippincott Company, East
Washington Square, Philadelphia, Pennsylvania 19105.

6 5 4 3

Library of Congress Cataloguing in Publication Data
Sweeney, Mary Anne.
   An introduction to nursing research.

   Bibliography
   Includes index.
   1. Nursing—Research. I. Olivieri, Peter, joint au-
thor. II. Title. [DNLM: 1. Nursing. 2. Research WY20.5
S974i]
RT81.5.S95   610.73'072   80-19193
ISBN 0-397-54263-1

The authors and publisher have exerted every effort to ensure that drug selection and dosage set forth in this text
are in accord with current recommendations and practice
at the time of publication. However, in view of ongoing
research, changes in government regulations, and the constant flow of information relating to drug therapy and drug
reactions, the reader is urged to check the package insert for
each drug for any change in indications and dosage and for
added warnings and precautions. This is particularly important when the recommended agent is a new or infrequently
employed drug.

Printed in the United States of America

Contents

Preface

This textbook was designed to provide the undergraduate student with a foundation for the study of nursing-related problems. The authors set out with two major objectives: to provide students with an understanding of the terminology and concepts necessary to effectively read research publications, and to demonstrate some of the steps of the research process. This book is unique in that it combines aspects of the three fields of nursing, statistics and computer science. This helps to provide a rounded picture of the scientific process within a particular discipline such as nursing. The authors' approach has been to write for the student who has had no previous background of study in these specific research-related disciplines.

The practitioners of both the present and future need to be familiar with the basic terminology and concepts of the scientific method in order to comprehend and incorporate research findings into their nursing practice. An ability to read, interpret, and integrate research information with clinical skills will be developed through an understanding of the information presented in the chapters of the text.

ORGANIZATION OF THE CONTENT

The text has been divided into six parts. Each part was constructed with different objectives in mind. This organization was set up to provide the reader with a logical grouping of ideas that have common themes that will help the learner integrate the key concepts of the text. A brief summary of the intended focus of each section of the book and the corresponding chapters follows:

PART I: FOUNDATIONS OF RESEARCH IN NURSING
    Part I contains four chapters that give the background of the research process with a nursing perspective.
    CHAPTER 1: RESEARCH AND THE NURSING PROCESS
            Objectives: (1) To review the historical development of research within the nursing profession
            (2) To provide students with an understanding of the current status of research in nursing
    CHAPTER 2: LEARNING RESEARCH LANGUAGE
            Objective: To introduce the basic terminology used in research publications
    CHAPTER 3: THE RESEARCH PROCESS
            Objective: To describe the steps involved in conducting the research process within a profession
    CHAPTER 4: READING AND CRITIQUING RESEARCH STUDIES
            Objectives: (1) To introduce the student to an actual research report
            (2) To identify the types of information needed to begin to critque a study

PART II: BEGINNING RESEARCH SKILLS
    Part II covers the more specific aspects involved in initiating an actual research project. The chapters present much of the information that is necessary for writing a study proposal.

    CHAPTER 5: STARTING TO DEVELOP THE RESEARCH PROBLEM
            Objectives: (1) To understand how nursing problems are identified by researchers
            (2) To introduce students to locating, utilizing, and writing up the literature related to a research topic
            (3) To be aware of the role of theory in the planning of research
    CHAPTER 6: DIFFERENT APPROACHES TO CONDUCTING RESEARCH
            Objective: (1) To develop an awareness of the varied ways in which research can be conducted

CHAPTER 7: IDENTIFYING HYPOTHESES AND SELECTING A SAMPLE
> Objective: To point out major factors that should be defined and explained in a study

PART III: GATHERING INFORMATION

Part III introduces the factors that must be considered by researchers when setting out to collect information from the subjects they are hoping to get answers from. It moves from the discussion of some generalized issues such as the ethical aspects of data collection, to the more practical aspects of what type of data collection instrument ought to be used.

CHAPTER 8: COLLECTING DATA: PLANS AND PROCEDURES
> Objectives: (1) To make students more aware of the importance of ethical and legal considerations when collecting data
>
> (2) To introduce the different kinds of data that might be useful in performing research
>
> (3) To present different techniques for collecting information

CHAPTER 9: SELECTING AND USING EXISTING INSTRUMENTS
> Objectives: (1) To make students more aware of the types and locations of the different data collection instruments that are available
>
> (2) To provide students with some criteria for selecting the most appropriate type of instrument for their studies

CHAPTER 10: DESIGNING YOUR OWN INSTRUMENT
> Objectives: (1) To provide students with a detailed description of how to design their own data collection instruments
>
> (2) To provide guidelines concerning what to do with the data after the instruments have been completed

PART IV: INTERPRETING INFORMATION

In order to make meaningful comments about the data that one has collected, it is necessary to analyze this information. The chapters in this part describe the ways in which data may be summarized and presented. In addition, an introduction to some of the techniques of statistical analysis is presented.

CHAPTER 11: AN INTRODUCTION TO DESCRIPTIVE STATISTICS
> Objective: To introduce students to terms used to describe data (the mean, the median, and frequency distributions)

CHAPTER 12: USING STATISTICS TO MAKE DECISIONS
> Objectives: (1) To provide students with some facility for using statistical techniques for comparing different groups
>
> (2) To provide students with a method for making estimates based on data that may be available

CHAPTER 13: PRESENTING INFORMATION IN GRAPHS AND TABLES
> Objectives: (1) To make students comfortable with finding, analyzing and interpreting information in graphs and tables
>
> (2) To provide students with the proper technique for constructing graphs and tables for their own use

PART V: USING THE COMPUTER

The computer is a powerful tool that will continue to have an influence on us for many years to come. The chapters in this part introduce some of the applications of computers in the field of nursing. Furthermore, the reader is introduced to the computer in a way that will encourage its use.

CHAPTER 14: APPLICATIONS OF COMPUTERS IN THE HEALTH PROFESSIONS
> Objective: To provide students with an overview and examples of the many applications of the computer in health-related professions

CHAPTER 15: TAKING A TOUR OF THE COMPUTER CENTER FACILITIES
> Objective: To introduce students to what a computer facility looks like and the different kinds of "computers" they may encounter in their careers

CHAPTER 16: USING THE COMPUTER AS AN AID TO RESEARCH
> Objectives: (1) To make students comfortable with using the computer as a tool in their academic or professional activities
>
> (2) To explain to students the ways in which they may use the computer

(3) To introduce students to writing simple instructions to get the computer to solve a problem
(4) To give students some facility with using computer programs written by others

CHAPTER 17: FINDING OUT WHAT COMPUTER RESOURCES
ARE AVAILABLE TO YOU
Objective: To provide students with a checklist of questions
to make it easier for them to find out about and
utilize available computer resources

PART VI: COMMUNICATING RESEARCH RESULTS
Research cannot be effective if the results are not communicated well.
In addition to providing guidance on this very point, this part presents, in
detail, an actual research study conducted by nursing students. Finally,
some suggestions for staying active in research are presented.

CHAPTER 18: ANALYZING AND INTERPRETING RESEARCH RE-
SULTS
Objective: To explain how to organize and review study results so that appropriate conclusions can be drawn
from them

CHAPTER 19: A DESCRIPTIVE STUDY OF AND BY UNDERGRAD-
UATE NURSING STUDENTS
Objective: To provide students with an example demonstrating the integration of the research, measurement,
and computer concepts covered in the text. This
section highlights some of the principles and
techniques utilized by undergraduate students in
carrying out an actual classroom assignment.

CHAPTER 20: GETTING ACTIVELY INVOLVED IN RESEARCH
Objective: To present a plan for active involvement in future
research endeavors

All of the sections of the book contain "Commentaries" on interesting
or humorous side-lights related to the chapter material. These commentaries
add a distinct flavor to the presentation of material in conjunction with the
pictures and other graphic devices used throughout.

The appendices supply various types of information such as outlines
for writing up research reports, suggestions for topics, bibliographies, varied
reference materials, statistical tables and answers to problems interspersed
throughout the text.

Many sources are given for continuing the learning process and for obtaining additional materials and information.

The authors recognize that nursing research, statistics, and computer science are indeed worthy of courses in and of themselves. And yet, all are significantly interrelated and necessary for a text dealing with the research process. Consequently, the authors have developed a modular approach to presenting the material so that it can be adapted to a variety of curriculum designs. It is important to note that the textbook is not intended to prepare nurses as statisticians or computer programmers. Each of these disciplines is approached from the viewpoint of the "user" rather than the theoretician.

ACKNOWLEDGMENTS

The effort to put together a substantative book on a topic as comprehensive as this involves the help and cooperation of many people.

The Advanced Clinical-Research Team at the Boston College School of Nursing was most helpful and supportive. Marion Heath, Marguerite O'Malley, Mary Ann Corcoran, Joyce Dwyer, Pauline Sampson, Jill Bloom, Cindy Doctoroff, Ronna Krozy, Ellen Freeman, and Barbara Hedstrom helped us often and without recognition.

Our sincere thanks to Mary Pekarski, Mary Ann Garrigan, and Marilyn Grant for their indispensible support and assistance. Our thanks also to Mary Dineen, Doris Schneller, Eileen Broderick, Jim English, Jeffery Johnson, Helen Manock, Donald McHugh, Patricia Regan, and Rita Olivieri.

Without Terri Quinton, Linda Dunn and Stephanie O'Leary, the manuscript would never have been typed. And finally, a special note of thanks to Karen Hoxeng and the staff at Lippincott.

Mary Anne Sweeney, R.N., Ph.D.
Peter Olivieri, Ph.D.

AN INTRODUCTION
TO NURSING RESEARCH

PART

I

Foundations of Research

The first part of this book has been organized to help the reader become more familiar with important background information about research. This kind of information is necessary in order to recognize what research is all about, to see how it relates to the nursing profession, and to understand some of the terminology and concepts that are common to most studies. In other words, the introductory chapters seek to dispel some of the normal apprehensions that occur whenever the word "research" is uttered. It is important to see research as a useful tool that can be utilized to enhance professional nursing practice by reading published study reports, cooperating with various phases of the projects of others, or actually planning and conducting a small study on one's own. The authors have long noted that the attitude of the neophyte researcher is a strategic factor in influencing the amount of time and effort one is willing to invest in learning about the research process. So read on! Research involves discipline, that's true, but it can also be exciting, interesting, and rewarding.

Part I contains three chapters that present background information about the research process and its relationship to nursing, and concludes with a reprint of a published study in the fourth chapter. This particular research study was conducted to gather information about the attitudes of undergraduate nursing students. This initial part of the book was written with the intention of providing a beginning framework for utilizing research information and as preparation for understanding the more technical aspects of the process that are covered in the later sections of the text.

CHAPTER

1

Research and the Nursing Profession

THE HISTORICAL DEVELOPMENT OF RESEARCH IN THE NURSING PROFESSION

It is surprising to most nurses to learn that the origins of nursing research can be traced to the nineteenth century. In fact, the first nurse to attempt to use facets of the research process as a basis for giving nursing care was a familiar figure in history, Florence Nightingale. This noted scholar sought to increase the clinically based level of knowledge of patient care by searching for factors that were related to varying recovery, morbidity, and mortality rates. She often noted the lack of accurately recorded health-related statistics as evidenced by the statement she made in 1859:

> The organization of a Statistical Department (of the Army Medical Department) has proved to be essentially necessary for the public service, by the simple fact that, during the first year of the Russian war, there was hardly a single trustworthy statistical return produced. Besides, statistics have never yet been applied to the solution of problems connected with the health and efficiency of the army.[1]

After her return from the Crimea, Miss Nightingale devoted much of her time to publicizing the lack of adequate health and medical facilities for the British soldier, utilizing statistics to clearly illustrate her case. She worked zealously to produce a report for Parliament entitled *Contribution to the Sanitary History of the British Army* that outlined various aspects of health problems and suggested reforms. Miss Nightingale was an avid collector of information through the use of interviews, questionnaires, and previously existing records. She was talented in handling numbers and in devising charts and graphs to demonstrate the relationship of the numbers to each other. The diagrams in Figure 1.1 were produced by Florence Nightingale to show the comparison of the relative mortality rate of males in Manchester, England with that of the British army in the Crimea between 1854 and 1856. This clever visual use of numbers dramatizes the situation and allows for rapid comparisons of varied types of information. Each wedge illustrates the mortality rate per thousand for each separate month, and thus enables the reader to compare the death rate of each month with those of the others, while at the same time comparing it with the death rate in the city of Manchester. This illustrative device also permits the reader to see the pattern for the entire two years at one glance.

Miss Nightingale wrote the following commentary to accompany the diagrams:

> *The Diagram of the Mortality of the Army* in the East consists of two parts, 1 and 2. Beginning with No. 1, the first monthly wedge of the mortality is that for April, 1854, about the middle of which month the British army arrived at Gallipoli, in good health. It went to Bulgaria in June. The three small wedges for April, May, and June show what comparative mortality was for the first quarter of the campaign. The dotted circle represents what the mortality would have been for the whole year if the army has been as healthy as men of the army ages are in Manchester, which is one of the most unhealthy towns in England. It will be seen that the average mortality for the first quarter was less than that of Manches-

DIAGRAMS OF THE CAUSES OF MORTALITY
IN THE ARMY IN THE EAST.

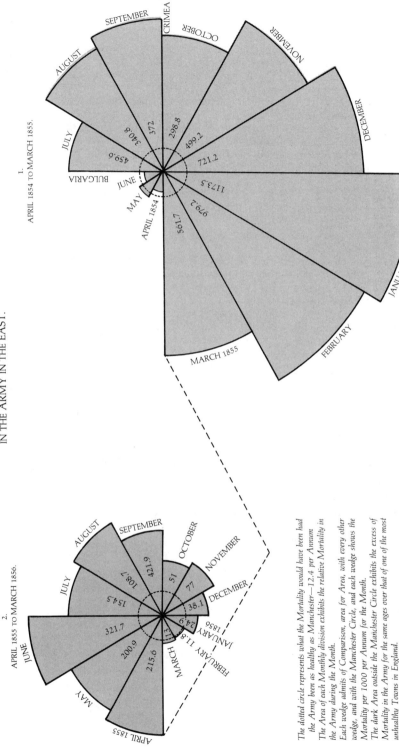

1.
APRIL 1854 TO MARCH 1855.

2.
APRIL 1855 TO MARCH 1856.

The dotted circle represents what the Mortality would have been had the Army been as healthy as Manchester—12.4 per Annum
The Area of each Monthly division exhibits the relative Mortality in the Army during the Month.
Each wedge admits of Comparison, area for Area, with every other wedge, and with the Manchester Circle, and each wedge shows the Mortality per 1000 per Annum for the Month.
The dark Area outside the Manchester Circle exhibits the excess of Mortality in the Army for the same ages over that of one of the most unhealthy Towns in England.
The figures show the Mortality per 1000 per Annum.

ter. The army was in Bulgaria in June, July, August, and during the first half of September. It will be observed that during this period the mortality rises immensely, far beyond, in fact, what it ever attains in Manchester.

The army landed in the Crimea on September 14, and sat down before Sevastopol in the beginning of October. During that month the health of the army improved, but the mortality was still enormous. It went on increasing in November, December, until January 1855, it exceeded the proportionate mortality from the Great Plague of London. It was very high in February, but declined in March and April. In May, 1855, (Diagram 2) Cholera appeared in its epidemic form, augmenting the mortality in June. The mortality thereafter subsided, month by month until March, 1856, it had very nearly returned with in the Manchester circle, which it did entirely in April, May, and June of that year; so that the army left the Crimea for England in a more healthy state and with a lower amount of mortality than it had when it set foot in the East, or, indeed, than it ever had before when stationed at home.

The first question which presents itself is—What can have been the cause of this? Health is known to depend on the observance of certain laws. Surely, before a picked body of men in the prime of life could have been cut off by a mortality greater perhaps than that of any pestilence on record, there must have been some very glaring disobedience to have these laws.[2]

The diagram in Figure 1.2 was constructed in a similar manner to illustrate the *causes* of the previously visualized rate of mortality in the Crimea during the same two-year period. Nightingale was an advocate of preventative health measures and used this device to show the tremendous loss of life caused by preventible diseases rather than by the actual wounds and ravages of war.

The famous nurse had done her work well—urging doctors, government officials, and members of Parliament to heed the importance of keeping accurate patient records. It is amazing to look at a report written almost a century and a quarter ago and see terms we tend to think of as modern ways of expressing numbers. The analysis of the numbers of sick and wounded in the hospitals of the Crimea for a nine-month period in 1854 through 1855 includes such headings as "percents per annum" and the "mean of Admissions and Discharges" as can be seen in Table 1.1. Miss Nightingale used some of the information on the mortality rate from the table to prepare the Diagram Representing the Mortality in the Hospitals at Scutari and Kululi. The percentage of cases treated (the far right-hand column in Table 1.1) was used to determine the numbers in the wedges of the diagram in Figure 1.3. More than a century ago, Miss Nightingale anticipated and clearly communicated the need for measuring outcomes of both medical and nursing

DIAGRAMS OF THE MORTALITY
IN THE ARMY IN THE EAST.

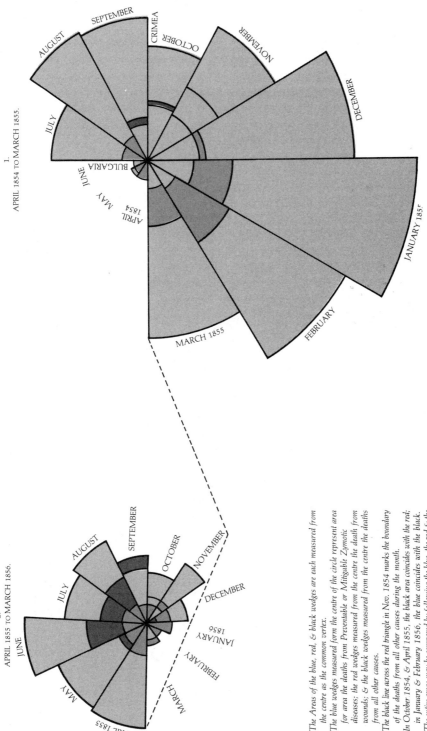

2.
APRIL 1855 TO MARCH 1856.

1.
APRIL 1854 TO MARCH 1855.

The Areas of the blue, red, & black wedges are each measured from
the centre as the common vertex.

The blue wedges measured form the centre of the circle represent area
for area the deaths from Preventable or Mitigable Zymotic
diseases; the red wedges measured from the centre the death from
wounds; & the black wedges measured from the centre the deaths
from all other causes.

The black line across the red triangle in Nov. 1854 marks the boundary
of the deaths from all other causes during the month.

In October 1854, & April 1855, the black area coincides with the red;
in January & February 1856, the blue coincides with the black.

The entire areas may be compared by following the blue, the red & the
black lines enclosing them.

Table 1.1

Analysis of the Weekly States of Sick and Wounded, from October 1, 1854, to June 30, 1855, in the Hospitals of the Bosphorus

Date	No. of Days	Sick Population of the Hospitals (Mean of Weekly Numbers Remaining)	Cases Treated (Mean of Admissions and Discharges Including Deaths)	Deaths	Mortality: Rate Percent per Annum on Sick Population	Percent on Cases Treated
1854						
Scutari						
Oct. 1–Oct. 14	14	1,993	590	113	148	19.2
Oct. 15–Nov. 11	28	2,229	2,043	173	101	8.5
Nov. 12–Dec. 9	28	3,258	1,944	301	121	15.5
1854–1855						
Scutari and Kululi						
Dec. 10 to Jan. 6, 1855	28	3,701	3,194	572	202	17.9
Jan. 7–Jan. 31	25	4,520	3,072	986	319	32.1
Feb. 1–Feb. 28	28	4,178	3,112	1,392	415	42.7
Kululi						
Feb. 1–Feb. 28	28	648	581	302	608	52.0
Scutari and Kululi						
Feb. 25–Mar. 17	21	3,779	1,621	510	235	31.5
Mar. 18–Apr. 7	21	3,306	1,650	237	125	14.4
Apr. 8–Apr. 28	21	2,803	1,190	127	79	10.7
Apr. 29–May 19	21	2,018	1,350	70	60	5.2
May 20–June 9	21	1,504	996	48	56	4.8
June 10–June 30	21	1,442	1,266	28	34	2.2

Source: F. Nightingale (attr.): A Contribution to the Sanitary History of the British Army During the Late War with Russia. London, J. W. Parker, 1859.

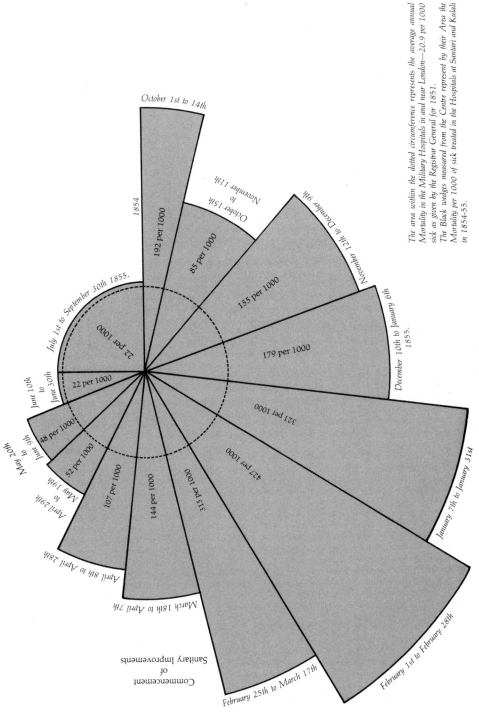

The area within the dotted circumference represents the average annual Mortality in the Military Hospitals in and near London—20.9 per 1000 sick as given by the Registrar General for 1851.
The Black wedges measured from the Centre represent by their Area the Mortality per 1000 of sick treated in the Hospitals at Santari and Kulali in 1854-55.

Figure 1.3. Diagram representing the mortality in the hospitals at Scutari and Kulali from October 1, 1854 to September 30, 1855. (Source: F. Nightingale (attr.): A Contribution to the Sanitary History of the British Army During the Late War with Russia. London, J. W. Parker, 1859).

care, a popular topic in the health-related journals of today.[3] It is interesting to note that many of the areas in need of further study mentioned by Miss Nightingale (such as environmental health hazards and communicable disease control) have been the focus of investigations within the past few years.

Commentary 1.1
Nightingale the Researcher

Florence Nightingale was the only person in England to emerge from the Crimean War with a professional reputation enhanced. Her historical role in the nineteenth century has assumed such great importance that she has been proclaimed to stand with Lister and Simpson for the magnitude of their work for the welfare of mankind. This unique role for a female of Victorian England has been created largely through her research endeavors. Dr. Irene Palmer, a Nightingale authority, notes that research involvement was a natural outgrowth of Miss Nightingale's keen intellect, multiple interests, and the following qualities:

· insatiable curiosity
· command of her subject
· familiarity with methods of inquiry
· good background in statistics
· ability to discriminate and abstract
· attention to detail
· expressive communication skills
· ability to record and codify observations

The following excerpt describes the influence of the famed nurse's research techniques on the medical field:

> Nightingale had a fantastic ability to codify her observations in a systematic way that made them useful to others. Story has it that she and John Snow were colleagues in the London Cholera epidemic of August 1854, and that the records Nightingale maintained on the origins of the victims helped Snow pinpoint the role of The Broad Street pump.

Miss Nightingale is perhaps best known for her irrefutable studies of the health status of the British Army at home, in the Crimea, and in India. She designed questionnaires, analyzed results, and presented conclusions which provided the basis for tremendous corrective reforms in health care.

> [In the course of investigating health care] in civilian hospitals, she had the extraordinary vision to propose a system of hospital record keeping and disease nomenclature. Although not adopted because of the expense involved, the Nightingale influence of a century ago can be seen in the standard nomenclature and system used internationally today.
>
> This nurse researcher utilized historical, explanatory, descriptive, comparative, and field methods in her investigative work.
>
> I. Palmer: Florence Nightingale: reformer, reactionary, researcher. Nursing Research 26, 2 (March–April, 1977): 84–89.

The direction of research efforts in the nursing profession has come full circle since those early days of concern with patient care problems and has, after many years of educationally oriented investigations, recently refocused on clinically based problems.

There is very little evidence of serious research endeavors during the formative years of nursing. The primary focus during the first half of the twentieth century was clearly on nursing education and the push to institute reforms. Nursing leaders (including M. Adelaide Nutting, Annie W. Goodrich, and Isabel M. Stewart) contended that nursing needed to break free from the hospital-based system and move into a college or university setting. They joined with prominent observers from outside the profession who called for the establishment of a solid theoretical foundation for nursing. Until the early 1920s, the profession had been concerned with increasing the quantity of nurses and establishing additional hospital-affiliated schools.

Commentary 1.2
The Beginning of Research in Nursing

A paper was recently prepared by M. Elizabeth Carnegie, Ed.D., to trace the historical development of research in the nursing profession. The early development of research was outlined as follows:

BEFORE 1900

Virtually nothing in the research area was recorded in the literature before the turn of the century. Linda Richards, reputed to be America's first trained nurse, began keeping complete written records at Bellevue which had been done sporadically before that time. This was one of many examples of nurses assisting medical authorities in collecting data. Nurses shared in the scientific investigations of the medical profession but conducted none on their own. Perhaps one reason was recorded in the *Diary of a Pupil Nurse, 1909:* "To say that any tendency to experiment and find another, perhaps better, way of doing things is distinctly discouraged is putting it mildly."

1900–1909

Five articles appeared in the literature (all written by nurses with a physician as co-author of one) which were based on studies. Topics varied from a study of care of Visiting Nurses for 500 cases of pneumonia (including statistics) to a study of morbidity and mortality due to unclean milk, to a study of the economic use of surgical supplies.

Other significant research reported during this period included:

"The Education and Professional Position of Nurses" (Nutting, 1907) was the earliest study of nursing education by an American nurse.

History of Nursing (Nutting and Dock, 1907) chronicling the milestones of nursing in two volumes.

Visiting Nursing in the United States (Walters, 1909) which was a survey sponsored by the American Nurses' Association.

1910–1919

A handful of articles based on studies were published by nurses. Most were concerned with procedures, equipment or supplies. Nurses agreed that educational standards were in need of upgrading and standardization. The Rockefeller Foundation offered support to Winslow and Goldmark for a firsthand study of nursing schools. The sample included nurses who were teachers and administrators of 23 schools, 49 public health agencies, and some private duty nurses. This was the beginning of the famed report *Nursing and Nursing Education in the United States* that was published in 1923. This was also the beginning of a far-reaching trend in nursing research: the entrance of non-nursing influence in terms of economic support and investigative personnel.

E. Carnegie: Historical Perspectives of Nursing Research. Nursing Archive, Special Collections, Boston University Libraries, 1976.

Between 1920 and 1950, large-scale studies were undertaken to investigate the quality of the learning process through which nurses were trained, as well as the type of work they became involved in after graduation. The Winslow-Goldmark Report of 1923 (Committee for the Study of Nursing Education) forcefully recommended the reorganization of nursing education and the movement into university settings. This study, which was initiated by the Rockefeller Foundation, was a force in encouraging the establishment of the early collegiate nursing schools, such as those at Yale and Western Reserve. Although only 2 percent of the basic nursing schools (27 of the 1,383 schools) were in university settings by the mid-1930s, the number of collegiate programs expanded to a total of 138 by the mid-1940s.[4]

Another large-scale study of nursing was organized during this time and was supported by the Russell Sage Foundation. Esther Lucille Brown, a noted sociologist, was the main investigator and published her report in *Nursing for the Future* in 1948. In her study, Dr. Brown attempted to answer two questions that she had heard frequently raised about nursing: (1) Can nursing develop a specific content of its own, thus establishing a larger claim to professionalism? and, (2) Will nurse educators ever engage in any considerable amount of research and writing that for some universities is the hallmark of the right to be included within the fraternity of higher education? The "Brown Report" (as the book was popularly called) provided an updated description of nursing practice and echoed the earlier studies in strongly recommending research development within nursing, as well as movement of the educational process into a university milieu.[5] Thus, this period of nursing history was characterized by the lack of a cohesive thrust regarding the level of education and the kind of preparation necessary for nursing practice. Although some leaders in the profession looked forward to strengthening the academic aspects of nurse preparation, the main body of the profession was divided on this issue. Assistance with this problem in the form of funding, providing the expertise to conduct studies about the profession, and the formulation of recommendations about the future education of nurses, came largely from non-nursing sources. Although a number of educational leaders within nursing recognized that nursing required a body of theoretical knowledge solely its own in order to attain professional status, the majority of nurses did not acknowledge this necessity for theoretical development. Finally, a decided trend toward conducting nursing education in university-based settings started to take shape in the early 1950s. The concurrent move toward recognition of the need for the development of an organized nursing theory by means of scientific research gained similar momentum.

It is important to note that the university-based location for nursing education provided a number of opportunities for nurses that were simply unavailable in a hospital-based environment. The university provided students with a broader, as well as a more in-depth, experience with liberal arts and basic sciences. Faculty were able to work closely with university colleagues from a variety of fields while located in a setting where advanced study, research, and publication were considered an important part of a teacher's role. Resources, such as university libraries, media centers, computer and statistical laboratories, consultation, and grants for funding research, were all more accessible on the campus.

By mid-century, The American Nurses' Association and the National League for Nursing both strongly recognized the need for research in all

Commentary 1.3
The Eye of the Beholder

In writing about our nursing heritage, Lucie Young Kelly summarizes the results of a number of studies conducted from the 1930s through the 1950s that describe how nurses see themselves, as well as how others see them.

Nurses generally were satisfied with their choice of a profession which they viewed as one requiring obedience to orders, exactness, and little intellectual stimulation. They felt unappreciated by the public and worried about being considered "faster" in sexual matters than other women.

Physicians could agree on little about nurses except that they did not spend enough time at the bedside, and they wanted the prestige of a professional and the hours of organized laborers. On a questionnaire designed to determine how they viewed the moral status of nurses (from saint to "loose woman") most remained noncommittal and checked the neutral category.

The public view of nurses varied according to social class:

1. The upper-class perspective—A skilled menial.
2. The middle-class perspective—Semiskilled or skilled individual who works a while before marriage or is widowed or divorced.
3. The lower-class perspective—A noble profession allowing a girl to make a good marriage and use her knowledge for the benefit of her husband and children.

The public was in agreement about one thing, since all levels did have serious questions about nurses' morality.

L. Kelly: Our Nursing Heritage: Have We Renounced It? Image 8, 3 (October, 1976): 43–48.

aspects of nursing. In 1955, the Commonwealth Fund donated a gift to the National League for Nursing that was to be used to support candidates for research training and education. The American Nurses' Foundation was established at about the same time as the research branch of the American Nurses' Association. This foundation sponsors and supports nursing research investigations through the allocation of grants. The U.S. Public Health Service joined the two nursing organizations by establishing the Nursing Grants and Fellowship Program in 1955. This action, in effect, made public funding available for research investigations and research training for nurses. The initiation of these three different kinds of support for research in nursing has had a profound, although little recognized, effect on the entire profession. Even though monetary support for nursing investigations has steadily increased over the past quarter of a century, it is still below the level necessary for adequate research activity. For instance, in fiscal 1972, less than $4,000,000 was allocated to research in nursing by governmental agencies, and this amount included traineeships for the education of advanced research students. In contrast, more than $40,000,000 was provided for medical research.[6] The problem exists in a similar proportion today.

The funding for research projects that became available in the mid-1950s did not provide the solution to the research dilemma in nursing. The available research support was not in great demand because nurses lacked the educational preparation necessary for conducting research. Many professionals felt that a graduate degree with specific coursework in research and related disciplines was a necessary prerequisite to receiving funding for research investigations. Thus, the relationship between nursing education and research in nursing has been a close one. The paucity of candidates seeking admission to graduate programs in nursing during the mid- and late-1950s was related to the fact that there were insufficient numbers of nurses prepared at the baccalaureate level. Although the number of students enrolled in college-based programs has been steadily increasing, less than 2 percent of the employed professional nurses held masters' degrees by 1960 and less than 7 percent held baccalaureate degrees.[7]

Two fairly recent studies of the nursing profession have once again highlighted the dual themes of the need for advancement in the educational preparation for nurses and the need for more research. In 1961, the Surgeon General's Consultant Group on Nursing reported statistics on the continued lack of nurses with advanced degrees. This finding was a major factor in obtaining increased government scholarship funding for the education of nurses. Much of the progress which has been made to date can be attributed to the availability of money for educational assistance. The most up-to-date nationwide study about the nursing profession was conducted jointly under the auspices of the American Nurses' Association, the National League for

Nursing, and several private foundations. This National Commission for the Study of Nursing and Nursing Education was directed by a social scientist, and the results have become popularly known by his name—The Lysaught Report. At the conclusion of the three-year study, the Commission presented recommendations for implementing change in nursing in terms of four priorities for action. The first and second recommendations to the profession involved research and were stated as follows:

1. Increase research into the practice of nursing and the education of nurses;
2. Improve educational systems and curricula based on the results of that research.[8]

The past has been characterized by research in nursing which has been largely conducted by non-nursing professionals. Studies have, for the most part, been supported and funded by non-nursing groups. Study highlights have consistently dealt with educational issues and have documented the lack of organized research activity and the lack of theoretical foundations for nursing practice. There are bright spots as well. National organizations in nursing are becoming more vocal about research, funding for research is becoming more available, more nursing groups (such as Sigma Theta Tau, the National Honor Society of nursing) clearly place a value on research in nursing. The nursing profession has now concluded its first century of existence and has reached a point where it can look forward to future progress in the development and utilization of research.

TRENDS IN RESEARCH EDUCATION

The educational preparation of nurses for research and research-related courses is quite variable. Prior to the early 1970s, there was an inconsistent pattern of including research courses in various curricula. Most graduate programs and some baccalaureate programs required students to study and undertake some form of research. Exposure to research in other types of nursing educational programs was sporadic. In response to this unstructured situation, in 1972, the National League for Nursing issued a formal statement which suggested that various nursing programs (including graduate, baccalaureate, diploma, associate degree, continuing education, and practical nursing programs) should offer students the opportunity to learn about research. This organization suggested that students should learn to interpret research, to learn its methods and significance, to be able to assess the findings, and to adapt those that have value into their everyday patient care.[9]

Educators have the task of determining the placement and content of research in each type of program.

The National League for Nursing, the major accrediting agency for nusing educational programs, has strongly recommended that baccalaureate

Commentary 1.4
A Sequential Plan for Learning About Research in Nursing

A planned sequence of research courses will provide for better learning experiences and increased mobility for nurses throughout the educational process. Nurses who are responsible for curriculum planning should work now to organize levels of research skills to enhance the differentiation between educational levels.

BACCALAUREATE LEVEL COURSES

Focus on research process rather than finding answers to major questions or problems. Concurrent theory and practical application of process. "Actual practice in conducting each step of the research process is as important as it is for clinical courses." Develop understanding through group analysis of simple research reports. An introductory course should be offered in the first or second year of the baccalaureate program. A second study may be built into one of the regular clinical courses. Students in associate degree and diploma programs should have an introductory research course. Prepares nurses to participate in ongoing research in clinical facilities with more understanding of their role.

MASTERS' LEVEL COURSES

Sophisticated presentation of the research process and research methodology. (Students enrolling in masters' programs who have not had an introductory level course should be required to take additional coursework.) Selection of more difficult nursing problems for study. Completion of a research project. More emphasis on obtaining meaningful results. Current research critiqued with depth by each student in written format. Prepares the nurse to assist in a major research project.

DOCTORAL LEVEL COURSES

Sophisticated, in-depth, course work. Individual design and completion of a research project. Discriminating analysis of published research. Prepares the nurse to design and conduct a major research project.

E. Treece: Articulation between courses in nursing research: the need and the process. International Nursing Review 24, 1 (January–February 1977): 11–14.

programs provide research experiences for nursing students, and seeks to assess the research-related aspects of the curriculum when conducting program reviews. The Commission on Nursing Research of the American Nurses' Association issued an official statement on recommended education in research that was published in 1976 in a pamphlet entitled *Preparation of Nurses for Participation in Research*. The Commission divided the areas of educational preparation into three categories: undergraduate education, graduate education, and continuing education. The specific recommendations for study at each of these three levels are as follows.[10]

Preparation for Research Within Undergraduate Education

An attitude of inquiry and an introduction to research should be initiated in the early phases of undergraduate education. A climate should be fostered in which the findings of research are sought and utilized in the provision of patient care. In addition to providing the nurse with a fund of usable scientific knowledge, undergraduate education should include both an introduction to and a beginning experience in the research process.

On the undergraduate level, education for research should prepare the nurse to read research critically and to determine its value to practice. It should also provide an understanding of the rights and responsibilities of participants in research as well as of the rights of subjects.

The preparation of nurse researchers involves supervised activities in an investigative program including observation of and participation in all phases of research, from the definition of a researchable problem through the dissemination and utilization of findings. This preparation must include participation in theory building and conceptualization, acquisition of investigative skills, experience in data reduction and analysis, practice in interpretation of results, competence in writing of research findings, and consideration of all aspects of the research experience.

The following topics are often covered:
A. The nature of inquiry
    1. Logic and the reasoning process
    2. Development of knowledge
    3. Significance of the research question
    4. Importance of theories in science
B. Introduction to research ethics
    1. Ethical issues in research
    2. Protection of human and animal subjects
    3. Place of boards of review
    4. Behaviors of researchers
C. Introduction to the research process
    1. Establishment of the knowledge base
    2. Identification of scientific methodology
    3. Identification and appropriate utilization of related resources
    4. Elements of critique
D. Introduction to research methodology
    1. Evolving or formulating a conceptual framework including statement of rationale
    2. Developing a problem statement
    3. Defining and operationalizing variables
    4. Development of methods or tools
    5. Development of a disciplined approach to data collection and processing
    6. Understanding of reliability and validity
    7. Interpretation of findings
    8. Interrelationship of design, analysis, and interpretation
    9. Dissemination of new knowledge
E. Utilization of research findings
    1. Necessary or sufficient conditions for generalization
    2. Recognition of other conditions where findings are not applicable
    3. Communication of results of utilization

Preparation for Research Within Graduate Education

Research education for the graduate student builds upon a previously gained background of knowledge, assumes development of an advanced knowledge base, and includes advanced study of methods in research. Graduate education emphasizes experience in the conduct of research under direction of an experienced precepter. It promotes an acceptance of the obligation to conduct, disseminate and apply research.

The following topics are often covered:
A. Philosophy of research
    1. Philosophy of science
    2. Utilization of inductive and deductive logic
    3. Human rights and ethics

       4.   Ethics of collaboration
       5.   Theory development and relation to research
  B. Conduct of research
       1.   Development of an advanced knowledge base and use of information retrieval systems
       2.   Design and implementation of research
       3.   Importance of replication
       4.   Entree into research settings
       5.   Development of methods or tools
       6.   Reduction, analysis, and presentation of data
       7.   Interpretation and significance of findings
  C. Advanced research methodology
       1.   Development and critique of design models appropriate to the question
       2.   Sampling techniques
       3.   Measurement and advanced statistics
       4.   Use of the computer in analysis
       5.   Depth in the art of critique
  D. Dissemination of findings
       1.   Professional writing/speaking
       2.   Application of findings

Preparation for Research Within Continuing Education

Continuing education toward the advancement of research in nursing is important in view of the rapidly changing knowledge base and the continued development of new methodology. Continuing education relevant to research must take several forms. Offerings of subject matter analogous to those listed above for undergraduate and graduate education should provide the opportunity for nurses to update their skills in research and to be introduced to the research process. Programs should be developed for nurse educators, nursing service administrators, and nurse practitioners, which will encourage improved climates supportive of open inquiry by nurse researchers and the furtherance of research in patient care.

Through sound programs of continuing education—including symposia, colloquia, and seminars as well as formal education—active nurse researchers will be able to extend their knowledge, improve their understanding of the substantive base of research, and incorporate new concepts and methods in research. The practitioner will be better prepared to function as a participant in and implementor of nursing research and its findings and to assess nursing interventions and patient outcomes within a research framework. The administrator will have an expanded information base for decision making related to the support and implementation of research studies and findings.

Excerpts Reprinted with permission of American Nurses Association, Kansas City, Missouri.

The recommendations of both the National League for Nursing and the Commission on Research of the American Nurses' Association deal with the present and future status of research-related education. The inclusion of the category of study labeled "continuing education" points up a partial solution to the present-day research dilemma in nursing. The vast majority of nurses practicing at this point have had minimal exposure to research-related coursework or experience in the course of their educational programs. Plans for "continuing education" programs in research and related subject areas, when coupled with a fairly standardized experience for new students in the profession, will be likely to produce results at a faster pace.

There is no set minimum level of educational preparation for planning and conducting research. A study was conducted by Jeanne Berthold in 1973 to determine whether the academic degrees held by nurses influenced the awarding of government research grants. It showed that the educational background alone was not a significant factor in acceptance or rejection of the proposals.[11] Still, many people consider that a doctoral degree is a necessary prerequisite to involvement in research. This stems from the fact that doctoral level educational programs require students to conduct independent research studies. The dissertation requirement has been utilized for many years to provide candidates the opportunity to demonstrate competence in research. Therefore, it is safe to assume that nurses with doctoral degrees have had basic educational preparation and personal experience with research. By the mid 1970's the percentage of working nurses with doctoral degrees was small (0.2 percent or 1,106 of the 778,470 employed nurses)[12] in comparison to the number of nurses employed in the United States. By 1980, the number of doctorally prepared nurses had grown to approximately 2,500.[13] Although this group of academically prepared individuals has contributed to the advancement of research in nursing, it has not yet made a large impact in this area for three reasons. The first stems from the limited size of the group. The second reason becomes apparent when it is noted that many of these nurses work in administrative, governmental, and educational settings and have limited involvement in everyday types of patient care problems. This has hampered the development of studies with a direct impact on patient care. This third reason for the lack of a unified impact on nursing research by these doctoral level nurses is the type of degree they possess. The previous lack of doctoral programs in nursing has led nurses to obtain degrees in allied fields, such as psychology, education, sociology, anthropology and biology. The diversity of interests represented by these other disciplines can enrich nursing research only if these scholars retain allegiance to scientific advancement in nursing, as well as in their adopted academic field.

Most nurses who now hold masters' degrees are familiar with the rudiments of the research process because research-related coursework and the completion of a thesis have traditionally been components of graduate level education. Since this master's level group also consists of a small percentage of the entire nursing population (3.2 percent or 24,885 of the 778,470 employed nurses),[14] the amount of academic exposure to the foundations of research of the majority of practicing nurses is uncertain, but likely to be limited. The nursing profession is attempting to deal with both sides of the problem through fostering a better research background for the students currently enrolled in nursing programs while encouraging continuing education programs for nurses, already graduated, who have had very limited contact with research. Formal coursework builds the foundation for knowledge, as well as the confidence required for conducting studies. Some educators recommend that this knowledge be combined with supervised practice in carrying out the research process. It is similar to learning in other areas of nursing: there is a need for direct exposure to real-life situations so that optimum learning can take place.

PROFESSIONAL COMMITMENT TO THE VALUE OF RESEARCH

As previously noted, it has been generally accepted that throughout the development of nursing, the value of research as an integral part of the profession has been overlooked. In 1974 the American Nurses' Association, the major professional organization for nurses, publicly recognized the need to firmly establish research as a priority for the entire profession. At that time, research in all areas of nursing practice was delineated as the principal thrust for the decade. The official statement put forth by the American Nurses' Association at its national convention was stated as follows: "All professional nurses should foster the initiation, dissemination, and utilization of research as an accepted and integral part of nursing practice, nursing services, and nursing education."[15]

The increased level of publicity for research will alert more practitioners to the value of using the results of scientific studies for updating knowledge and everyday clinical practice. Health care centers are recognizing the need for research and showing strong support for nursing-related studies. This is a great achievement for nursing since it will provide clinical role models for students to emulate. The inclusion of research in baccalaureate programs has placed additional emphasis on the development of research projects by nursing faculty. In fact, most of the research carried out in nursing was conducted by the faculty of university programs. Of the 108 authors who published studies in *Nursing Research* in 1973, 75 percent were nurses. Of this group of nurses, 93 percent were on the faculties of university nursing programs.[16] Commentary 1.5 shows this trend to be fairly constant. The university setting provided a climate for research and facilitated the utilization of the expertise of co-investigators in other disciplines. Thus, this three-pronged emphasis on the need for research within a nursing framework will gradually result in a more clearly defined set of values about research within all the facets of the profession.

Commentary 1.5
Who Publishes Nursing Research and What Type?

The main journal for communicating research findings in the nursing profession is *Nursing Research.* The editor's report for the articles published in 1976 contained the following information:

AUTHORS

Of the 116 authors, 76 (66 percent) were nurses. The remaining non-nurse authors were members of a wide variety of disciplines. Thirteen fields were represented with sociologists, psychologists, and educators comprising nearly half. The vast majority (80 percent) of authors were employed by universities. The second largest group of authors (9 percent) were employed by hospitals.

AREA

Nearly half (46 percent) of the 59 articles were clinical studies. The majority were medical-surgical in focus which was a change from the majority of maternal-child studies of previous years. The most prevalent nonclinical articles were in the area of attitude or behavior of health workers.

RESEARCH APPROACH

Descriptive—42 articles (71 percent). Experimental or quasi-experimental—12 articles (20 percent). Historical—4 articles (7 percent). Review of literature only—1 article (2 percent).

M. Carnegie: Editor's Report, 1977. Nursing Research 26, 1 (January–February 1977): 3.

PRIORITIES FOR RESEARCH

The early studies in nursing were, for the most part, educationally oriented. Varied aspects of education and administration have been explored throughout the past few decades. These studies have done such things as compare students in different types of basic nursing programs, identify effective behaviors or other characteristics of nursing faculties, and explore the effectiveness of staffing patterns in clinical settings. The focus has been largely on the nurse. There are a number of explanations for the development of studies within this area. Initially, nurse investigators sought to utilize research methodologies and tools that were already in existence. Since the investigators were located primarily in educational settings where similar studies were being conducted on students in other disciplines, they found it comfortable to carry out this type of research because a pattern or model existed. A large number of more or less captive subjects were available in classrooms and a large amount of information about these students was on record from routine admission and testing procedures. Many studies that described the personality characteristics of nursing students or predicted their academic success were planned and executed.

Attempts at planning and conducting patient-oriented investigations were less prevalent because of the large number of problems that resulted from contending with hospital routines and varied patient care factors. There was a clear lack of available models that could be used to measure the results of nursing care and this, too, influenced the paucity of clinically based studies.

The current emphasis of the professional organizations on research involves the delivery of nursing care. The American Nurses' Foundation has recently highlighted the focus of professional research in this area by funding only those proposals that show a clear intention to deal with clinical patient-related facets of nursing. The improvement of patient care through the research process is closely tied with the consumer-oriented health care atmosphere currently prevalent throughout the entire health care system.

Since nursing is both a scientific discipline and an applied art, the research focus has been difficult to define. Nurses who have already participated in research studies have been able to select areas of study that have been vastly different in nature, yet still applicable to nursing. The Commission on Nursing Research of the American Nurses' Association set up a list of priorities for the 1980's to guide members to study areas of nursing that are considered crucial for the advancement of scientific knowledge in the profession. The priorities were set up to generate knowledge that would help to guide nursing practice in the following areas:

1. Promoting health, well-being, and competency for personal care among all age groups.

2. Preventing health problems throughout the life span that have potential to reduce productivity and satisfaction.
3. Decreasing the negative impact of health problems on coping abilities, productivity, and life satisfaction in individuals and families.
4. Ensuring that the care needs of particularly vulnerable groups are met through appropriate strategies.
5. Designing and developing health care systems that are cost-effective in meeting the nursing needs of the population.
6. Promoting health, well being, and competency for personal health in all age groups.[17]

COMMUNICATION OF RESEARCH RESULTS

The main vehicle for communicating about nursing research studies has been a journal that was founded in 1952. *Nursing Research* mirrors the development of research within the profession. This has been reflected in the roster of investigators who have published reports in the journal since its inception, and in the subject matter of the reports. Most of the researchers who published in the early years were physicians, psychologists, and sociologists. By 1973 the 108 authors consisted of one sociologist, two physicians, ten psychologists, and 95 nurses.[18] The dramatic decrease of non-nursing authors has shown that the nursing profession is finally developing a body of research scholars of its own.

There is a crucial need for research in nursing to be translated into interesting and accessible formats. Studies need to be reported in a fashion that can be readily understood by the large body of practitioners involved in direct patient care even though they may not be well versed in research terminology. Research results will be more easily carried over into practice when communicated through a variety of widely read publications that were not formerly research-oriented. The *Journal of Nursing Education, Nursing, Nursing Outlook,* and *Journal of Nursing Administration* are a few examples. The recent appearance of research-related articles in such a variety of publications is viewed by many nurses as a sign of progress. This is important because a study published in *Nursing Research* in the spring of 1975 confirmed what many nurses had long thought about the communication of research results: that nursing research findings were neither widely read nor transferred from publication into practice.[19] A perusal of a number of nursing journals published outside the United States shows that the development of research in nursing is in no way restricted to this country. Widespread publication of research information and results will be a major factor in further strengthening the position of research in nursing.

Commentary 1.6
Cross-Cultural Nursing Research

Patinhara Pokkiarath Bhanumathi conducted a research study to compare the conceptions of nurses in India and the United States about the "sick role" of the patients in the two diverse cultures. She based her study on social science research that has been carried out in this area, and reasoned that such a study was important to the profession since nurses seek both employment and educational opportunities in different countries with varying cultures. She states specifically that, "Planning patient care depends on the nurses' understanding of the patient as a unique person which in turn rests on their expectations of patient behavior. Caring for patients with varying cultures and working with nurses belonging to different cultures present problems for any society."

The researcher had an idea that "sick role expectations" would vary between an actively oriented culture (the United States) and a passively oriented one (India). A brief exploratory study was conducted to find out if these differences actually did exist, and to determine fruitful areas for further study.

The following statements represent some of the differing viewpoints that were obtained from 60 staff nurses who were actively engaged in direct patient care in each of the two cultures studied:

AMERICAN NURSES' VIEW

They expect sick individuals (both acutely and chronically ill) to be as independent as possible. They expect patients not to worry. They expect the chronically ill to ask for help if they need it.

INDIAN NURSES' VIEW

They exempt a sick person from his normal social role responsibilities. They treat acutely and chronically ill persons as dependent individuals. They feel the obligation to do everything for the sick person. They expect patients to want pity. They do not expect patients to take an active part in trying to get well. They see careless and wrong living habits to be predominant factors in causing illness.

P. Bhanumathi: Nurses' conceptions of "sick role" and "good patient" behavior: a cross-cultural comparison. International Nursing Review 24, 1 (January–February 1977): 20–24.

RESEARCH AND PROBLEM SOLVING

Problem solving is a process used to deal with a specific problem that is an immediate irritant in any kind of setting. Nurses are expert in applying problem-solving techniques to their clinical practice. In fact, this has been the normal mode of dealing with problems encountered in the process of giving patient care. It should be noted that knowledge about nursing care was originally transmitted by teaching students a variety of standardized techniques or skills that had, at best, a questionable scientific basis. The procedures were often rigidly enacted, and it often seemed as if things were "always done this way." As new situations developed for which there were no set procedures, and as creative and daring practitioners arrived on the scene, the use of problem-solving techniques became even more widespread.

The clinical nurse first identifies a patient problem that is affecting the delivery of health care and verbalizes this problem to herself and possibly to some of her coworkers. Additional information is gathered about the problem, and possible ways of handling the situation are devised. One of these possible solutions is put into practice, and the results are eventually analyzed to see if the particular solution worked. In the event that it did not work, another of the possible interventions is tried until one is found that provides the solution to the patient care problem. These commonsense solutions are usually shared with other members of the staff through patient care conferences, nursing rounds, or perhaps in writing by noting the new method of treatment and its results in the Kardex or progress notes. If the solution to the problem works in a number of different instances, this new patient care information could be shared with greater numbers of nurses through publication of the information. The results of clinical problem-solving exercises have been transmitted to the main body of the profession by such widely read publications as the *American Journal of Nursing* and *Nursing Clinics of North America*. Most often, however, the information (in the form of a nursing procedure) remains within one group of nurses or one health care agency. Since it is applicable to one particular situation, it does not contribute to the advancement of nursing theory.

Nursing theory can best be advanced through conducting organized research. This is a very different approach from problem solving. The main difference between research and problem solving is the purpose for which each process is utilized. Problem solving is an acceptable way to devise one or more solutions in a particular situation. Research is utilized to obtain knowledge that is generalizable or that goes beyond individual situations. Although it may be tempting to use research to solve administrative problems, to answer questions of value judgment, or to produce solutions to immediate problems, research has as its goal the search for truth in a scientific or systematic manner. The scientific approach consists of an orderly process, based on sound theoretical formulations, that delineates a number of steps to be followed in gathering information about a general problem area. The process through which the investigator proceeds has been set up to provide objectivity and some measure of confidence that the study results will be a valuable addition to the professional knowledge base. The research process is an established method of inquiry that is utilized in the same way by all disciplines. The subject matter of the problem being investigated may be within the theoretical province of one professional discipline, such as nursing, but the manner in which the study is approached and conducted should be understandable to scientists in all fields.

Scientific research is defined by Kerlinger as systematic, controlled, empirical, and critical investigation by hypothetical propositions into the presumed relations among natural phenomena.[20] According to this definition, research is enacted by following a prescribed set of steps and procedures in order to assure objectivity and decrease bias. Second, the scientist must write down his propositions so that they may be communicated to others and checked against reality.

Some authors have tried to distinguish between nursing research and research in nursing. They describe "nursing research" as the study of the care process and the problems encountered in the practice of nursing. "Research in nursing" is defined as the study of the profession itself and of the various characteristics of its practitioners.[21] These are fine distinctions that may become more meaningful after an understanding of the research process is more fully developed. For the remainder of this book *nursing research is defined as the application of the scientific method of critical investigation to the study of all nursing problems with the goal of expanding the theoretical basis of nursing through the discovery of new knowledge.*

NURSING RESEARCH IN CLINICAL SETTINGS

More research has been conducted into the characteristics of nurses and the nursing profession as a whole than has been carried out on the activities of nurses or just what it is that nurses do for patients. One goal of planning and conducting research in any professional discipline is the discovery of knowledge (facts and relationships between phenomena) that can be organized into meaningful theories and subsequently taught to new students who desire membership in that professional group. A theory is a set of interrelated constructs (concepts), definitions, and propositions that present a systematic view of the phenomena by specifying relations among variables, with the purpose of explaining and predicting the phenomena.[22] Thus, theory could be used to assist nurses in systematically assessing nursing problems in patient care situations and in predicting the outcomes of specific interventions.

Much of the care of the nursing profession is involved with nurse-patient interactions in dealing with health care problems. The activities of nurses in dealing with health care problems can be roughly classified according to the "nursing process." This nursing process consists of the five phases of assessment, nursing diagnosis, planning, intervention, and evaluation.[23] This system is an organized framework to look at the nurse's approach to health care situations. It can be used to provide documentation for nursing actions, as well as a source of potential research problems. The nursing process delineates a professional mode of behavior and should not be confused with research. However, it is precisely this clinically oriented aspect of nursing that has received the least amount of research attention to date. Although there are a number of substantial reasons for this situation (from lack of expertise in planning this type of research to a lack of ways to measure the effects of nursing care), the problem is one that needs to be addressed by all levels of nurses.

This can be effected in two ways according to the background of the nurse. The first is to ensure that the main body of practitioners are introduced to the research process so that they can read and utilize research results in their practice. The second way is to encourage the nurses who have some degree of research knowledge to gain expertise through planning and conducting studies that involve nurses and their clients. The theories upon which much of nursing practice is based have been largely borrowed from other disciplines. Knowledge about what nursing does for patients can only be advanced through conducting relevant, precise, clinically based studies. In this era of consumer-oriented accountability, it is becoming increasingly important to be able to define the nursing care being rendered and its related effects. Research, the controlled method of study, is one way to document results of nursing care. It should be made clear that the results of just one research study are looked upon as tenuous conclusions. Research findings need to be shown as true in varied studies before a great deal of weight is placed on them. Even though it takes time to build up a body of knowledge, the utilization of the research process provides a measure of assurance that the accumulated information is substantial.

The next chapter is designed to help the reader become more comfortable with research. It was set up to explain some of the terms most often used in communicating about the research process so that the studies which follow will be more easily understood.

REFERENCES

1. F. Nightingale (Attr.): A Contribution to the Sanitary History of the British Army During the Late War with Russia. London, J. W. Parker, 1859, p. 11.

2. *Ibid.*, pp. 6–7.

3. F. Nightingale: *Notes on Hospitals*. London, Longman, Green and Co., 1863, pp. 171–176.

4. L. Simmons and V. Henderson: Nursing Research A Survey and Assessment. New York, Appleton-Century-Crofts, 1964, p. 21.

5. E. L. Brown: Nursing for the Future. New York, Russell Sage Foundation, 1948, p. 150.

6. J. Lysaught: An Abstract for Action. New York, McGraw-Hill, 1970, p. 85.

7. Facts About Nursing. New York, American Nurses' Association, 1960, pp. 109, 116.

8. Lysaught, An Abstract for Action, p. 155.

9. E. Carnegie: The research attitude begins on the undergraduate level (Editorial). Nursing Research 23, 2 (March–April, 1974): 90.

10. American Nurses' Association Commission on Nursing Research: Preparation of Nurses for Participation in Research. Kansas City, Missouri, American Nurses' Association, 1976.

11. J. Berthold: Nursing research grant proposals. What influenced their approval or disapproval in two national granting agencies. Nursing Research 22, 4 (July–August, 1973): 292–299.

12. Facts About Nursing 76–77. Kansas City, Missouri, American Nurses' Association, 1977, p. 11.

13. A. Jacox: Strategies to promote nursing research. Nursing Research 29, 4 (July–August, 1980): 216.

14. Facts About Nursing 76–77, p. 11.

15. ANA convention '74. American Journal of Nursing 74, 7 (July, 1974): 1274.

16. E. Carnegie: The shifting of research emphasis and investigators (Editorial). Nursing Research 23, 3 (May–June, 1974): 195.

17. Commission on Nursing Research: Generating a scientific basis for nursing practice: Research priorities for the 1980's. Nursing Research 29, 4 (July–August, 1980): 219.

18. Carnegie, Shifting of research emphasis, p. 195.

19. S. Ketefian: Application of selected nursing research findings into nursing research practice: a pilot study. Nursing Research 24, 2 (March–April, 1975): 89–92.

20. F. Kerlinger: Foundations of Behavioral Research. New York, Holt, Rinehart & Winston, 1973, p. 11.

21. S. Gortner: Research for a practice profession. Nursing Research 24, 3 (May–June, 1975): 193.

22. Kerlinger, Foundations of Behavioral Research, p. 9.

23. H. Yura and M. Walsh: The Nursing Process. New York, Appleton-Century-Crofts, 1978.

CHAPTER

2

Learning Research Language

LANGUAGE AND CUSTOM

"RESEARCH is a term which came into English from the Old French root word *cerchier*, meaning to search or seek, and the prefix *re*, meaning again. Research is reflective seeking or intensive search with a view of becoming certain."[1] It is but one part of the overall process of inquiry that is the cornerstone of any learned profession. The various words that are used to express the same idea as the word INQUIRY give a good indication of the different types of skills utilized in the research process:

Inquire	Explore	Seek a clue
Seek	Trace	Hunt
Frisk	Ferret	Pursue
Look for	Unearth	Examine
Scan	Fathom	Disect
Scrutinize	Probe	Winnow
Reconnoiter	Grapple with	Thresh out
Rummage	Analyze	Interrogate[2]

Research can be much more easily understood once the reader becomes familiar with the words and abbreviations customarily used in writing about the research process. There are new words to learn that are applicable only to research procedures, and there are more commonly used words that have new, specific meanings when used in a research setting. It is similar to learning a new language, and "catching on" to it now will help to make the rest of the book more understandable.

When reading research reports and articles, you'll notice that there are certain customary styles used in presenting the information. Much of the information is written in the passive rather than the active voice. In addition, the *past tense* is used when writing about the research. This may seem logical when reading published reports of completed studies, but sometimes becomes a problem for novices the first few times they write a research report. Even if you are planning the way you *will* eventually collect the information for a study, the writing you do to explain the process should be in the past tense, just as if it has already occurred. This process, incidentally, prevents rewriting of the report when the project has been completed!

TERMINOLOGY

Also, in writing a report, the individuals conducting the study never use first person pronouns, such as "I," "we," or "us." They are referred to in the report as RESEARCHERS, INVESTIGATORS, AUTHORS, or some such familiar term. Likewise, the people or things being studied are not referred to by means of pronouns, but are called SUBJECTS (often abbreviated as the lower case letter *s*), PARTICIPANTS, OR RESPONDENTS. The POPULATION (often designated by a capital N) is the total possible membership of the group being studied. Since it is not always feasible or desirable to collect information from the total group, a small portion of the whole population is often selected for use in a study. This microcosm of the population is called the SAMPLE (often designed by a lower case *n*). The use of symbols, such as N or *n*, has become customary to conserve space and avoid repetition throughout a study. Whenever the notation n=70 appears in a research report, the author is talking about information from a sample of 70 subjects who have been selected from a larger group by a process called SAMPLING. This important sampling (or selecting) process can be conducted in a variety of ways. Since the sampling process determines the subjects who are included in the actual group being studied, it will have an effect on the accuracy of the results of the study. Although sampling will be covered in detail in later chapters, it is important to know that there is a major distinction between RANDOM methods in which everyone in the group has an equal chance of being included in the sample, and NONRANDOM methods of sampling that are less systematic about choosing members of study groups. For instance, the random method is similar to the practice of lottery-type drawings in which each individual's name is written on a piece of paper and placed in a drum. While only one name is selected from the drum by an unbiased individual, all of the participants are satisfied that they had an equal chance of being chosen. Such is not the case with the nonrandom methods in which candiates are chosen with less precision. One example of a nonrandom sampling method involves asking for VOLUNTEERS to represent a group. Thus, a random sample of 2,000 nurses (n=2,000) from the population of 800,000 active practitioners would be theoretically REPRESENTATIVE of the total group. This randomization would make the study results GENERALIZABLE to the entire population of nurses. If the same study were conducted on a sample of 2,000 nurse volunteers who sought participation on their own, results could only be safely generalized to the volunteer, nonrandom group involved. Although the volunteers could be representative of all the 800,000 practicing nurses, there is more of a possibility that they may not be.

Two additional terms are used when talking about the subjects who take part in a research project. The HAWTHORNE EFFECT was first described in the early studies in industrial settings (the Hawthorne plant of the Western Electric Company) to explain a phenomenon that takes place whenever humans are involved in experiments. The Hawthorne effect generally means that people's behavior will change in some way when they know they are being watched or observed by researchers. Investigators should plan their studies carefully to avoid the influence of the Hawthorne effect on study results as much as possible. On the other hand, the HALO EFFECT refers to judgments made about subjects by observers or raters. Subjects may be rated consistently high or low on the basis of the impression they give the observer, rather than being rated solely on the factor being studied. The Halo effect can also be used to describe the response of an individual when answering written questions. A questionnaire that measures an attitude toward a particular nursing procedure would structure the questions so that a nurse with a favorable attitude would have to agree with some items and disagree with others. People are naturally reluctant to disagree with all items (or vice versa), so the variety in the type of response increases accuracy. Thus, it should be noted that subtle changes in behavior can occur as a result of participation in a research project. Since this may affect both subjects and observers, it should be an important aspect of the planning and preparation for research projects. Elaborate schemes to lessen the impact of uncharacteristic or inaccurate responses have resulted in the coining of further research terminology. For example, the DOUBLE-BLIND method of interacting with subjects describes the familiarity of both the subjects and researchers with the specific factors being studied. In this instance, the people carrying out the procedures are not aware of the exact type of treatment they are administering to each subject. In one study, for example, the nurses who administered various pain killing drugs to patients used a medication labeled A, B, or C according to a set routine as ordered by the doctor conducting the experiment. The nurse remained "blind" or unaware of the specific medication name or dosage. This eliminated the possibility that the nurse would transmit clues to the patients about the effectiveness of the drug. Since both nurse and patient are "blind" (hence a double-blind) to the type of medication and exact dosage of drugs A, B, or C, the researcher should be able to get a more objective idea of the potency and action of each drug. There are various steps researchers can use to collect information with the least amount of ERROR possible. Error can result from a variety of sources (the sampling process, the mistakes a subject makes in filling in an answer sheet, the statistical procedures utilized) and careful planning is required so that researchers can keep the margin of error low.

The use of symbols (various letters from our familiar alphabet, as well as a few from the not-so-familiar Greek alphabet) and abbreviations is common throughout research reports. The common symbols need to be learned, since they are like a type of shorthand used to save time and space and are not usually explained in the text. The symbols listed below are among those utilized most often.

n = sample	X = score
N = population	$\overline{X}$ = mean score
H = hypothesis	Σ = total or sum of a number of scores
r = correlation	> = greater than
p = probability	< = less than

The opposite is true of abbreviations. Each abbreviation is initially identified in a study by being placed in parentheses immediately following the full name of the organization or title for which it stands. Thus, after the abbreviation has been identified to the reader, it can be used in place of spelling out the full name throughout the remainder of the report. For example, in writing about the American Nurses' Association (ANA), the author would identify the abbreviation in this manner the first time the organization is mentioned in the paper, and then refer to the group as the ANA for the rest of the report.

The research study begins with the formulation of a RESEARCH PROBLEM that evolves from one or more questions the researchers have set out to answer. Their choice of using a research framework rather than using problem-solving techniques indicates that they wish to expand the knowledge base for this topic, and that they wish to seek answers in as objective a manner as possible. The term research problem is used to describe the topic area that is of general interest to the researchers, and need not be what is thought of as a "problem" in the sense of a difficult situation. The researchers hope to conduct their project to obtain EMPIRICAL information on the subject. This term is generally used to mean factual information obtained through research experience and observation. In order to find answers for the research questions, the investigators must concoct an overall plan for conducting the study that is called the RESEARCH DESIGN. The design is like a blueprint that outlines the way in which they will gather the necessary information on the topic. There are a number of different kinds of overall designs that the researcher might use. The more specific plans for enacting the study are usually grouped under the heading of RESEARCH METHODOLOGY. The methodology is similar to the steps cited in a procedure manual since the specific measures and the way in which they are used are explained. Thus, the use of a specific test or questionnaire to collect desired information in a study is one aspect of research methodology.

The authors need to be very specific about defining various terms that are used in the study, by providing OPERATIONAL DEFINITIONS. For instance, the researchers need to define the term nurse in the manner in which it applies to their project (not a dictionary, but rather an active definition) such as the following:

nurse   in this study refers to currently licensed registered nurses who have baccalaureate degrees. These nurses have accrued a minimum of two years of clinical experience in nursing since graduation, and are currently assigned to a full-time position on a medical-surgical unit.

The key factors influencing the study also need to be carefully defined. These factors, or VARIABLES, are classified according to their relationship to the problem being investigated. The INDEPENDENT (also called treatment or stimulus) VARIABLE is generally used to identify something the researchers are introducing into the situation so that they can study and measure its effect. Since the independent variable is under the influence of the researcher, it can be applied in varying degrees that can be measured. For instance, in clinical nursing studies, this could be a new method of carrying out a procedure. If a new method of giving a patient a bed bath were devised, this "new bath procedure" could be an independent variable in a study designed to measure its effect on patients. One group of patients (Group A) would receive their bath according to the "new bath procedure." Thus, patients in Group A would be listed as members of the EXPERIMENTAL or TREATMENT GROUP. A similar group of patients (Group B) would receive the standard bed bath in the usual manner in order to provide the contrast with the experimental group. The patients in Group B who are receiving the bath in the usual manner are members of the CONTROL GROUP. The word control in research parlance means that nothing extraordinary has been allowed to influence this group, and it is considered the standard against which a difference or a change is measured.

The DEPENDENT VARIABLE is the term used to label the effects or the factors that the researchers are measuring. Suppose the researchers wanted to know more about the effect of the different bath procedures on the patient's body temperature. The dependent variable being measured in this instance would be the body temperature. EXTRANEOUS VARIABLES are other factors that may effect the study outcome that are important enough to be controlled or tabulated in some way. In the bed bath study, both the time of day of administering the bath and the amount of room heat could influence the body temperature. Both factors in that situation could be controlled by the researchers. The previously cited examples are ENVIRONMENTAL types of extraneous variables. The other type, ORGANISMIC, refers to characteristics of the subjects that may influence the study results, such as the patient's age. There are usually a wide variety of extraneous variables present in each research situation when human subjects are used.

After the researchers have defined the research problem that they are going to study, they formally state the relationship of the variables they expect to find in this particular situation. This statement may take the form of a question, but is written more often as a declarative sentence. This statement of expected relationship between variables is very often an "educated guess" based on results of similar studies that have been conducted in the past. This statement is called a HYPOTHESIS (often designated by a capital H). Often, there is more than one hypothesis that the researcher wishes to study. The plural of this term becomes HYPOTHESES, and when multiple statements are utilized, they are numbered for clarity, usually with a subscript number included after the symbol H. An example of a second hypothesis in the bath study would be stated as follows:

H_2: Females in both study groups will have a greater decrease in body temperatures after experiencing the bath procedure than will males in both study groups.

The design of the study also suggests the type of DATA or information the investigator needs to collect from the subjects in the study. The word data is the plural form (researchers are generally working with multiple pieces of information) and often causes grammatical problems. The correct use, when describing the collected information, is to say that *data were* tabulated. The investigator has the opportunity to choose the method of collecting the necessary data from a variety of possibilities. The use of information which has been previously collected and tabulated is a common research practice and makes use of what is called EXISTING DATA. Nursing studies of this type utilize sources such as administrative records and patient charts for gathering information. Data can also be collected by INDIRECT means such as observation of subjects. There are two general ways in which observers can be utilized to collect data. PARTICIPANT OBSERVERS are the ones who actually take part in the interaction that is being studied. They participate right along with the study subjects. NONPARTICIPANT OBSERVERS are the ones who watch and record an interaction without actually taking part in it. In many studies that utilize nonparticipant observers, the observers are not even in the same room as the subjects, but are required to watch the designated behavior through a two-way mirror. DIRECT collection of information from subjects is carried out by using devices, such as tests, questionnaires, or various machines, to elicit answers from subjects. This eliminates the necessity of having the information pass through some indirect source, such as observers. Researchers can collect information by using one or any combination of the methods they choose as most appropriate for the situation. The dependent variable indicates the type of information that is sought (for example, body temperature) and the researcher needs to determine exactly how he will go about collecting the data to QUANTIFY or measure it.

The type of information needed by researchers should be viewed in relation to the overall time frame in which it is available. The type of study that requires previously recorded information (and therefore requires looking back into the past) is termed RETROSPECTIVE. Studies that measure some characteristic at one point in time (usually the present) are called CROSS-SECTIONAL. LONGITUDINAL studies collect specific information from a group of subjects at various intervals over a lengthy period of time that extends into the future. A PROSPECTIVE study is one that has been designed to study a particular problem (such as factors affecting heart disease) by following the subjects over a span of time to see the relationship of specific variables (such as smoking behavior and exercise patterns) to the development of heart-related problems. A COHORT study takes a group of subjects with a similar background and follows them by taking measures of different variables over an extended time.

Both the type of data that are required to answer the original question and the time frame in which the research is conducted will influence the study SETTING. The setting is where the action of data collection takes place, whether it is a LABORATORY setting (subjects placed in a special environment the researcher has created), a FIELD SURVEY (subjects in their natural environment), or any number of conventional sites, such as classrooms or health care centers.

One of the most important decisions the researcher must face involves the selection of the instrument that will be used to collect data. The INSTRUMENT is the device used to record the information obtained from subjects. There are many kinds of instruments, including questionnaires, interview guides, rating sheets, performance checklists, mechanical devices, and various types of paper and pencil tests. Several properties of the instruments must be considered when deciding which one to use. Two of the most crucial are the RELIABILITY and VALIDITY of the measuring device. A reliable instrument will produce consistent results on repeated use. In the study of body temperature, a thermometer in proper working condition would give consistently accurate readings of the degree of body heat when used repeatedly during the testing. A valid instrument is one that gives a meaningful, relevant measure of the desired commodity. The thermometer gives a relevant or appropriate indication of the degree of body heat at a given time, and this quality makes such an instrument useful in this situation.

Once the researchers have selected an instrument that is appropriate for collecting the data they want, they must try it out to see how well it works. A "dry run," or practice session, in using an instrument is called a PRETEST. Most of the time the subjects used for a pretest are similar to, but not the same as, the ones who will eventually be part of the sample group. A PILOT STUDY is more extensive than a pretest. It is the conduction of a small-scale study that includes an analysis of the results. Pilot studies are often carried out to assist researchers in refining the overall design, the statement of the hypotheses, or the specific aspects of the methodology. They are most useful in the preliminary planning stages of large-scale projects.

After the data are collected, they must be arranged in some type of meaningful form so that the researchers can make some statements about what they've found. The main section of a study that pertains to STUDY RESULTS presents the major findings of the original research problem. The hypotheses will be either ACCEPTED (as true) or REJECTED according to what has been found. In this section the researchers often refer to the level of STATISTICAL SIGNIFICANCE of the findings. This phrase has a particular meaning in research language. It has to do with the statistical properties of the study results (the degree of accuracy with which they may be viewed), and will be covered in later chapters. The investigators then draw CONCLUSIONS directly from the findings. The INTERPRETATIONS of the results (roughly how the researchers view the relationship between the problem and the results) precede RECOMMENDATIONS or suggestions for further study. Research results are always considered to be tenuous and open to verification through further investigation.

The direct duplication of a research study, or REPLICATION, is often carried out to confirm findings of a study or to expand knowledge in the area. This may be attempted by repeating the original study while using a different kind of sample. Therefore, the research results of one or two studies would not be said to "prove" something, and research writers must be cautious in using absolute words. It is far better to write that "the present research study supports the following theoretical stance . . ." than to purport that "the present research study *proves* the following theoretical stance." Caution should always be used in writing about results of all kinds of investigations. In a similar vein, the writers should not use affective words such as "the researchers *feel* or *believe*." The information reported should be documented from acceptable sources rather than presenting a personalized account. FOOTNOTES are utilized to point out the authors and sources of the ideas or statements that need to be documented. The exact format for presenting the information needed in the footnotes can vary, but each should contain the essential information about the originator of the idea and the location in which it was recorded. The investigators should provide the reader with a comprehensive list of all their sources of information. This BIBLIOGRAPHY is placed at the end of the study and precedes the appropriate APPENDICES. An APPENDIX contains information that is considered to be supplemental to the material in the main text. The study involving the new type of bed bath would most likely include a lengthy detailed description of the new bath procedure in the appendix rather than in the main text of the report. Appendices are labeled alphabetically. A reader would be directed to find this supplemental information by instructions placed in parentheses within the main text, such as (See Appendix A).

One of the final steps of a research project entails the formulation of an ABSTRACT. The abstract is a brief (usually 100 to 200 words) resume of the entire study. This condensed version of the project is placed at the beginning of the study and is the abbreviated summary that is available for listing in library reference sources. For example, abstracts of different types of psychologically oriented studies are placed together in a volume called *Psychological Abstracts*. Investigators can quickly scan the abstracts and identify the studies they want to locate to examine in greater detail.

In summary, the research terminology that should be familiar to you at this point includes the following:

RESEARCHERS	HAWTHORNE EFFECT
INVESTIGATORS	HALO EFFECT
AUTHORS	DOUBLE-BLIND
SUBJECTS	ERROR
PARTICIPANTS	RESEARCH PROBLEM
RESPONDENTS	EMPIRICAL
N	RESEARCH DESIGN
n	RESEARCH METHODOLOGY
POPULATION	OPERATIONAL DEFINITIONS
SAMPLE	VARIABLES
SAMPLING	INDEPENDENT VARIABLE
RANDOM	EXPERIMENTAL GROUP
NONRANDOM	TREATMENT GROUP
VOLUNTEERS	CONTROL GROUP
HYPOTHESIS	DEPENDENT VARIABLE
HYPOTHESES	EXTRANEOUS VARIABLES
H	ENVIRONMENTAL EXTRANEOUS VARIABLES
PARTICIPANT OBSERVERS	
NONPARTICIPANT OBSERVERS	ORGANISMIC EXTRANEOUS VARIABLES
EXISTING DATA	INSTRUMENT
INDIRECT DATA COLLECTION	RELIABILITY
DIRECT COLLECTION	VALIDITY
QUANTIFY	PRETEST
RETROSPECTIVE STUDIES	PILOT STUDY
CROSS-SECTIONAL STUDIES	STUDY RESULTS
LONGITUDINAL STUDIES	ACCEPTED/REJECTED
PROSPECTIVE STUDIES	STATISTICAL SIGNIFICANCE
COHORT STUDIES	CONCLUSIONS
STUDY SETTING	INTERPRETATIONS
LABORATORY SETTING	RECOMMENDATIONS
FIELD SURVEY	REPLICATION
BIBLIOGRAPHY	FOOTNOTES
REPRESENTATIVENESS	APPENDICES
GENERALIZABLE	ABSTRACT

Most of these terms will be used throughout the following chapters and a working knowledge of them will make research procedures less difficult to understand. The following chapter utilizes many of these terms while explaining the usual steps of the research process.

REFERENCES

1. C. B. Williams: A Research Manual for College Studies and Papers, 3rd ed. New York, Harper & Row, 1963, p. 1.

2. P. Roget: Roget's Thesaurus of Synonyms and Antonyms. New York, Galahad Books, 1972, p. 87.

CHAPTER

3

The Research Process

UNDERTAKING THE RESEARCH PROCESS

Research is a purposeful activity that is done to add to scientific knowledge. The research process consists of a number of steps that are carried out to accomplish this purpose. The logical, orderly nature of the research process can truly be appreciated after some experience in utilizing these steps in conducting a study of a meaningful research problem. The research process provides a means of organization much like a road map. The exact route is left up to the discretion of the investigator, but broad landmarks are provided for finding the general or overall direction.

The research process is a progression of steps that constitute the skeleton of various types of studies in a multitude of disciplines. The general process is the same for conducting research in philosophy, psychology, or nursing. This fact will become more important to you as you read research reports in your chosen professional field and in other academic disciplines as well. After a working knowledge of the basic research steps is mastered, the PROCESS recedes into the background as the CONTENT of the study is highlighted. It is often interesting to note how readily the student with rudimentary research knowledge is able to transfer the newly acquired skills in reading about the research process to another field and thus easily broaden his or her background. The process of carrying out research (as well as being able to read, critique, and utilize study results) has long been listed as a function of a true professional. Once the member of a profession has acquired knowledge and skills in research, it becomes quite an easy task for him or her to read research in other disciplines. Thus, this skill fosters a sound interdisciplinary sharing of ideas with those inside, as well as outside of, the profession.

An understanding of the research process requires the professional to first adapt a positive attitude toward research. This attitude consists of the following components.

A Search for the Truth

The person undertaking a research project should aim to discover facts or new relationships in as unbiased a manner as possible. The occasional lack of honesty in the reporting of study results that is highlighted by the media stems from a very small percentage of professionals engaged in scientific research. Investigators seek to end up with a report of their work that clearly and accurately describes the procedures that were carried out. The researcher attempts to list all of the biases and limitations of the study in as candid a manner as possible in order to prevent misunderstanding of the study results. The reader, although realizing that the researcher is aiming to present an accurate picture of the study, has the responsibility of evaluating the work with a critical eye so that only results of sound studies will be utilized in professional practice. Research findings that are uncovered through an objective process will stand up to the scrutiny of and replication by fellow scientists. Objectivity, rationality, and open-mindness are thought to be ingredients in this truth-seeking process, and should be each investigator's goal. The amount of research that has been conducted on scientists or researchers to substantiate the presence of these particular qualities is very limited. In an article in *Psychology Today*, Dr. Michael Mahoney calls for an examination of the members of a scientific community, especially in the areas of objectivity, rationality, intelligence, open-mindness, and humility.[1] Whether the presence of these characteristics can be substantiated or not, the beginning researcher should aim for them.

Patience

Research takes time as well as objectivity. Although some steps of the process can be executed more rapidly than others, the entire venture is likely to require a considerable expenditure of time and energy. Time schedules for research projects often reflect the slow, but orderly pace at which a project proceeds. Novice researchers can overcome some of the initial impatience they often feel by setting up a schedule of deadlines for various stages of the project. This schedule should be considered tentative, however. Such a time schedule provides a list of accomplishments that can be checked off as the study progresses. It also provides a pattern for estimating time allocations for future projects since individual work rates vary widely from person to person. Flexibility, adaptability, and a willingness to revise and update work are highly valued assets in many phases of research.

Ability to Accept Criticism

As much as it may be uncomfortable or even painful to have parts of a project or report critically analyzed by an objective reader, it is a necessary part of conducting research. The first step entails getting ideas, procedures, conclusions, or whatever into written form. It is often helpful to set the "write up" aside for a few days so that you can reread it from a fresh vantage point and make any necessary alterations. Then seek consultation from someone with expertise in the field, and be open to constructive suggestions that may well improve the quality of the project.

Willingness to Revise

The wise researcher knows that the initial step in writing a report or devising an instrument should be considered a working copy or rough draft. Some steps of the process imply the necessity for change. For instance, the pretesting of instruments implies that the finished version will be the result of a "trial-by-fire" and thus an adaptation of the original design. Rewriting for the purpose of attaining greater clarity is a common aspect of scholarly writing, and not the sign of ignorance (or worse) as many beginning researchers are apt to think.

Sharing

Research is more apt to be carried out by a group of people than by an individual working alone. Even individual projects that are undertaken to fulfill degree requirements, such as doctoral dissertations (usually considered to be examples of singular, original research), are carried out with provisions for consultation by a committee of experts in the field. It is usually more stimulating and more enjoyable to be able to converse about various aspects of the project with someone who has a working knowledge of the study and who has a reason to be as interested in the project as you are. The theme of sharing also includes professional consultation. Since it is difficult to be proficient in all the areas a research study may involve (for example, statistical analysis or test construction), it is important to note that assistance from experts in various fields may be necessary. Consultation is a common and often desirable part of research.

Attention to Detail

The study must be recorded and reported clearly and explicitly enough to provide for easy replication by another scientist. All phases of the study should be described with concise explanations of the plans and procedures that were followed. Vague, ambiguous statements should be replaced by precise, sufficiently detailed communication. The documentation of sources of information utilized in a report, such as in footnotes or bibliographical references, should be cited correctly with regard to both style and content.

Interesting

Research can be enriching, stimulating, and even fun. A lot of effort should be put into finding just the right topic. You'll be more motivated to read various studies if the topic is one that commands your interest. You'll probably put more effort into creating a really good study if intellectual challenge and curiosity are present to spur you on. The level of interest in the material may even show through between the lines in the written report. Although report writing is a task that demands self-discipline from most people, the interest you have in the subject is bound to affect your attitude. Many students find their curiosity is aroused by studies dealing with such ordinary human events as sexual practices, dating patterns, social interactions, and various aspects of death and the dying process. Contrary to popular opinion, research does not need to be stuffy, highbrow, esoteric, or boring in order to be worthwhile. The account of the particular historical research study summarized in Commentary 3.1 clearly demonstrates this point.

Commentary 3.1
No Such Historical Figures in Nursing . . . That We
Know of . . .

The curiosity of one of the faculty of the Boston College history department was stimulated while watching a late-night TV horror movie about Dracula. Dr. Raymond McNally noted that many of the geographical references mentioned in the film (and later in Bram Stoker's novel, *Dracula*) were authentic locations, such as names of towns, the Borgo Pass, the Carpathian mountains, and, above all, a place called Transylvania. He subsequently discovered that the setting for the tale was modern-day Romania, and began to wonder if some historical basis existed for the vampire legend, since some of the facts seemed real.

A colleague, Dr. Radu Florescu, was a logical addition to the unusual historical research project since he was already familiar with the locale and folklore of his native land. Both scholars worked to uncover the story of "an authentic human being fully as horrifying as the vampire of fiction and film—a 15th century prince." A Fulbright scholarship and other research support assisted them in uncovering a story which they relate as follows:

> [This] is a complex story, for it involves a 15th century prince known in his time as both "Vlad Tepes" and "Dracole"; the fictional Dracula created by Bram Stoker in 1897; and the beliefs of the Romanian peasants in Transylvania and Wallachia both today and in the 15th century. The complex story brings up many questions. Was the real Dracula a vampire? Did the peasants of his time consider him a vampire? What connection is there between the real prince and the vampire-count created by Stoker? What do the Romanian peasants believe today about Vlad Tepes and vampires? And have we been dealing simply with "history" or are there mysteries here beyond the reach of historical research?

R. NcNally and R. Florescu: In Search of Dracula. New York, Warner Paperback Library, 1972.

THE ORGANIZATION OF THE RESEARCH PROCESS

The research process remains fairly constant even though the approach to the research, the type of research, or the purpose for undertaking the research may vary. Thus the steps of basic and applied research may be similar even though there may be wide variation in the underlying objectives of each kind. BASIC RESEARCH is often defined as pure research that is carried out to advance knowledge in a given area. It is done to build up or add to existing theories in a specific discipline. APPLIED RESEARCH is carried out to add to professional knowledge in real-life situations. Nursing is a prime example of a profession in need of research in both the theoretical (nursing science) and applied (clinical practice) aspects of the field. The research steps may be altered or tailored to fit a particular study and, although some steps are routinely omitted in certain types or projects, the main elements are recognizable. The series of steps in the process may be more easily remembered if they are placed within an overall framework. Most studies can be subdivided into three main areas under which the steps can be classified. The three main distinctions in organizing the research process are (1) defining the problem area, (2) explaining the methodology of how the study was carried out, and (3) analyzing and presenting the study results. Although the step-by-step description of the research process varies somewhat according to the source of explanation, the following twelve steps listed by Abdellah and Levine present a comprehensive picture of the research process.[2]

THE STEPS IN THE RESEARCH PROCESS

1. Formulate the problem
2. Review the literature
3. Formulate the framework of theory
4. Formulate hypotheses
5. Define the variables
6. Determine how variables will be quantified
7. Determine the research design
8. Delineate the target population
9. Select and develop method for collecting data
10. Formulate method of analyzing the data
11. Determine how results will be interpreted (generalized)
12. Determine method of communicating results

The steps of the research process do not have to be utilized in the exact order in which they are listed and, in fact, often overlap. The various aspects of each of the steps will be explained throughout the remaining chapters of the text. They have been listed here to give some guidelines about the usual sequence in which the steps are enacted. The relationship of the three general areas of a research project to the twelve specific steps in the research process can be visualized in Figure 3.1.

The next chapter presents the report of a research study that was carried out on two groups of nursing students. You can locate most of the twelve

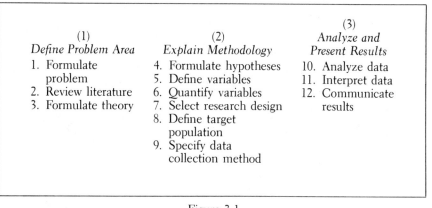

Figure 3.1

Diagram of the Relationship Between the Three Main Aspects of Research and the Specific Steps of the Research Process

steps of the research process within the study even though some are easier to find since they are more clearly labeled than others. The study has been reproduced to provide an actual example of the implementation of this process. The chapters immediately following the study will trace the development and actualization of these steps in greater detail.

REFERENCES

1. M. Mahoney: The truth seekers. Psychology Today 9, 11 (April 1976): 60–65.
2. F. Abdellah and E. Levine: Better Patient Care Through Nursing Research. New York, Macmillan, 1965, p. 91.

CHAPTER

4

Reading Research Studies

PREPARATION FOR READING A
RESEARCH STUDY

Now that you have some familiarity with the language of research, as well as the steps involved in the research process, it is important to start using that new knowledge right away. This chapter has been set up to provide you with an opportunity to practice using this knowledge by actually reading a published nursing research study. Keep a paper and pen handy to jot down any words or phrases that may still be unfamiliar. The extra effort expended in looking up the terms noted in this way will greatly increase your facility with research-related materials. You may not have had the opportunity to read through a research study before, and it is important to note that it may not be as awesome or incomprehensible as you had imagined. If you have had previous experience in reading research reports, you should note that your understanding of research can be enhanced by each new study you become familiar with. Novice researchers should make a definite point of finding a number of studies that pique their curiosity and then reading them from start to finish slowly and thoroughly. Each study is unique. Each investigator utilizes different aspects of the steps of the research process that are most applicable to the particular subject being studied. Familiarity with several different studies will highlight the varied approaches that can be used to accomplish the goal of obtaining objective, scientifically based knowledge.

The study you are about to read was undertaken to find out more about the factors that influence a person's attitude about death. Nursing students are likely to have more contact with death than other students on campus since they have educational experiences both in the classroom and in the clinical area with terminally ill patients. The researchers wanted to investigate whether these educational experiences made a difference in the attitudes these students held about death and the dying process—to try to measure the effect of this educational experience in nursing, the researchers decided to find out the attitudes of two groups of students. They needed one group that was completing a program in nursing seniors in a baccalaureate nursing program and a similar group of students who had not yet been exposed to this educational experience (freshmen in the same baccalaureate nursing program). The attitudes of the two groups about death would be different if the nursing education had had an impact in this area.

The abstract is presented first, and as you can see, it summarizes the entire project. It would be most helpful if you would read the abstract first, and then proceed through the entire study. Keep reading, even if you are not exactly clear about some parts of the study, because it is important to get an overview of the entire process. Look at the tables as you read each section, since they do expand on the material that is written. After completing the study, read the abstract again since it presents a good summary of the highlights of the study and should help you to remember important points.

A RESEARCH EXAMPLE

ATTITUDES OF NURSING STUDENTS TOWARD THE DYING PATIENT

Rosalee C. Yeaworth · Frederic T. Kapp · Carolyn Winget

A questionnaire to measure attitudes toward death and dying persons was administered to 108 freshmen and 69 seniors in a baccalaureate nursing program. Compared to freshmen, the responses of senior students indicated greater acceptance of feelings, more open communication, and broader flexibility in relating to dying patients and their families. These differences were statistically significant (p = .01). A nursing curriculum is described which provided experiences in caring for dying patients; classes on loss, grief, and death; small group discussions and the availability of one-to-one counseling for students who take care of dying patients.

Our society has a proclivity to deny, avoid, or ignore death. Hospitalizing seriously or terminally ill persons, isolating the elderly in retirement villages, and removing geriatric patients to nursing homes enables the community and the family to avoid interaction with the dying person. On the other hand, health care personnel of hospitals, nursing homes, and retirement complexes are confronted with situations where they must interact with dying persons, yet their previous training has rarely prepared them to cope with the realities of death. Defensive behavior such as indifference, hostility, or detachment toward persons who are terminally ill or dying are often the consequence.

A difficult but constructive alternative to these dehumanizing approaches to patient care is to come to grips, work through, and deal with feelings about death so that one's own anxieties do not block the process of helping the dying person. Kübler-Ross (1969) has emphasized that individuals must take a hard look at their own attitudes toward death and dying before they can be helpful with terminally ill patients without feeling anxiety or other discomfort.

Of the various categories of health professionals, nurses play a pivotal role in facilities for geriatric and terminally ill patients. In the course of their professional duties, they have a potential for much constructive interaction with patients, clients, and staff. Because of her leadership role, the nurse acts as a model for a variety of other personnel. Therefore, it is imperative that nurses become aware of and deal with their attitudes toward death and dying and realize how such attitudes affect their practice (Quint, 1967). Ideally, development of this awareness should begin early in the professional educational program.

The considerable body of literature in the area of death and dying has been mainly philosophical, theoretical, or anecdotal (Browning and Lewis, 1972; U.S. National Institute of Health, N.D.). Recently, studies on the attitudes of the dying patient toward his own death have appeared. But, little research has been devoted to the attitudes of health care personnel and how they may affect or modify the management and treatment of terminally ill patients. Golub and Reznikoff (1971) compared attitudes of graduate nurses and nursing students toward death. Because of similarities between the two groups, they concluded that "nurses appear to acquire common attitudes early . . . and these may remain comparatively stable throughout their nursing career" (p. 508). Their study did not attempt to ascertain what changes occurred during the educational program.

For the purpose of this study, attitude was defined as a complex, structured psychological tendency to respond in a consistent way to social objects or situations. Attitudes consist of cognitive, affective, and behavioral components. The instrument used for this study, like most attitudinal scales, relied on subjects' reports in regard to affective and behavioral components.

The curriculum of the nursing college which was the setting for this study included various learning experiences designed to assist students to become aware of and understand their feelings and beliefs about death and dying. Some of the earliest clinical placements for students were in extended care facilities, where facing dying patients was very much a reality. Collaborative teaching efforts included lectures, small group clinical conferences, assigned experiences with dying patients, as well as one-to-one counseling of students by faculty. The program was designed to shape attitudes toward working with dying patients and their families.

This research at the University of Cincinnati Medical Center was supported in part by a grant from the American Cancer Society (Ohio Division).

PURPOSE

The purpose of this study was to ascertain whether there were differences between freshman and senior nursing students on attitudes or beliefs about death and dying.

METHOD

SETTING. The College of Nursing and Health is an autonomous college of the University of Cincinnati, a municipal, state-affiliated university which offers a four-year program leading to the degree of Bachelor of Science in Nursing. Students have clinical experiences in a variety of settings, including two hospitals which are units of the Medical Center, affiliated private hospitals, a veterans hospital, extended care facilities, and community and industrial health clinics.

SUBJECTS. The entire freshman and senior classes of nursing students in the College of Nursing and Health of the University of Cincinnati during the academic year, 1972–1973, were the subjects for this study. Demographic data for the 108 freshmen and 69 senior students are given in Table 1. With the exception of two men in the

Table 1
Demographic Data for Two Groups of Nursing Students

Data	Freshman Nursing Students (N = 108)		Senior Nursing Students (N = 69)	
	N	(%)	N	(%)
Sex:				
Female	106	(98.0)	69	(100.0)
Male	2	(2.0)	0	(0.0)
Race:				
White	97	(89.8)	68	(98.6)
Black	11	(10.2)	1	(1.4)
Age:				
Under 20	99	(91.7)	0	(0.0)
20–25	2	(1.9)	56	(81.1)
26–35	2	(1.9)	11	(15.9)
Over 35	0	(0.0)	0	(0.0)
Not answered	5	(4.6)	2	(2.9)
Religious affiliation:				
Catholic	38	(35.2)	23	(33.3)
Jewish	4	(3.7)	2	(2.9)
Protestant	52	(48.1)	37	(53.6)
Other/Not answered	14	(13.0)	7	(10.1)
Intensity of religious belief:				
Strong	39	(36.1)	14	(20.3)
Moderate	49	(45.4)	38	(55.1)
Weak	13	(12.0)	13	(18.8)
None/Not answered	7	(6.5)	4	(5.7)

freshman class, all subjects were women. Eleven of the freshmen and one of the seniors were Black. Over 90 percent of the freshman students were under 20 years of age and 81 percent of the seniors were in the age range of 20 to 25. In both classes about one-third of the students were Catholic and about half were Protestant. Senior nursing students reported less intensity of religious belief than freshmen, although this difference was not statistically significant.

INSTRUMENT AND PROCEDURE. An interdisciplinary team composed of a social worker (the executive director of Cancer Family Care) and faculty both from the College of Medicine and the College of Nursing and Health worked together to devise the "Questionnaire for Understanding the Dying Person and His Family." Members of the research team had had varying amounts of experience with dying patients and in conducting teaching sessions for medical students or nursing students in their work with the dying patient.

The questionnaire has three sections. Part I includes 50 items that are answered on a five-point scale from strongly agree to strongly disagree. Thirty-three of these items are weighted so that responses indicative of flexibility in interpersonal relations, desire for open communication around critical issues, and "psychological-mindedness" in relation to patients and families of dying persons are assigned a low score. Items contributing to an overall profile of rigidity of attitudes, i.e., focusing primarily on physical needs during terminal illness, and showing a lack of insight into psychological factors influencing the self and others, are scored on the high end of the continuum. Item construction was designed to minimize a "halo effect" in responding by using both positively and negatively worded items on similar content issues. Within the questionnaire, items are randomly distributed.

Examples of questions are:

> Regardless of his age, disabilities, and personal preference, a person should be kept alive as long as possible.
> Dying patients should be told they are dying.
> The dying patient is best served by a matter-of-fact focus on medical issues.
> Fear of death is natural in all of us.
> If a patient talks about his fear of death, his doctors and nurses should reassure him that he has little to worry about.
> Patients are better off dying in a hospital than at home.

Part II deals with experiences with death and dying, both in one's personal life and in one's professional training—i.e., had one experienced death in one's immediate family, and if so, at what age? Had other close relatives died, and if so, what was subjects' age at the time of that experience? Attitudes toward funerals and autopsies as well as attitudes toward educational experiences about death are tapped. Two sentence-completion tasks that deal with the self's facing death are also included.

Part III requests demographic data on the respondent.

All questionnaires were administered during the fall quarter of the school year by faculty of the College of Nursing and Health.

In addition, senior students were asked how their education had influenced their attitudes:

Had they ever taken care of a dying patient? Had they sought help in dealing with feelings about working with a dying patient? What part of such care was most stressful? How had feelings been handled? What components of the educational process had been most helpful? Did they believe more learning experiences about death, dying, and suicide were needed?

Data were subjected to chi-square analysis and the t-test.

RESULTS

A score was assigned to each subject on the basis of the 33 weighted items in Part I, and means were computed for the two groups of students. The range of possible scores was from 33 to 165. The results are given in Table 2.

Data gathered from Part II of the questionnaire, regarding death in the student's personal life, are given in Table 3. About ten percent

Table 2
Mean Scores of Two Groups of Nursing Students on Attitudes toward the Dying Patient and His Family Based on Scores on Part I of the Questionnaire

Class	Range	$\overline{X}$	SD
Freshman (N = 108)	57–98	78.68	8.52
Senior (N = 69)	51–83	67.77	7.61

$t = 8.69, p < .001$

Table 3
Experiences with Death among Family Members for Two Groups of Nursing Students from Part II of the Questionnaire

Experiences with Death	Freshman Nursing Students (N = 108)		Senior Nursing Students (N = 69)	
	N	(%)	N	(%)
Death in immediate family:				
Parent	3	(2.8)	12	(17.4)
Sibling	7	(6.5)	3	(4.3)
More than one	0	(0.0)	1	(1.4)
None	98	(90.8)	53	(76.9)*
Age of student at time of death of parent or sibling				
Under 5	3	(2.8)	1	(1.4)
6 to 10	2	(1.9)	2	(2.9)
11 to 16	3	(3.8)	5	(7.2)
Over 16	0	(0.0)	6	(8.7)
Not applicable	98	(90.8)	53	(76.8)
Not answered	2	(1.9)	2	(2.9)
Death of other close relative:				
Yes	85	(78.7)	54	(78.2)
No	23	(21.3)	13	(18.8)
Not answered	0	(0.0)	2	(2.9)
Age of student at time of death of close relative:				
Under 5	5	(4.6)	2	(2.9)
6 to 10	29	(26.9)	16	(23.2)
11 to 16	32	(29.6)	18	(26.1)
Over 16	11	(10.2)	18	(26.1)
Not applicable	23	(21.3)	13	(18.8)
Not answered	8	(7.4)	2	(2.9)

* $\chi^2 = 5.45$, $p < .02$, 1 df (categories combined)

of the freshman nursing students reported some experience with death of an immediate family member (parent or sibling); for seniors this proportion rose to over 20 percent. A number of senior students had experienced a relatively recent death (i.e., after age 16), while none of the beginning student group reported this experience. About three-fourths of each class reported the death of a close relative, not in the nuclear family, and the age at which this experience occurred was similar for the two groups.

As indicated in Table 4, freshmen, as compared to seniors, reported more experiences with deaths among friends from all causes except for that ascribed to acute illness, where the proportions were similar. These differences were not statistically significant.

Table 5 shows the categorization of responses to the task of completing the sentence, "I would/would not want my family to know I have a fatal illness because. . . ." A higher percentage of freshmen indicated they would not want their families to know (19 percent com-

Table 4
Experiences with Death of Friends of Two Groups
of Nursing Students

Type of Death of Friend	Freshman Nursing Students (N = 108)		Senior Nursing Students (N = 69)	
	N	(%)	N	(%)
Suicide	9	(8.3)	2	(2.9)
Accident	48	(44.4)	22	(31.9)
Acute illness	19	(17.6)	13	(18.8)
Chronic illness	16	(14.8)	6	(8.7)
Old age	18	(16.7)	8	(11.6)

Table 5
Replies of Two Groups of Nursing Students to the Sentence Completion
Task: "I (Would/Would Not) Want My Family to Know I Have
a Fatal Illness Because. . . ."

Category of Response	Freshman Nursing (N = 08)		Senior Nursing (N = 69)	
	N	(%)	N	(%)
Would not want family to know because:				
Concern for needs of parents	2	(1.9)	2	(2.9)
Concern for needs of self	12	(11.1)	3	(4.3)
Concern for mutual needs: parents and self	6	(5.6)	1	(1.5)
Unclassified	0	(0.0)	1	(1.5)
Subtotals	20	(18.6)	7	(10.2)
Would want family to know because:				
Concern for needs of parents	25	(23.1)	16	(23.2)
Concern for needs of self	17	(15.7)	13	(18.8)
Concern for mutual needs: parents and self	22	(20.4)	23	(33.3)
Idea of facing reality, being honest	9	(8.3)	5	(7.3)
Parents right to know	11	(10.2)	1	(1.5)
Unclassified	0	(0.0)	2	(2.9)
Subtotals	84	(77.7)	60	(87.0)
No answer/undecided	4	(3.7)	2	(2.8)
Total[1]	108	(100.0)	69	(100.0)

[1] Numbers rounded to total 100 percent

pared to ten percent). Of those students who indicated that they would want their families to know, a higher proportion of freshmen than of seniors introduced the idea that their parents had a right to know about the fatal illness (ten percent of freshmen and two percent of seniors).

Table 6 shows the categorization of responses to the task of completing the sentence, "If I learned today that I had a fatal illness, I would probably. . . ." Overall, there were significant differences in how the two groups of students responded to this task ($\chi^2 = 17.85$, 5 df, $p < .01$). More freshmen than seniors emphasized doing something. Freshmen and senior students who emphasized "doing" were split fairly evenly between those who would continue living as usual and those who would begin to appreciate life more and do all the things they had always wanted to do. More freshmen mentioned behavior related to religious beliefs, i.e., pray, read the Bible, go to church.

Replies to the additional questions given only to senior students were used for immediate feedback to faculty members planning senior curriculum. These replies, however, did suggest that a change in attitude had resulted from the educational process.

Sixty-five of the 69 senior students had nursed a dying patient. Forty-one indicated that lectures had been helpful in preparing them

Table 6
Replies of Two Groups of Nursing Students to the Sentence Completion Task: "If I Learned Today That I Had a Fatal Illness, I Would Probably. . . ."

Category of Reply	Freshman Nursing Students (N = 108)		Senior Nursing Students (N = 69)	
	N	(%)	N	(%)
Emphasis on emotional responses	12	(11.1)	21	(30.5)
Emphasis on "doing":				
Continue as usual	20	(18.5)	6	(8.7)
Appreciate life, do things always wanted to do	22	(20.4)	8	(11.6)
Religious or altruistic doing	7	(6.5)	1	(1.4)
"Unclassified doers"	6	(5.6)	3	(4.3)
Combination of emotional and doing	24	(22.2)	16	(23.2)
Emphasis on intellectual, accepting response	9	(8.3)	4	(5.8)
Unclassified others	2	(1.9)	4	(5.8)
No answer or don't know	6	(5.5)	6	(8.7)
Total	108	(100.0)	69	(100.0)

$\chi^2 = 17.58$, 5 df, $p < .01$

to work with the dying patient and his family; 28 believed actually caring for dying patients was helpful; and 15 indicated that clinical conferences were helpful. Thirty-seven seniors indicated that they had sought help with their feelings by talking with a classmate, 35 by talking with a faculty member, and 23 by talking with other personnel involved in the dying patient's care.

DISCUSSION

The mean score of the seniors on the 50 items of Part I was significantly different from the mean score of the freshmen. The seniors' responses indicated greater acceptance of feeling, more open communication, and less use of stereotyped atitudes. Their replies to the two open-ended questions of Part II followed this same pattern.

Since this research design was cross-sectional, whether the differences in scores represented attitudinal changes that occur during professional socialization might be questioned. This issue cannot be resolved within the limits of this study; however, the senior students indicated they believed their professional education had influenced their attitudes.

These seniors were the first class to complete a new integrated curriculum which stresses small group learning and encourages faculty-student interaction. This class began clinical experiences in the sophomore year at extended care facilities. Coordinated with such experience was a formal class on loss and grief, using Engel (1962) as a primary reference. This was followed by a class on death and dying for which Kübler-Ross (1969) was the primary reference. Concomitant clinical conferences were held with small groups of students when patients with whom they were working died or were near death. About one-half of the seniors took advantage of individual faculty counseling in dealing with their feelings and attitudes about a dying patient. A nursing faculty member who served as mental health integrator was on call for consultation with other faculty as well as for counseling students.[1] As students moved into pediatric units where they were faced by deaths of children and acute care areas where sudden, unexpected deaths were encountered, further clinical conferences were held and individual counseling continued to be avail-

[1] The faculty member who was available for counseling and who conducted many of the clinical conferences was Fern H. Mims. Her position as mental health integrator was made possible by a grant from the National Institute of Mental Health—NIMH 5 TO 2MH06352.

able. Thus, the base of information presented in didactic classes was reinforced by clinical experiences and small groups or one-to-one discussions.

Significantly more of the seniors than freshmen reported experiences with death of family members. Unexpectedly, more freshmen than seniors indicated that they had experienced the death of a friend. This could be a result of chance. Or, perhaps the younger students, having had less experience with death, included the death of any acquaintance in their responses; while seniors, having had more experiences with death, tended to respond only to the death of close friends.

The differences in the responses of the two groups on the open-ended questions relating to self were consistent with the differences manifested on the attitudinal items. More seniors than freshmen would want their families to know if they (the students) had a terminal illness because they believed mutual support and sharing were important. More seniors indicated that they would react on an emotional level if they knew that they had a terminal illness. Thus, compared to freshmen, seniors were more accepting of feelings and more aware of the importance of being able to share their feelings with significant others. These attitudes could be the result of having had the experience of working with a dying patient. Freshmen relied more on religious beliefs to cope with their anxieties about death than did seniors.

As with any study that compares senior and freshman students, verbal facilitiy cannot be discounted as a factor accounting for some of the differences in scores. After four years of exposure to faculty values and to learning experiences, it could be argued that the senior students were more aware of how faculty would want them to respond. Several things should have reduced the probability of students' giving answers which they believed the faculty wanted: 1) The questionnaire was developed by a committee that was not directly involved in teaching the nursing students. 2) The faculty member who administered the questionnaire to the senior students had not done any of the clinical supervision or teaching that would relate to the area of death or dying, nor was she in any way involved in grading senior students. 3) Students were assured that feedback in relation to the results of the study would be reported as a group to preserve confidentiality for individuals.

The overall findings suggest that important shifts in attitudes about death and dying can result from the nursing education. A longitudinal study is needed to verify these findings as well as well-designed, observational studies to determine whether such attitudinal changes are reflected in subsequent professional behavior. In addition, future research, using an instrument such as presented here, should incorporate assessment of faculty attitudes and those of students.

REFERENCES

Browning, M. H., and Lewis, E. P., comps. *The Dying Patient: A Nursing Perspective.* New York, Educational Services Division, The American Journal of Nursing Co., 1972.

Engel, G. L. *Psychological Development in Health and Disease.* Philadelphia, W. B. Saunders Co., 1962.

Golub, Sharon, and Reznikoff, Marvin. Attitudes toward death; a comparison of nursing students and graduate nurses. *Nurs Res* 20:503–508, Nov.–Dec. 1971.

Kübler-Ross, Elisabeth. *On Death and Dying.* New York, Macmillan Co., 1969.

Quint, J. C. *Nurse and the Dying Patient.* New York, Macmillan Co., 1967.

U.S. National Institutes of Health. *Selected Bibliography on Death and Dying,* by J. J. Vernick. Washington D.C., U.S. Government Printing Office, n.d.

This article originally appeared in *Nursing Research* 23 (1): January–February 1974 and is reprinted with permission © 1974 by American Journal of Nursing Company.

UTILIZING RESEARCH INFORMATION

Now that you have finished reading the research study, there are additional points you should consider about this report, as well as any further studies you read. These points are presented to provide you with the proper framework in which to visualize a study and to utilize the information it presents.

One of the first tasks of the reader involves identifying the framework in which the study should be placed. This consists of the following steps:

1. Identify the date on which the study was published. As a general rule of thumb, it takes approximately one year for an article to reach print after it has been submitted for publication, depending on the backlog of articles for each particular journal. Since it has taken some months for the planning, execution, and actual writing of the study, it may be assumed that the information you are reading was gathered at least one and a half years before the publication date of the article. This knowledge enables you to put the study into historical perspective according to the events

that were happening within society in general, as well as those within the profession, at the time it was conducted. Studies that were carried out several decades ago can still provide useful information if they can be seen in this perspective. The study you have just read was published in early 1974. The two-year period preceding the appearance of this article was characterized by a great popular concern with the subject of death and with dying patients. It is also a good idea to recall the societal influences that may have affected the subject's responses. For instance, nursing students would most likely have read the popular books of the time such as *Love Story* and have seen numerous television specials on the subject of death while the study was being conducted. Research involving attitudes and reactions of members of the health professions toward the dying process were just beginning. A number of more detailed studies have been published since this one appeared.

2. Note the type of journal in which the article appears. *Nursing Research* was one of the few professional publications in nursing which published research reports in this form in 1974. The identity of the journal is perhaps more of an issue in related disciplines (such as psychology) that have a large variety of journals of varying quality which are publishing reports.

3. Note the information provided about the authors of the report. Does the educational background or the employment site of the researchers seem to contribute to their understanding of the problem area? A pitfall of some of the nursing studies conducted in the past was the inexperience or lack of involvement of the researchers with actual aspects of nursing. It can be easily noted that the three authors of the study you have just read come from different educational backgrounds and that nursing is one of them.

4. Look at the list of references at the end of each study. Try to get a sense of the quality of the information the researchers have used in constructing their study: factors such as the reputation of the writers in that particular field, the relevancy of the works to the problem being studied, and the spread of dates of publication of the articles cited. This study on attitudes of student nurses toward the dying patient seems to fare well when measured against these factors.

After placing the study in the proper framework, the reader should take steps to utilize the information contained in the study. This process is begun by undertaking the following steps:

1. Restate the problem investigated and specifically the purpose of the study in your own words. Then summarize the results of the study in a sentence or two. In this way you can crystallize the information you have read and use it to increase your level of understanding.

2. Evaluate the overall relationship between the study problem and results. Do the findings seem realistic or feasible? Does your background knowledge and common sense indicate that this information could be true?

3. Think up similar ways the study could have been carried out. Let your imagination and creativity loose to dream up alternate plans for finding answers to this problem. This could include such things as using new techniques of gathering information, gathering other types of information, or changing the composition of the subjects studied. There are always many possible suggestions for change.

4. Translate the results of the study into terms that are meaningful in your professional work. How could this information be utilized in a practical way when interacting with other health professionals, when giving nursing care to patients, or when fostering your own professional identity? The new knowledge needs to become personalized if it is to have lasting impact.

It is important to start thinking about the study just as soon as you have stopped reading it. The ways to think about the study that have just been described are but a start in the process of active participation in the research process. This is the first step in becoming an intelligent consumer of research as suggested in a textbook by Mayo and LeFrance.[1] Guidelines, such as those proposed by Downs and Newman,[2] should be utilized when some degree of expertise in reading research has been established. The final chapter of this book will present more detailed guidelines for critiquing and evaluating research studies. Active participation starts with the questions you have thought of while reading the study and continues with the suggestions and alternate plans you formulate when thinking about the overall project. Active involvement in research can lead to intellectual stimulation, an increased willingness to consider alternate ways of approaching problems, and an increase in objectivity. You will feel more confident about your abilities to undertake a small research project after you read several research studies in this active way. The next chapter explains how the research process is initiated to begin the study of a research problem.

REFERENCES

1. C. Mayo and M. LaFrance: Evaluating Research in Social Psychology. Monterey, California, Brooks/Cole Publishing Company, 1977, pp. 1–18.

2. F. Downs and M. Newman: A Source Book of Nursing Research. Philadelphia, F. A. Davis Co., 1977, pp. 1–12.

PART

II

Beginning Research Skills

The second part of this book covers some of the more specific aspects of initiating and starting to carry out an actual research project. Each research study begins with the selection of a topic. Chapter 5 contains an explanation of this selection process and, in addition, gives guidelines for utilizing professional literature in developing the topic. Practical tips are given for locating relevant articles from the vast amount of published material available, and for documenting the sources of information when they are utilized in writing a literature review. Guidelines for identifying a theoretical or conceptual basis for the study are covered as well.

Chapters 6 and 7 cover the various ways in which research can be conducted and assist the reader in identifying the important factors that need to be specified whether one is conducting or critically analyzing research studies.

CHAPTER

5

Starting to Develop the Research Problem

SELECTING THE PROBLEM

The first step in undertaking any research project is to identify a general topic that is appropriate for further study. The opening statements of a study are usually not precise, but rather generalities that set the stage for the story to unfold. There are many times during the course of a day when each one of us says, "I wish I knew more about this idea," or "I wonder why this way of doing this treatment seems to work better," or "If I changed this procedure and had all the nurses do it my way it would be interesting to see what would happen."

We have all read the apocryphal story of the falling apple which led Newton to the discovery of the laws of gravity. The point of the story is well taken—events that stimulate thinking in certain areas can lead to all kinds of learning experiences. Some of the best research ideas stem from simple thoughts or questions that we all produce on a regular basis rather than from the mysterious experimental research laboratories we picture in our minds when we think about research.

Some scientists state that the research problem stems from an "irritant" in a situation, but they usually mean that it stems from an incident in which they have been stimulated to think seriously about something. In the most simple terms research problems stem from ideas we want to know more about (in general, basic research) or from a desire to find improved ways of doing things (such as in applied research).

The problem is usually thought of in generalized global terms. It is very common in the beginning stages of a study to have a nebulous or undefined set of thoughts about the subject. Confusion is a routine part of the initial stage of defining a topic for a research study and should be considered a normal occurrence. Many investigators believe that the process of defining the problem for a study is the most difficult stage of the entire research venture. The problem or topic defines the general focus of the study and sets the tone for the remainder of the project.

There is considerable variation in the way in which researchers define the problems of studies. There is no one "correct way" to effect this process within any given discipline. Kerlinger uses a question-type format for delimiting research topics as he explains in the following statement. "A problem, then, is an interrogative sentence or statement that asks: What relation exists between two or more variables? The answer is what is being sought in the research."[1] The statement of the problem in the type of study Kerlinger advocates would give the reader background information about the general topic and would then lead to the posing of a research question. This characteristic way of defining the research problem is presented in Figure 5.1.

Other scientists view the statement of the problem as an abstract process in which the researcher defines the topic through a logical, narrative process that presents information about the problem but does not result in the development of a recognizable "question" as such. This method begins with a statement of the general problem in its broadest terms and gradually narrows the focus as it proceeds. This type of approach to defining the research problem often concludes with a declarative statement regarding the purpose of the particular research project. The problem is both broad and applicable to many different types of studies. The statement of purpose that follows the

Statement of A Research Problem in an Interrogative Form

Cancer of the breast is one of the major illnesses affecting women in this country. The American Cancer Society (1974) estimated that in 1975 there would be 89,000 new cases of breast cancer and 33,600 deaths, making breast cancer the leading site of cancer incidence and death in American women. While there is an 85 percent five-year survival rate when diagnosis and treatment occur early, by the time most women discover a lump, 60 percent already have lymph node involvement, reducing the survival rate to 40 to 45 percent. Thus, the earlier detection is made, the better the long-term prognosis.

While screening with mammography in cancer detection clinics has shown that tumors can be identified at a nonpalpable stage, widespread screening is not feasible at this time, nor is it indicated for all age groups. What remains for early detection, then, is monthly breast self-examination (BSE) supplemented by yearly physical examination. Despite the simple, quick, cost-free BSE procedure, it appears that many women do not practice this behavior with any regularity. The Gallup Organization's study (Women's attitudes, 1974) of over 1,000 women revealed: Most women overestimate the prevalence of breast cancer, believe that the majority of breast lumps are malignant, are confused as to the causes of breast cancer, and fear and panic in relation to the topic. While there was an increase since 1970 in awareness of BSE (four out of five women had heard of it) and an increase in claims of monthly practice (23 percent claimed to practice BSE monthly), the lack of regular practice by a majority of women appeared to result from ignorance of the importance of BSE, fear and anxiety, and lack of knowledge about or confidence in how to do it.

Another contributing factor is the general lack of acceptance of preventive medicine. Health professionals have focused so long on illness and medical care that it is a difficult task to reorient the consumer to take steps to keep well.

BACKGROUND OF THE STUDY

This investigation focused on the question: What are the health beliefs about breast cancer and BSE and the extent of BSE practice in a selected group of adult women in a selected suburban community?

Source: M. Stillman: Women's health beliefs about breast cancer and breast self-examination. Nursing Research 26, 2 (March–April, 1977): 121–122. Reprinted with permission.

Figure 5.1

exposition of the general problem of the research study is specific, clear, and definable. An example of this technique of presenting the research problem can be viewed in Figure 5.2. It is accompanied by the diagrammatic representation of this refining process in Figure 5.3. It should be clear that the

---

Statement of A Research Problem in a Declarative Form

As the number and diversity of psychiatric facilities have increased in the past decade, roles and functions of nurses in these settings have required nursing educators to explore new means of providing learning experiences for students and practitioners of psychiatric nursing.

Whether this educational preparation is to be directed toward intensive individual care, family interaction, or group work, a central focus common to all *initial* psychiatric nursing experience is the nurse-patient relationship. Knowledge and skills inherent in the therapeutic individual relationship are fundamental in the provision of a therapeutic milieu, working with auxiliary staff and with interdisciplinary team members.

The nurse-patient relationship is based on an application of behavioral theories and implemented through use of self, expressed in purposeful communication (American Nurses' Association, 1967). Although knowledge of abstract concepts is required to create and maintain helpful relationships, the complex skills that are behavioral expressions of these concepts are difficult to describe and teach.

Modern technology provides techniques for isolating identifying, and demonstrating concepts. Videotaped student-patient interviews have been used in psychiatric nursing for students to learn by viewing their own behavior and for peer and instructor critique (Muslin and Schlessinger, 1971; Muecke, 1970; Berger, 1970). Although demonstration by role model has been advocated (Maeger, 1968), its use has been infrequently reported.

The visual and audio model of expected behavior, placed in the context of real life situations, should be an excellent tool for teaching abstract concepts and their application in practice. Since patients' first contacts in the hospital are frequently with nurses, and in view of the importance of these initial contacts, it would seem an essential learning experience for students to be able to offer these patients a degree of empathic understanding on this first contact.

Purpose. The purpose of this study was to identify verbal and nonverbal behaviors that facilitate empathic communication on initial interactions between an experienced psychiatric nurse and a psychiatric patient using a videotape of the interactions.

Source: E. Mansfield: Empathy: concept and identified psychiatric nursing behavior. Nursing Research 22, 6 (November–December 1973): 525. Reprinted with permission.

Figure 5.2

Diagram of the Steps Involved in Refining the Narrative Presentation of the Research Problem Contained in Figure 5.2.

Psychiatric nursing roles and functions have recently changed.

↓

Educators should update students learning experiences but keep the central focus on the nurse-patient relationship.

↓

Nurse-patient relationship = abstract concepts and skills difficult to describe and reach.

↓

Abstract communication concepts can be recorded on videotape to assist student learning.

↓

Videotaped interview by educator role models should provide an excellent device for teaching communication skills.

↓

Students who learn communication skills from videotapes of educators should be skillful in initial nurse-patient contacts.

↓

Purpose of study

Figure 5.3

authors have started with sweeping, broad generalities and have gradually narrowed the focus by limiting the *options on each subsequent step*.

It should be noted that the original idea that initiates the steps of the research process may become altered or modified during this refining of the problem. A number of things may cause this change to occur. The definition of the problem necessitates a preliminary review of the literature on the general topic in order to determine the amount and kind of research that has been completed in the area. Both the available literature and further independent thinking about the subject may lead to new directions. Suggestions for further study located in the research reports of others may open up new avenues of investigation. Consultation with experts in the field and with peers may provide a different slant to a general topic. Input from many sources is a necessary part of the formulation of a problem if the study is to proceed in a meaningful fashion. The very practical constraints of time, money, expertise, and overall feasibility may combine to place restrictions on a problem and limit the ground that can be covered in a single study. It is helpful to start out with the notion that a problem is often defined in terms that are too large for any single study, and proceed with the attitude that your study will contribute to a limited portion of this generalized topic.

The search for a problem should take many of the following points into consideration:

1. Start out with general topics within the professional realm in which you have a genuine interest. Chances are that you have already been doing some reading in this area because it intrigues you. Have you found yourself attracted to articles and books on specific topics, such as the natural childbirth process, personality characteristics of nurses, death and the grieving process, or various aspects of human sexuality? Try not to pick something foreign to your whole existence or something in which you have little interest. In cases where you have a limited say in determining the general problem (for example, when you are employed as part of a team and the topic is predetermined), there is usually sufficient leeway to allow for incorporation of interests in various parts of the study to make it interesting from a personal standpoint.
2. Write out your rough ideas about the problem. This may alleviate some of the confusion that is often present in the beginning, and you will be able to see the project develop as the problem is streamlined.
3. Talk to colleagues about your topic. This will not only provide opportunities to clarify your own thinking, but may result in added knowledge from the input of others. Researchers usually undertake collaborative projects, and communication about the problem in research group discussions is often one of the most productive ways to accomplish the task of delineating the topic.

4. Consider whether the problem is appropriate for the type of study you want to undertake. Does the problem imply the study of something that is possible to measure? Is the problem suitable for research or is it an administrative decision, a trivial matter, a soon-to-be-outdated method of caring for patients? Could such a study be carried out within the time limits of the situation?
5. Locate a published study that deals with the general problem even though it probably isn't exactly what you had in mind. Reading the study will give you a general idea of the steps others have taken in this area, and what the productive areas and pitfalls may be. Such a study may also suggest some practical ways of carrying out a similar study.

The general problem needs to be defined before a review of literature is undertaken in order to give direction to the literature search. A preliminary review will lead to further refinement of the problem into practical, manageable terms. Once the problem has been refined and a purpose for the study has been defined, the next step entails a thorough search of the literature for relevant information and theoretical material that has been written about the topic. Although the introductory part of a research project entails the first three steps of the research process listed in Chapter 3, the steps are often enacted in a flexible, as well as combined, form. The three initial steps, which include defining the research problem, reviewing the literature, and formulating the theoretical framework, are all present in the introductory part of a research study. They may be combined into one section (as often happens in published articles) or may be written up separately in a formal research report. In other words, the written description of the problem may be clearly labeled as a chapter (in a formal report) or a section (of a published article) or may not be demarcated at all if it is integrated with other parts of an article. (See Appendix A for an outline of the format of a typical nursing research paper. Note that the problem is clearly labeled in this type of report.) Regardless of the style of the write-up of the study, the first step in initiating the research process involves the identification of this topic.

REVIEW OF THE LITERATURE

Purpose

The review of the literature is undertaken to enable the researcher to become a subject matter "expert" on a particular problem. Selection of a research problem is actually the first step in the review of the literature since it gives direction to the library search. Since there are very few topics available on which little or nothing has been written, the review of relevant literature is conducted for a number of important reasons:

1. To gain a scholarly breadth and depth of knowledge about the problem.
2. To find examples of ways in which other researchers have conducted studies on this topic. A general picture of the state of research on the specific topic will let you know what has not been covered by previous investigators in the field.
3. To locate instruments that could be used to collect data for the study. This could include using the instrument just as it is, adapting it for the particular study, or using it as a pattern for one that you are devising from scratch.
4. To find a thrust for your study by examining "suggestions for further study" at the end of a research report. If you are still trying to refine the problem, these suggested directions for research can be very helpful since they are being written by investigators who have studied the general topic in some depth.
5. To ascertain the amount of material that has been produced relating to this problem, to identify the leading writers in this area, and to obtain some direct quotations that can be used in your write-up.
6. To discover various points of view of different schools of thought regarding the problem.
7. To find out if the study you are thinking about has previously been carried out by other researchers.
8. To locate information about the problem other than written material. This could include such things as photographs, slides, filmstrips, taped interviews, and various memorabilia (such as historical nursing uniforms and equipment).
9. To find the original, primary source material.
10. To decrease anxiety about doing research. A trip to the library to read several related articles or studies is a step in the right direction if you are having trouble refining the problem or even if you have been unable to select one. Reading several articles will make you feel like you've accomplished something and may provoke further ideas about the subject.

Searching through the literature can be interesting and exciting. It is usually a fairly comfortable process for novice researchers since there are very few students undertaking a research project for the first time who are not familiar with the library and how it operates. The search for useful materials and literature can be more rewarding if both time and energy are conserved. In order to accomplish this step of the research process most easily, it is crucial to develop an organized system of collecting and recording the information.

Organization

The first step requires that you get a system organized before you ever set foot in the library. All the indexes, journals, and "stacks" can make a mildly disorganized person veritably dizzy, so it's best to plan in advance. The important aspect is that you should feel comfortable with the system so that you can keep it operating throughout the entire literature search. The following suggestions describe one such system, but can be modified according to your own preferences.

1. Acquire note cards and make sure they are the only things you have to write on when you actually get to the library. It is far too tempting to use a scrap of loose paper or a back page in a notebook to jot something down. The cards are uniform in size, able to be resorted in various orders, and are easily filed for later use once the project ends. Many bookstores carry notebooks made up of index cards that can be easily removed by tearing along a perforated line. This provides a handy way of keeping these bibliography cards all together while you are in the early stages of the library search.

2. Decide on the technical format of documenting reference sources in the research project and learn the accurate way of writing the bibliographical information. Use this style consistently on each card for citing information about each particular source. Record the complete bibliographical data on each card and be sure to include the following:

   Periodicals: author, title, name of publication, volume, page numbers, and date.
   Books: author, title, edition, place of publication, publisher, date, page numbers of direct quotations. It is both time-consuming and frustrating to have to return to the sources to gather overlooked pieces of information in order to complete the citation.

   The bibliography card should also include a notation on the whereabouts of the source (such as *International Nursing Index*) which tipped you off about the existence of the article or book. This should also include a full citation of the name of the source, volume, year, and page numbers. This information may be necessary for two reasons. First, you will be able to return to the source of the reference if you need to check it. Second, the article may not be in your school library, and the librarian needs the verification of the source of information from the index in order to make out an interlibrary loan request. If you record the information on the bibliography cards in this manner, you can put the cards into alphabetical order when you have finished writing the paper, and the bibliography will be completely ready for typing.

3. Plan to read each article as if you will never get a chance to read it again. Summarize (annotate) the content on the bibliography card and write out direct quotations that you think sound useful or colorful. Be sure to use quotation marks so that you will remember later that this statement was a quote, and put page numbers where the information is located at the end of the quote. The summary should be written in sufficient depth to allow you to paraphrase the information in the later write-up. Make a note if the study or article contains an interesting instrument or method of collecting data from subjects. A sample of such a bibliography card can be seen in Figure 5.4.

4. Write out a bibliography card with the appropriate heading for all sources that look like they might be pertinent to your problem. If you find that the title has been misleading or for some reason you can't use the information, don't throw the card out. Make a notation on the card such as "reference contained nothing useful" and keep it with your collection to prevent you from looking up the same material again at a later time. It is not uncommon to become a little confused about titles or journals when looking up a large number of references.

5. Be aware of new sources of finding references and be prepared to expand your collection. Don't set a limit on your references or decide you will pursue only those listed in the card catalogue or an index or two. Some of the best sources of new citations are overlooked this way. Remind

---

Sample of an Annotated Bibliography Card

Kee, Joyce L. and Gregory, Ann P. "The ABC's of Fluid Balance and mEq's in Children." *Nursing 74*, June 1974, pp. 28–36.

Source: International Nursing Index 1974. Vol. 9. Pg. 649.

The article emphasizes the clinical manifestations of a dehydrated pediatric client. It begins by giving percentages of children's water content vs an adult's. "At birth, the newborn baby's body water content is 70% to 80% of his weight, whereas an adult's is 20% less. By age 2, the child's fluid drops to the adult's 50–60% of body weight level." (pg. 28.)

The authors continue by citing the threats to fluid balance.
1. *Dehydration*
The younger the infant the smaller his fluid reserve. He needs a proportionately larger fluid intake and output because of an increased body surface, increased metabolic.

Figure 5.4

yourself to constantly check the reference lists at the end of articles or books and put headings on new cards as you discover new sources.

6. Make photocopies of articles that you consider to be key references or ones that you think you may quote extensively.

7. If you are not sure of how to gauge the standing of a reference in its field, develop a system to keep track of how often it is quoted or used in bibliographies of related articles. This is a rough gauge of the importance other writers place on the value of the work.

8. Make a list of all the key words under which you could find information related to your topic in indexes or catalogues. This will enable you to locate articles relating to your topic that have not been classified under the exact words you use when referring to the problem.

LOCATING LIBRARY MATERIALS

Reference Materials

Once you have devised a system of recording references, it is time to actually go to the library and find out a lot of what there is to know about this subject that you have selected as a problem. Since each library has its unique features, you may need to refresh your memory about the services provided at the one you choose to use. However, there are a number of special features a library might have, such as interlibrary loans (a system in which your library can obtain copies of articles it does not have in its collection from another member library), special collections, microfilm files, and computer searches of the literature. You should seek out specific information on these special features. Orientation to the library's services could save time and energy in the long run.

Most libraries contain a standard set of book sources, indexes, abstracts, pamphlet indexes, and specialized ways of locating information that you can manage on your own. Figure 5.5 is a selected list of the common sources of health science literature that are available in a university nursing library. These sources provide the key to obtaining some of the vast amount of literature currently available in the health fields.

Computer Searches

Computerized literature searches are becoming more prevalent for use in supplementing certain manual searches since they can save time and energy when conducting a search for information. An "on-line" search can

Selected Sources for Locating Health Science Literature*

This abbreviated listing is highly selective and is based on one nursing library's usage patterns. It makes no attempt to include directories, handbooks, and statistical sourcebooks.

1. INDEXES (BOOKS)
    The card catalog of the library.
    U.S. National Library of Medicine, Current Catalog. (1966–date). Washington, D.C., Government Printing Office. Supersedes National Library of Medicine Catalogue 1955–1965, Armed Forces Medicine Library Catalog 1950–1954.
    Cumulative Book Index. (1898–date). New York, H. W. Wilson Company.
    Books of the Year. In: January issue of American Journal of Nursing.
    Books in Print. Annual, New York, R. R. Bowker.
    Medical Books and Serials in Print. Annual, New York, R. R. Bowker.

2. INDEXES (Periodicals. Sometimes includes books and other materials.)
    Annual or cumulative indexes to one serial title (such as: *American Journal of Nursing, Nursing Outlook, Nursing Research, Public Health Nursing*).
    International Nursing Index. (1966–date). New York, American Journal of Nursing Company.
    Nursing Literature and Allied Health Literature Index. (1965–date). and its annual cumulation, *Cumulative Index to Nursing and Allied Health Literature.* Glendale, California, Glendale Adventist Medical Center.
    Nursing Studies Index 1900–1959 by Virginia Henderson and others. Vol. 4 Philadelphia, J. B. Lippincott Company, 1963–1972.
    Index Medicus and its annual cumulation, *Cumulated Index Medicus.* (1960–date). Washington, D. C., National Library of Medicine. Includes *Bibliography of Medical Reviews.*
    Hospital Literature Index and its 5-year cumulations, *Cumulative Index of Hospital Literature.* (1945–date). Chicago, American Hospital Association.
    Education Index. (1929–date). New York, H. W. Wilson Company.
    Social Sciences Index. (1975–date). New York, H. W. Wilson Company. Supersedes in part *Social and Humanities Index.*
    Readers Guide to Periodical Literature.

* Selected from the Boston College School of Nursing Library Handbook, Compiled by Mary L. Pekarski, Librarian. Reprinted with permission.

(Continued)

Figure 5.5

3. ABSTRACTS (Periodicals. Sometimes includes books and pamphlets.)
    Abstracts of Hospital Management Studies. (1965–date). Ann Arbor, Michigan, University of Michigan, Cooperative Information Center for Hospital Management.
    Abstracts of Reports of Studies in Nursing. In: last section of each issue of *Nursing Research*. (1960–1978). New York, American Journal of Nursing Company.
    Abstracts of Studies in Public Health Nursing, 1924–1957. In: *Nursing Research*, 8: 45–115, Spring, 1959. New York, American Journal of Nursing Company.
    Nursing Abstracts. (1979–date). Forest Hills, New York.
    Psychological Abstracts. (1927–date). Washington, D.C., American Psychological Association.
    National Technical Information Service (NTIS). Weekly Government Abstracts: Health Planning. Springfield, Virginia., NTIS.
    ERIC (Education Research and Information Center).
    Current Index to Journals in Education (CIJE). (1969–date).
    Resources in Education (RIE). (1966–date).
    Resources in Vocational Education AIM/ARM. Project, Center for Vocational Education, Ohio State University.

    Other abstracts include *Biological Abstracts, Chemical Abstracts, Excerpta Medica, Medical Care Review, Nutrition Reviews* and *Sociological Abstracts*.

4. SPECIAL SUBJECT INDEXES AND ABSTRACTS
    There are many special indexes and abstracts that cover only one subject and often include books, pamphlets, periodicals and sometimes audiovisuals such as *Nutrition Reviews*; "Abstracts of Current Literature" in *Rehabilitation Literature*; "Classified Bibliography on Geriatrics and Gerontology" in each issue of the *Journal of Gerontology* with separate bound volume cumulations; and *Bibliography on Death, Grief and Bereavement, 1845–1973*, compiled by Robert Fulton and published by the University of Minnesota Center for Death Education and Research.

5. INDEXES (Government documents and other pamphlets.)
    MEDOC: a computerized index of U.S. Government documents in the medical and health fields. (1968–date).
    Monthly Catalog of Government Documents. U.S. Government Printing Office. (1937–date).
    "Pamphlets" In: *Cumulative Index to Nursing and Allied Health Literature*.
    "Publications of Organizations and Agencies" In: *International Nursing Index*.
    American Nurses' Association. *Catalog of Publications*.
    National League for Nursing. *Publications Catalog*.

(Continued)

Figure 5.5 (cont.)

6. INDEXES, ABSTRACTS (Dissertations)
    Dissertation Abstracts International. (1938–date).
    International Directory of Nurses with Doctoral Degrees. New York, American Nurses Foundation, 1973.
    "Dissertations" In: *International Nursing Index*. (1974–date).

7. INDEXES (Audiovisuals)
    Comprehensive Nursing Audiovisual Resource List, 3 V. Farmington, Connecticut, University of Connecticut Health Center, 1979.
    Health Sciences Audiovisual Resource List, 1978–79. 3 V. Farmington, Connecticut, University of Connecticut Health Center, 1979.
    National Library of Medicine Audiovisuals Catalog. (1977–date). Washington, D.C.
    "Audiovisual Materials" In: *Cumulative Index to Nursing and Allied Health Literature Index*. (1961–date).

Bibliographies at the end of relevant articles or book chapters can be helpful. Nurses are urged to develop regular library browsing habits to compensate for the time lag between publication of the journal and its citation in an index. Many of these indexes can be searched by computer, and their specialized data bases are described in Figure 5.6.

Figure 5.5 (cont.)

generate an immediate printout that includes the following information: author, title, length of article, data, journal location, and in some instances, an abstract of the article. If large numbers of articles are involved, it may be less expensive to have the references listed "off-line," which entails a three-to-five-day wait. There are a number of different bibliographic data bases available for such a mechanized search of the literature that might be useful for the health professional. An example of some of the available data bases that may be of interest to nurses and pertinent information about them are listed in Figure 5.6. The most widely known computer-based service in the health professions is MEDLINE. The anacronym MEDLARS (Medical Literature Analysis and Retrieval System) was changed to MEDLINE (the abbreviated MEDLARS On-Line) by the National Library of Medicine when the system was initiated in 1971. Computer terminals are available in many hospital as well as university libraries, and can be utilized for assistance in a literature search

Commentary 5.1
A Handy Reference Source

A bibliography compiled by Susan Taylor covers over 1,000 items published in English on nursing research from 1950 to 1974. The broad classifications consist of some of the following topics:

Development, Trends, Need for
  Nursing Research
General Articles
Textbooks
Research Process
Nursing Science/Theory
Areas for Study
Research Climate/Stimulation
Grantsmanship
Ethics
Communication of Research
Evaluation/Critique of Research
  Reports

Clinical Research
Interdisciplinary Research
Research Personnel/Roles
Research Attitude
Education
Organizations/Agencies
Position Statements/Reports on
  Research
Articles on Conferences/
  Workshops/Seminars
Proceedings of Conferences
  Workshops/Seminars

S. Taylor: Bibliography on nursing research, 1950–1974. Nursing Research 24, 3 (May–June 1975): 207–225.

for a minimal charge. The following example illustrates the way in which a physician was able to utilize MEDLINE for the well-being of a patient.

> MEDLINE (the hospital library's computer terminal) was found to be extremely useful in determining the therapeutic approach to an unusual intraocular tumor. Conservative management would have dictated removal of the eye. A review of the world literature suggested an alternate approach which preserved the eye and vision while resulting in total excision of the tumor (Stephen H. Rostler, M.D.).[2]

The computerized search can provide the researcher with valuable information when it is used in the proper circumstances. A computer search is best utilized when the topic of the search can be specified precisely. The researcher may need to undertake a manual search if the topic is not defined completely and accurately since the librarian running the search will need to know the key concepts of your topic in order to effectively use the system. The computer can play a key role in a search when limiting factors are

Computerized Data Bases Related to Health Science Literature*

This is a selective listing of data bases of potential interest to nurses. New data bases are constantly being developed, check with a librarian for more current information.

EDUCATIONAL, PSYCHOLOGICAL, AND SOCIAL SCIENCE DATA BASES

ASI (AMERICAN STATISTICS INDEX). Publications represented involve the entire spectrum of social, economic, and demographic data collected and analyzed by all branches and agencies of the U.S. Government, and a selection of the scientific and technical data developed and published by those agencies. Coverage: Comprehensive (1973–date); selective (1966–date).

CHILD ABUSE AND NEGLECT. This data base consists of ongoing research project descriptions, bibliographic references, and service program listings. The bibliographic file includes books, journal articles, government and research reports, and conference proceedings. There are over 7,000 citations in the file. Coverage: (1965–date).

CIS (CONGRESSIONAL INFORMATION SERVICE). Information emanating from the work of almost 300 committees and subcommittees of the U.S. Congress in the areas of public service programs and policies, raw materials and consumer products, industry, technology, legal questions and interpretations, national and international government policies and events, and conservation. All Congressional hearings and reports are included.

ERIC. The complete file of education and related material from the U.S. Office of Education. It consists of material from *Research in Education* (education research reports and projects) and *Current Index to Journals in Education* (an index covering more than 700 journals of interest to Educators). Coverage: (1966–date).

EXCEPTIONAL CHILD EDUCATION RESOURCES (ECER). Covers published and unpublished literature on all aspects of the education of handicapped and gifted children. The file contains over 23,000 citations and is a valuable supplement to the ERIC data base. Coverage: (1966–date).

LANGUAGE AND LANGUAGE BEHAVIOR ABSTRACTS (LLBA). Provides selective coverage to the world literature on speech and language pathology; produced by Sociological Abstracts, Inc. Coverage: (1973–date).

* Reprinted with permission from *Computer Searches* compiled by Marilyn Grant, Reference Librarian, Boston College Libraries, 1979.

(Continued)

Figure 5.6

PSYCHOLOGICAL ABSTRACTS. Coverage of the world literature in psychology and other behavioral sciences from over 900 journals; technical reports, monographs and scientific treatises are also monitored for possible inclusion. Coverage: (1967–date).

SOCIAL SCISEARCH ®. Produced by the Institute for Scientific Information (ISI). Over 1,000 journals from all areas of the social sciences are covered completely and over 2,200 journals from the physical and natural sciences are covered selectively. (*The method of citation searching is used*; it is possible to find out which researchers are citing a particular author[s] work. This is based on the theory that if an author cites a particular work, then there is generally a subject relationship between the two pieces or research.) Coverage: (1972–date).

SOCIOLOGICAL ABSTRACTS (SOCABS). Over 95,000 citations from the world's sociological literature. Coverage: (1963–date).

HEALTH SCIENCE DATA BASES

EXCERPTA MEDICA. Provides worldwide coverage of over 3,500 biomedical journals. In addition to covering all fields of medicine, *Excerpta Medica* also has wide coverage of drug and pharmaceutical literature and related health sciences (environmental health, forensic science, health economics, hospital administration, and public health). Coverage: (June 1974–date).

MEDLINE. Covers all areas of biomedical literature, including nursing. There are several subfiles in the system. MEDLINE and BACKFILES (BACK66, BACK69, BACK72, BACK75) contains almost 3,000,000 citations from over 3,000 biomedical journals; Coverage; (1966–date). CATLINE covers books and technical reports cataloged by the National Library of Medicine since 1965. CANCERLIT contains over 159,000 documents on all aspects of cancer (human and animal studies, agents, tumors); Coverage: (1963–date). CANCERPROJ, with over 16,000 records, has information concerning on-going cancer research projects, protocols, or clinical trials. EPILEPSY contains over 24,000 epilepsy-related documents. Coverage; (1945–date). AVLINE contains over 7,000 references to audiovisual materials supportive of biomedical, dental and nursing education; Coverage: (through 1979).

BIOETHICS. Based on literature acquired and indexed by the Kennedy Center at Georgetown University. The file contains over 7,000 records dealing with ethical issues of interest in biology and medicine. Coverage: (1973–date).

HISTLINE. Contains over 35,000 records relating to the history of medicine and related health sciences.

(Continued)

Figure 5.6 (cont.)

NATIONAL HEALTH PLANNING INFORMATION CENTER (NHPIC). NHPIC is a central comprehensive source of information on health planning with a special nursing component. The Center's files are computerized and literature searches are available on request.

NATIONAL INSTITUTE OF MENTAL HEALTH (NIMH). Covers mental health literature from about 950 journals, symposia, and government reports. The file contains over 300,000 records. Coverage: (1969–date).

SCIENTIFIC AND TECHNICAL DATA BASES

BIOSIS PREVIEWS. Provides worldwide coverage of life sciences literature from *Biological Abstracts* and *Bioresearch Index.* The data base covers journal articles, books, theses, book reviews, seminars, symposia, translation journals, and nomenclatural rules. Coverage: (1969–date).

CA CONDENSATES. This data base is derived from *Chemical Abstracts* and covers documents in all areas of chemistry and chemical engineering. Includes patents of 26 countries, conference proceedings, dissertations, government reports, books and comprehensive chemical reviews, and journal articles from over 14,000 periodicals. Coverage: (1970–date).

ENVIROLINE. Contains citations concerning key environmental literature, including reviews of environmental books and extracts from the daily *Federal Register.* (It is produced by Environment Information Center, Inc.) Coverage: (1971–date).

SCISEARCH. Produced by the Institute for Scientific Information (ISI). Contains all the records printed in *Science Citation Index* and additional records from the *Current Contents* series not included in the printed version of *Science Citation Index.* About 2,600 journals from all areas of the sciences are covered completely. The method of citation searching is used. Coverage: (Jan. 1974-date).

MULTIDISCIPLINARY DATA BASES

COMPREHENSIVE DISSERTATION ABSTRACTS. Covers virtually every American dissertation accepted at an accredited institution since 1861. There is also some coverage of Canadian dissertations. The on-line data base is updated monthly, giving more current information available than the printed source. Coverage: (1861-date).

FOUNDATION DIRECTORY. Describes nearly 3,000 foundations that either have assets of $1 million or more, or make grants of $100,000 or more annually. Provides information on the foundation, location, structure, personnel, financial data, purpose, and activities. The file, which contains one year's data, is kept current through semiannual revisions.

(Continued)

Figure 5.6 (cont.)

FOUNDATION GRANTS INDEX. Contains information on grants awarded by more than 400 major American philanthropic foundations. Grants to individuals and grants under $5000 are not included. Coverage: (Jan. 1973–date).

NTIS. The complete *Government Reports Announcements* from the National Technical Information Service covering a broad range of disciplines from over 240 government agencies. Coverage: (Jan. 1964–date).

SSIE. Smithsonian Science Information Exchange, Inc. contains abstracts and indexed data describing supported research projects (grants, contracts, in-house projects) from over 1,300 government agencies and private organizations that support or conduct research. (It is not based on published literature. Instead of providing references to documents, it gives the name and address of the person[s] and or institution[s] involved in the research. The data base covers all subjects.)

Figure 5.6 (cont.)

involved in defining the topic so that only relevant literature will be located. For example, this process occurred when a nursing student requested a computer search of the literature to help locate articles on teaching diabetic patients for a clinical project she was planning. In just a few minutes time, she found that of 4,752 articles on diabetes mellitus, there were 36 that were appropriate for her project. The actual printout for this computerized search can be seen in Figure 5.7.

Types of Literature Sources

There are usually two types of literature sources that are classified according to the origin of the information. Primary source material is information provided directly by the subject under study. This type of information includes diaries, letters, interviews, eyewitness accounts, speeches, documents, and papers authored by the subject. It may also take the form of autobiographies or other books written by the subject. Primary source information is particularly valuable in providing information that has not been colored by the intervention of a second party, and can be useful in stimulating new ideas about the subject. Researchers should strive to locate primary material when undertaking a project because it provides the most unbiased raw material. An example of primary source material is the letter that appears in Figure 5.8. This letter, handwritten by Florence Nightingale, is part of the set that is owned by the Nursing Archives at Boston University.

A Computer Search of the
Literature on Teaching Patients About Diabetes

PLEASE TYPE IN YOUR TOPIC OF INTEREST
diabetes mellitus
NUMBER OF CITATIONS FOUND: 4752
DO YOU WISH TO REFINE THIS TOPIC WITH ADDITIONAL
KEY WORDS?
yes
PLEASE LIST ADDITIONAL KEY WORDS
patients/education
NUMBER OF CITATIONS FOUND: 42
DO YOU WISH TO REFINE THIS TOPIC WITH ADDITIONAL
KEY WORDS?
no
DO YOU WISH TO LIMIT YOUR LIST TO ENGLISH LANGUAGE
ARTICLES?
yes

1
AU—SALZER JE
TI —CLASSES TO IMPROVE DIABETIC SELF-CARE.
SO—AM J NURS 75(8):1324–6, AUG 75

2
AU—GOELLER J
TI —DIABETIC TEACHING IN A 200-BED HOSPITAL.
SO—DIMENS HEALTH SERV 52(6):44–5, JUN 75

3
AU—ENGLE V
TI —DIABETIC TEACHING: HOW TO WIN YOUR PATIENT'S
    COOPERATION IN HIS CARE.
SO—NURSING (JENKINTOWN) 5(12):17–24, DEC 75
CONTINUE PRINTING? (YES/NO)

USER:
yes
PROG:

4
AU—BAYER M
TI —DIALOGUE ON DIABETES.
SO—NURS CARE 8(9):20–1, SEP 75

(Continued)

Figure 5.7

5
AU—WEST TE
TI —A GUIDE FOR PATIENTS: THE CARE OF DIABETES DUR-
    ING ILLNESS.
SO—NURS MIRROR 142(17):53–4, 22 APR 76

6
AU—FEUSTEL DE
TI —NURSING STUDENTS' KNOWLEDGE ABOUT DIABETES
    MELLITUS.
AB—THIS STUDY INVESTIGATED WHETHER SENIOR NURS-
    ING STUDENTS ABOUT TO GRADUATE FROM BAC-
    CALAUREATE PROGRAMS WERE KNOWLEDGEABLE
    ENOUGH ABOUT DIABETES MELLITUS TO TEACH DIA-
    BETIC PATIENTS AND THEIR FAMILIES. THE SAMPLE
    CONSISTED OF 144 VOLUNTEER SUBJECTS FROM FOUR
    COLLEGES IN A METROPOLITAN AREA. A STUDENT WAS
    CONSIDERED ELIGIBLE TO TEACH DIABETIC PATIENTS
    IF HE COULD ANSWER ALL QUESTIONS CORRECTLY ON
    A 34-ITEM INSTRUMENT. THREE ADDITIONAL QUES-
    TIONS DEALT WITH EXTRACURRICULAR CONTACT
    WITH DIABETES: WAS THE STUDENT DIABETIC? HAD HE
    A DIABETIC IN THE IMMEDIATE FAMILY? HAD HE
    TAUGHT DIABETICS? NONE OF THE PARTICIPANTS AN-
    SWERED ALL QUESTIONS CORRECTLY: ONE STUDENT
    SCORED 31 CORRECT ANSWERS. ONLY TWO QUES-
    TIONS WERE ANSWERED CORRECTLY BY ALL STU-
    DENTS. THE STUDY INDICATED THAT THE GRADUAT-
    ING STUDENTS WERE NOT PREPARED TO DO DIABETIC
    TEACHING.
SO—NURS RES 25(1):4–8, JAN–FEB 76

7
AU—HASSELL J
AU—MEDVED E
TI —GROUP/AUDIOVISUAL INSTRUCTION FOR PATIENTS
    WITH DIABETES. LEARNING ACHIEVEMENTS AND
    TIME ECONOMICS.
AB—PATIENTS WITH DIABETES RECEIVING INSTRUCTION
    IN GROUP CLASSES UTILIZING AUDIOVISUAL TEACH-
    ING TECHNIQUES ACHIEVED SIGNIFICANTLY HIGHER
    POST-TEST SCORES THAN THOSE TAUGHT INDIVID-
    UALLY IN THE TRADITIONAL BEDSIDE MANNER. IN
    ADDITION TO THE SIGNIFICANTLY GREATER LEARN-
    ING, THE DIETITIAN'S TIME WAS REDUCED BY 100 PER

(Continued)

Figure 5.7 (cont.)

CENT, BASED ON CLASSES OF EIGHT PATIENTS. THE STUDY WAS CONDUCTED BY RANDOMLY ALLOCATING FORTY-FIVE QUALIFIED PATIENTS TO CONTROL OR EXPERIMENTAL GROUPS, PRE-TESTING THEM USING A QUESTIONNAIRE-INTERVIEW, GIVING BEDSIDE OR CLASS DIETARY INSTRUCTION, AND POST-TESTING, USING THE SAME QUESTIONNAIRE. VARIOUS PERSONAL CHARACTERISTICS OF THE PARTICIPANTS, AS WELL AS DATA RELATING TO THE DIABETIC STATE, WERE ALSO EXAMINED FOR POSSIBLE RELATIONSHIPS TO TEST SCORES AND TO ONE ANOTHER.
SO—J AM DIET ASSOC 66(5):465–70, MAY 75

Note: AU stands for author
      TI stands for title
      AB stands for abstract
      SO stands for the source in which the article is located.
      The variety of journals represented gives an indication of the breadth of sources scanned during this search of the literature.

Figure 5.7 (cont.)

Secondary source information is material provided by someone other than the original source. This type of information, although it often saves a great deal of time in locating data, must be utilized with sufficient caution. An example of secondary source information is the biography of Florence Nightingale written by Cecil Woodham-Smith. Although the author had access to primary source documents, such as the letter, diaries, and various scientific papers written by the famous nurse, the book is a secondary source since it is Woodham-Smith's analysis of Miss Nightingale's life. It is not unheard of for biographers to err, although the following account of deliberate misrepresentation of facts is an extreme example:

Since 1928, a biography of Horatio Alger, written by Herbert R. Mayes, has served as the standard reference work on Alger, with historians and scholars solemnly quoting it for more than 40 years. In June 1974, Mayes revealed that he had written the book as a satire, had filled it with contradictions and absurd fabrications, and invented events and occurrences totally from his imagination, with not one shred of evidence to prove his assertions had he been challenged. In all these years, no one checked the facts—the principles of

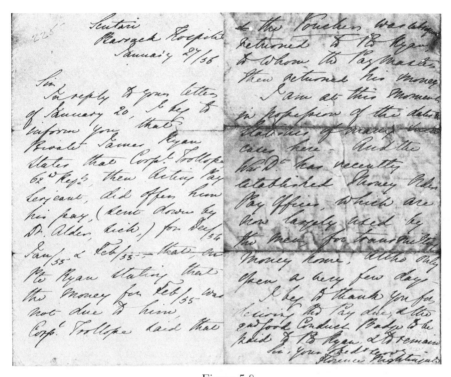

Figure 5.8

Primary Source Material: An Original Nightingale Letter Reproduced with permission from Nursing Archive, Special Collections, Boston University Library.

> internal criticism regarding that book were totally ignored by untold numbers of "scholars" (Holy Horatio!, 1974).[3]

A newspaper reporter's account of a historic event obtained by conducting interviews (as opposed to an article written directly by the person involved) is a secondary source of information since it has been colored in some way by the reporter. It is better in the same sense to read the original reports of research studies than to rely on secondhand summaries or interpretations that may appear in the literature review of a related study. Writers can sometimes use "poetic license" to view the results of the research report within their own frame of reference.

After the sources of information have been located and read, and after appropriate notes have been recorded, it is time to begin the process of writing a summary of the information for the formal research paper.

WRITING A REVIEW OF THE LITERATURE

After reading the references available about the problem being investigated, the author of a research study comes to a point at which it is necessary to put the information in writing. The purpose of this step in the research process is to create an accurate picture of the information you have found on the subject. One of the first questions usually asked by students at this stage is, "How do I know when to stop reading and start writing?" This is a difficult question to answer because the situations can vary widely according to both the problem being studied and the amount of literature available on the particular topic. In general, the researcher should feel confident about the breadth and depth of the reading that has been completed on the subject matter. The researcher who finds that there is an overabundance of material available on a given topic can limit the search in several ways:

1. By further refining the problem under review. For example, the topic of "smoking and health problems" could be narrowed to "health problems among adolescents who smoke."
2. By selecting an appropriate historical date for a cutoff time for the review. There is an abundance of literature that has been written on trends in nursing education. The researcher could select a "landmark date" (such as 1965 when the American Nurses' Association position paper was put forth as the official position regarding nursing education) and review the trends identified since that time. The researcher may decide to select a particular period for review, such as the trends in nursing education from 1960 to 1970. Often a brief history of the overall state of nursing education prior to the landmark or the arbitrarily selected date would be included to give the reader a full picture of the situation.
3. By checking the bibliographical references in the main or substantial works on the topic. The valuable, comprehensive, "classic" references are usually cited in a number of different works.

The researcher who finds very little material related to the topic should check that the subject headings selected are broad enough to include appropriate information. The Nursing Thesaurus for the *International Nursing Index* provides an excellent source for generating additional headings or guide words. The researcher who locates few references after exhausting various methods of seeking related literature should include this fact in the formal report. It is important to let the reader know that the amount of literature available was limited, rather than creating the impression that a cursory search was enacted.

Before beginning to write the review of literature, it may be helpful to look briefly at the bibliography cards to form an overall impression of the sources to be utilized. The researcher should attempt to utilize the literature to present a succinct, readable version of the topic. The following factors should be kept in mind when writing the review of literature.

Document sources of information

The reader of the literature review should be able to identify readily the source from which the information was obtained. It is standard practice to utilize both direct quotations and paraphrasing of the content of an author's work, but in both types of utilization the author needs to be given credit. There are a number of formats that can be used to document the credit. The researcher should adopt one system and use it throughout the entire paper. Some examples of resources that fully explain methods of documenting credit in scientific papers are:

1. Turabian, K. *A Manual for Writers of Term Papers, Theses, and Dissertations*. 4th ed. Chicago: University of Chicago Press, 1973.
2. *Publication Manual of the American Psychological Association*. 2nd ed. Washington, D.C.: The American Psychological Association, 1974.
3. *A Manual of Style*. Chicago: University of Chicago Press, 1969.
4. Sherman, A. *The Research Paper Guide*. Connecticut: Pendulum Press, Inc., 1970.
5. Cordasco, F. and Gatner, S. *Research and Report Writing*. 7th ed. New York: Barnes & Noble, 1963.
6. Hook, L. and Gaver, M. *The Research Paper*. 3rd ed. Englewood Cliffs, NJ: Prentice-Hall, 1962.
7. Lester, J. *Writing Themes and Research Papers: A Complete Guide*. Chicago: Scott, Foresman, 1967.
8. Lylerly, R. *Essential Requirements of the College Research Paper*. Cleveland: World Publishing Company, 1966.
9. Markman, R. and Waddell, M. *10 Steps in Writing the Research Paper*. Woodbury, NY: Barron's Educational Series, 1965.
10. Roth, A. *The Research Paper: Form and Content*. Belmont, California: Wadsworth Publishing Company, 1966.
11. Williams, C. *A Research Manual for College Studies and Papers*. 3rd ed. New York: Harper & Row, 1963.

The "Turabian method" (the format proposed by the first reference listed) is probably the most widely used method of documenting sources in college term papers. Numbers are used in superscript throughout the prose to identify the sources of the information mentioned. The bibliography includes the documentation of all sources of information (some literature may have served as background information and may not have been directly quoted in the write-up) utilized in preparing for and conducting the study.

Writing Style

Scientific papers should be written in a clear, formal style. The best of ideas will not be conveyed to the reader if the writing style is hard to comprehend. One of the greatest difficulties in reading research reports in various disciplines is the flagrant use of "jargon" or words that have meaning for only those initiated into that profession. The author should strive to write a summary of literature that is clear to readers unfamiliar with both the discipline and the particular study. A number of excellent resources are available for individuals who need assistance in presenting written material in a clear, orderly, yet uncomplicated manner such as:

1. Strunk, W. and White, E. *The Elements of Style*. New York: Macmillan, 1972.
2. Perrin, P. *Writer's Guide and Index to English*. 5th edition. Illinois: Scott, Foresman, 1972.
3. Wykoff, G. and Shaw, H. *The Harper Handbook of College Composition*. 4th ed. New York: Harper & Row, 1969.

Quotations

The exact words of other writers can be utilized in a review of literature to provide color or vividness that might add to the interest value of the paper. The words of well-known individuals in a particular field may be included to add weight or authority to the presentation. Perhaps you have found a statement that sums up a situation better than one you could write to put the same idea into words. A word of caution should be added in the event that a researcher is tempted to oversubscribe to the use of quotations. Too many or too lengthy quotations may detract from the readability of the presentation.

Controversial Issues or Conflicting Information

It is not uncommon to find a number of research studies reported on a related topic that present different or conflicting findings. The same lack of unanimity holds true for controversial issues in which two or more "schools of thought" can be easily located in the literature (for example, the issues of euthanasia, abortion, or the merits of transplant surgery). The review of the literature should present information on both sides of the issue rather than the one the researcher favors most. The inclusion of information on various aspects of a problem is another attempt to keep the research as unbiased as possible.

Interest Level

There is no reason for a review of literature to be dull or uninteresting. The use of words that are esoteric or hard to understand does not add to the scientific merit of the paper. The use of footnotes within the text allows for greater readability, as well as documentation. For instance, if you had located three different studies that came to the same general conclusion as a result of the research, you would not have to explain each study separately and provide repetitious information to the reader. You could combine remarks about three studies into one statement in the paper, such as: *Studies conducted by Regan,*[11] *Manock,*[12] *and O'Malley*[13] *have similarly concluded that baccalaureate nursing students demonstrate higher levels of academic achievement than baccalaureate students majoring in other professional fields.* Although you are presenting the material you have gleaned from the writings of others, you can summarize, paraphrase and put much of this section in your own words. The reader can look in the listing of footnotes for complete citation of the studies by each of the three authors (the footnotes would be appropriately numbered 11, 12, and 13).

Subheadings

The researcher can often use subheadings to divide the review of literature into sections to increase clarity and maintain interest level. This use of subheadings throughout this part of the paper can be useful in the organizational steps as well. The completed bibliography cards can be grouped according to similar themes or content and each section can be written independently. This can be a great help in reducing the task to more manageable proportions. A lengthy or involved review of literature is often concluded with a brief summary to focus the reader's attention on the important highlights.

THE THEORETICAL FRAMEWORK

At the same time researchers are gathering references from the current literature about their general problem, they need to locate a systematized body of knowledge that pertains to their work. The very foundations of thinking and acting in an intelligent, professional manner can be ascribed to the utilization of theoretical information. Theory is generally considered to be the organization of related knowledge that has been explained, critiqued, and found to be consistently true. Theories are used to understand complex operations since they put numerous ideas together so that many facets of the information can be utilized simultaneously. It not only helps researchers to understand present information, but helps them to predict how new phenomena will fit into the general scheme.

The review of the literature provides the investigator with the written viewpoints, observations, experiences or earlier studies completed within this topic area. It is not unusual to find disparate, conflicting, or insubstantial information as a result of reviewing journals and other periodicals. Often articles can be thought-provoking even when they are not specifically pertinent to the problem being studied. However, the researcher needs to stabilize the foundation of the work by locating or developing a substantial framework of knowledge that encompasses the limited territory of the study being enacted. Even though the basic theory upon which a study is based is open to change or alteration as new knowledge becomes available, it provides a safe home base for the venture out into the world of scientific investigation.

The task of the individual conducting a research study consists of locating and utilizing an appropriate theory for the study that is being drawn up. It does not encompass the devising or "inventing" of a theory. As Margaret Hardy writes:

> The development of adequate theories to describe, explain, predict, and control phenomena is a slow process and requires the cooperative effort of many persons. Knowledge is not acquired by one person in isolation but results from the cumulative efforts of many persons over a long period of time.[4]

Theories are developed by refining ideas and subjecting them to constant scrutiny by testing and retesting. In other words, theory grows from research. Although many individuals may contribute to the development of a theory, it often becomes popularized or associated with the name of one individual. Most nurses are familiar with such theories as Maslow's theory of motivation, or Erikson's theory of the stages of psychosexual development.

There are few nurses who have become well associated with theories since one of the biggest problems facing the entire profession is the limited amount of existing theory. The information that is used for professional practice, as well as for the education of new nurses, is composed of a dearth of theoretical knowledge that nursing can call its own. Much of this knowledge base is a patchwork of theory borrowed from the psychosocial, biological, and physical sciences. The same situation holds true for the theoretical base of the current research being conducted in nursing—the theory is often "borrowed" from the discipline most closely allied with the problem of the study. Researchers should scrutinize the problem and purpose of their study in order to pinpoint the most appropriate theoretical basis. In order to do this, they need to define the generalized or overall factor they are studying rather than its specific aspects. The purpose of the study presented in Figure 5.2 is very specific with regard to the particular aspects of the project undertaken by this psychiatric nurse. The theoretical basis of this investigation should encompass the generalized or broad area under study. Another way of identifying this area would be to name the broadest reference classification under which the particular study could be listed. A second reading of the purpose should be undertaken in order to make this determination. It seems that the overall topic of investigation in this instance focuses on therapeutic nurse-patient interactions with emphasis on the component of empathy. A further excerpt from the study demonstrates that the theories of a number of psychologists who have completed prior work in this area (such as Rogers and Truax) were utilized in constructing this particular theoretical framework. The theoretical framework of the study is presented in Figure 5.9.

Nursing will undoubtedly develop numerous theories as research progresses in testing out the ideas upon which the theories will be based. Then nursing theories, like theories of other disciplines, will be available to all scholars and professionals desiring to use them. The availability of theory will act as a stimulus in fostering more in-depth research. It would be wise to note that most theories are recorded in the texts of books (for instance, the theories of Rogers and Truax cited previously) rather than in journal articles. Occasional deviations from this rule of thumb may result from a perusal of journal articles in the nursing field. The article encapsulated in Commentary 5.2 was designed to organize disparate pieces of knowledge about one aspect of nonverbal communication, and create a useful framework for nursing studies. Because of the limited amount of available theory in nursing, it is important to trace the origins of theoretical development since, as a professional, you may encounter nursing knowledge in any of its stages. It is, therefore, important to understand the process through which ideas must pass in order to become recognized theories (and later—scientific laws or principles). CONCEPTS have often been labeled the "building blocks of theories since they are abstractions that are used to observe and classify the properties of phenomena being studied. The term "nonverbal behaviors" (as utilized in the statement of purpose in Figure 5.2) constitutes a concept since it represents a variety of methods of communication that do not utilize the spoken word. When enough knowledge is gathered to make statements that relate two or more concepts, we term these statements PROPOSITIONS. The way we

An Example of A Theoretical Framework

Theoretical Framework. Rogers' work formed the theoretical framework of this study. According to Rogers, experiences inconsistent with the self are perceived as threatening; the more numerous these are, the more the self must maintain itself by rigid organization.[1] These experiences, under certain conditions, may be perceived, examined, and assimilated. On acceptance and integration of these experiences, the individual becomes more accepting of others. As the individual accepts these experiences, he substitutes former distorted values with a continuing valuing process of his own.

Rogers' theories of personality and psychotherapy have been based on research that has consistently demonstrated the importance of empathy as one of the "facilitative conditions" in therapeutic interactions.[2,3] Levels of these conditions—empathy, congruence, and positive regard—that are offered to the patient and perceived by him as present in the interaction are associated with the patient's improvement or deterioration.

1 Rogers C., Client-Centered Therapy: Its Current Practice Implications, and Theory Boston, Houghton Mifflin Co., 1951.
2 Rogers C., Dymond R., eds., Psychotherapy and Personality Change: Co-ordinated Research Studies in the Client-Centered Approach Chicago, University of Chicago Press, 1954.
3 Rogers C., "The Necessary and Sufficient Conditions of Therapeutic Personality Change." Jour Consult Clin Psychol 21 95–103, 1957.

E. Mansfield: Empathy: concept and identified psychiatric nursing behavior. Nursing Research 22, 6 (November–December 1973): 526.

Figure 5.9

Commentary 5.2
A Touchy Subject

Kathryn Barnett has succeeded in an attempt to organize the ideas and research findings of scientists in a variety of disciplines regarding TOUCH, and has grouped the phenomena together in a way that will be meaningful in a nursing context. She justifies the need for recognizing important means of nonverbal communication within nursing by the following statement:

> Touch as a way of conveying meaning has been used
> since the beginning of mankind. Every known culture has

assigned some meaning to the act of touch. It is used between parent and child, between lovers, and between friends to convey love, kindness, empathy, and a multitude of other meanings. It has been used extensively in the medical disciplines—from the time of the witch doctors to the present-day practitioner of medicine. Modern practitioners of medicine, as well as researchers in many of the behavioral disciplines, have come to regard the area of touch as a means of communication as a valid field for research. In the light of that realization and on the assumption that the health team if obligated to meet the total needs of the patient throughout his stages of illness this investigation was undertaken.

The concepts of touch from various fields of study have been categorized into five areas affecting nursing. Each of these areas should provide the stepping stones for future research endeavors by nurses:

1. Mechanics of Communication
2. Touch as a Means of Communicating
3. Touch as a Basis for Establishing Communication
4. Touch as a Means of Communicating Emotions
5. Touch as a Means of Communicating Ideas

K. A. Barnett: A theoretical construct of the concepts of touch as they relate to nursing. Nursing Research 21, 2 (March–April 1972): 102–110.

test out the accuracy of these relationships is to form HYPOTHESES, or precise statements of relationship that can be evaluated for their predictive powers through objective research. As the progression of knowledge becomes increasingly complex, an organizational process results in the cataloguing of information about the concepts, propositions, and hypotheses. Either a CONCEPTUAL MODEL, which tangibly outlines the shape of the existing knowledge, is constructed or a CONCEPTUAL FRAMEWORK is designed which is defined as a "more loosely organized set or complex of ideas . . . that provides overall structure."[5] In either case, the knowledge is not as tightly organized as in a THEORETICAL FORMULATION. This organized, systematic yet still tentative area of knowledge advances to the refinement of a THEORY once sufficient evidence of its accuracy is amassed. Roy touches on the depth of knowledge involved in a theory when she describes it as "the working insides of a model."[6] The final progression is to the level of a SCIENTIFIC LAW or PRINCIPLE. This classification is used to describe an irrefutable relationship between variables that have withstood the scrutiny of repetitive investigations. A diagrammatic representation of this process of theory development can be found in Figure 5.10. It is important to remember that nursing theories by nature will generate large numbers of related hypotheses that will make this whole knowledge-building process seem less formidable.

As long as the eclectic approach is necessary in utilizing theory in relation to research projects, nurses will be required to use organized knowledge from related fields. This is especially true when one considers that it is highly unlikely that inexperienced researchers would identify an area of study that was completely unique and previously unknown to man. A search of an appropriate allied field is likely to yield a useful theory base. Careful attention must be paid to relating this knowledge base to the mainstream of nursing, however, to avoid a splitting-off effect.

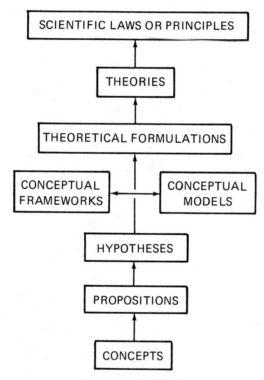

Figure 5.10. The components of theory development.

ORGANIZING THE INTRODUCTORY
SECTIONS OF THE STUDY

The organization of the introductory parts of a formal research study is not set up according to a number of steps that must be executed in a specific order. The process is flexible in that it can be tailored to meet the requirements imposed by the topic or by the experience or depth of knowledge possessed by the investigator. The definition of the problem, review of literature, specification of the theoretical base of the study, and all of the steps in between are often carried out in the overlapping order implied in Figure 5.11. The beginning researcher should not become too discouraged if the process of identification of the research problem requires several preliminary literature reviews before moving to the next stages. As Figure 5.11 clearly points out, the use of practical and clinical judgment is a key factor in the crucial beginning stages of this process. The nurse needs to translate the articles, the areas of inquiry, and theories to relevant situations in professional nursing.

Just as there are no set rules to govern the development of the introductory sections of a research project, there are no set rules to guide the writing up of this process. Occasionally, research articles clump all three sections under a heading of Introduction. Some reports treat the three main

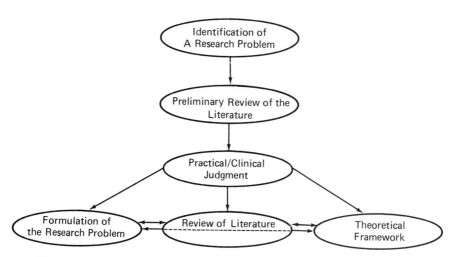

Figure 5.11. Development of the introductory sections of a research study.

areas as separate sections labelled Introduction, Review of the Literature, and Theoretical Framework. Others may combine the Review of Literature, and the Theoretical Framework, while keeping the development of the Problem as a separate section. Published articles often condense and combine the various introductory sections to conserve on space with little regard for identifying labels. When reading published research studies, it may be helpful in the beginning to label the three elements of the introductory section until you become skilled at recognizing them in any format.

REFERENCES

1. F. Kerlinger: Foundations of Behavioral Research. New York, Holt, Rinehart & Winston, 1973, p. 17.

2. Nurse Educator II, 2 (March–April, 1977): 8.

3. T. Christy: The methodology of historical research: a brief introduction. Nursing Research 24, 3 (May–June, 1975): 191.

4. M. Hardy: Theories: components, development, evaluation. Nursing Research 23, 2 (March–April, 1974): 105.

5. C. Peterson: Questions frequently asked about the development of a conceptual framework. Journal of Nursing Education 16, 4 (April, 1977): 25.

6. J. Riehl and Sr. C. Roy: Conceptual Models for Nursing Practice. New York, Appleton-Century-Crofts, 1974, p. 3.

CHAPTER

6

Different Approaches to Conducting Research

This chapter presents the kind of general information a researcher needs to consider once the introductory sections of the study have been completed. The areas that will be covered are the research approach, design, and setting. Each aspect concerns certain characteristic qualities the investigator can use to give form to her study. These strategic aspects need to be delimited prior to making the "nitty gritty" decisions covered in later chapters, such as "what questions" to ask from "what number" of people. The decisions made regarding these general areas of research approach and design are natural extensions of the definition of the problem. They continue to give substance and direction to a process that has already begun taking form. They guide the researcher to a point at which specific decisions can be made that will blend in logically with the study they are creating. The approach design and setting of a study are like important route signs on major highways. The specific questions (such as the number of people to get for a good sample) are analogous to rest stops and exit ramps along the main highway. They will be explained in later chapters.

A VARIETY OF APPROACHES TO RESEARCH

The "research approach" is the formal name for the general direction the researcher will travel in order to discover new information about the problem. The approach is a very generalized plan that is used as a guideline for finding answers to the problem or to the question that was initially posed. Once researchers have identified the general problem and inspected the relevant literature, they are well on their way toward selecting the approach they will utilize in conducting their own study. This holds true since the nature of the problem will limit the types of appropriate ways to proceed with the study, and the literature will usually suggest ways of achieving this goal that have been tried out by previous investigators. The investigator who is concerned with discovering the effects of a certain nursing procedure on a group of patients will obviously attempt to discover this information in a very different fashion from someone concerned with investigating the historical origins of nursing education in the United States.

There are six distinct ways to approach the study of a research problem. Each of the six types of research approach has its own particular time orientation, various ways of obtaining information, and different methods of organizing the intermediate steps in the study of the problem. Although the researcher's objective of obtaining scientific knowledge remains the same in each instance, the manner in which the objective is accomplished will vary considerably. The six approaches to the study of a research problem are the following: philosophical, historical, case study, methodological, survey, and experimental.

Philosophical Approach

The philosophical approach entails research into the thoughts or ideas that are important to a particular group or profession. Although this type of research is the least prominent of the six approaches to nursing, it is a necessary field of exploration within any profession. Despite the fact that studies of this nature are for the most part quite abstract and theoretical, some nurses are beginning to utilize their interests and skills in this intellectual area. Some examples of philosophical research in nursing have been recently published and include aspects of ethical considerations of patient care, decision making in nurse-patient relations, and the judgment process in nursing.

Historical Approach

The goal of historical research is to obtain facts from the past in order to make conclusions about this evidence. Interpretations are often made that relate to presently existing problems. Each profession has its share of founders, leaders, and achievements. The chronicling of these individuals and the events that shaped the profession are often overlooked while emphasis is placed more on present and future problems. Within the main body of the nursing profession there are a dearth of historiographers whose main focus is the collection, organization, and written analysis of data from the past. The historiographer seeks to document happenings that have already occurred, and to set the record straight in the event that the traditionally accepted version is incomplete. Commentary 6.1 contains an example of the latter in which the traditionally held version of events is placed in question by the surfacing of new documents.

Commentary 6.1
Will the Real "First Nurse" Please Stand . . . ?

Linda Richards (New England Hospital for Women and Children, 1873) has been traditionally known as the "first trained nurse" in the United States. She has been recognized as such by inclusion in the American Nurses' Association Nurses Hall of Fame. Documents have been recently uncovered which indicate that Harriet Newton Phillips was educated as a nurse at the Woman's Hospital of Philadelphia in 1863. Little of her career is known other than the facts that she practiced nursing in the community, received $4.00 per week for her services, and volunteered in the Civil War as well as working as a missionary among the Indians. With regard to her nursing education, the author states the following:

> We can assume that the training of Miss Phillips began with the female medical students entering October, 1863 and was completed in March, 1864, a six month course. The lectures included Anatomy and Physiology, Materia Medica, Chemistry, and the practical arts of nursing determined by the notes from Florence Nightingale.

> The author states that it is possible to pay tribute to Linda Richards for her accomplishments while recognizing Harriet Newton Phillips as the first trained nurse. She advocates documentation of our nursing heritage rather than fostering a myth. Since history is only as reliable as the documentation we can obtain, it must be kept open and subject to change as much as possible.
>
> Joan Large: Harriet Newton Phillips, the first trained nurse in America. *Image* 8, 3 (October 1976): p. 49–51.

The discovery of facts contained in the past is analogous to undercover work. Christy[1] compares the historical researcher with a sleuth in stating that the historiographer must go where the material is and needs the curiosity, perseverance, tenacity, and skepticism of the detective. This type of study most often utilizes primary source material, such as letters, diaries, official records, and eyewitness accounts. This information has not usually been compiled with research purposes in mind, but must be selectively used by the investigator to suit his purpose. For example, in 1934 Durkheim in his famous volume *Suicide*[2] was able to utilize actual death records (collected by the countries involved for legal purposes) for his data base. He was then able to relate the fluctuating suicide rate with sociological factors in effect in the society during each interval studied.

In 1972, Lois Monteiro was able to utilize the Nursing Archives at Boston University as the center for uncovering historical information about a nursing figure. In an article entitled "Research Into Things Past: Tracking Down One of Miss Nightingale's Correspondents," the author utilizes six letters sent by Florence Nightingale to an acquaintance between 1877 and 1892. This data base was utilized to shed light on Miss Nightingale's ideas about professionalism, and to highlight several of her personality characteristics.[3] Indeed, it was shown that some of these influences from the past can still be felt in the nursing profession even at this late date. With approximately 12,000 other original Nightingale letters in existence, there are numerous other possibilities of research in this vein. Many of the official documents of the former nursing leaders in this country such as M. Adelaide Nutting and Isabel M. Stewart await the perusal of a scholar-detective.

The recording of past events can serve to illuminate the growth of status of the nursing profession in relation to society at large. The nurses who find themselves concerned with the role of nursing within a political structure, such as the health care delivery system, could profit in many ways by reading a historiographer's account of a similar set of events from the past. The struggle waged by nurses in obtaining official rank from the U.S. Army is encapsulated in Commentary 6.2.

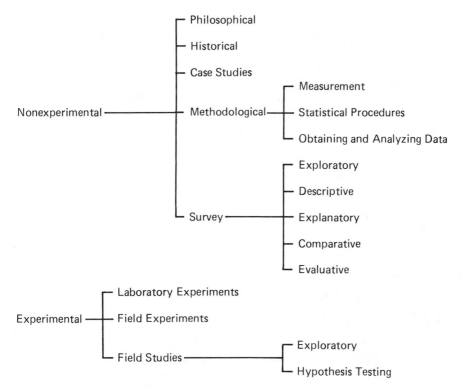

Figure 6.1. Classification of types of research according to nonexperimental and experimental designs.

Commentary 6.2
Aye Aye Sir . . . er . . . Ma'am

Philip Kalisch has published historical research that chronicles the struggle of nurses for official designation of military rank. The Army Nurse Corps was established as early as 1901, but with unclear status within the military structure. Although some questions had been raised about awarding rank to nurses, the wholehearted efforts in this direction began in 1917. M. Adelaide Nutting began contacting officials about the severe handicap the lack of rank placed on Army nurses in their efforts to carry out their work as they left for Europe in the midst of World War I. The professional component of the Army Medical Department consisted of 21,500 nurses (without rank) and 31,000 physicians (with rank).

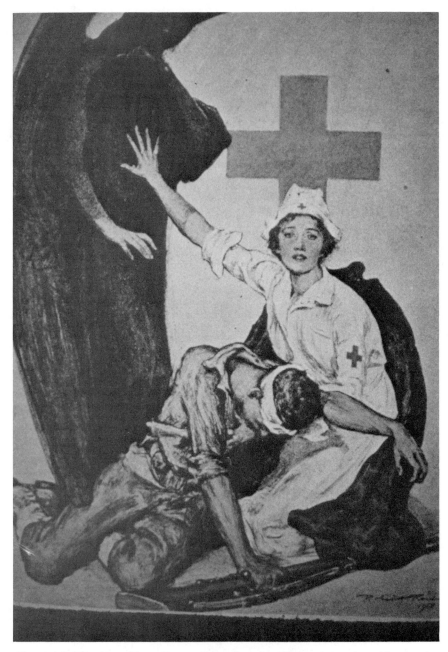

Figure 6.2. The Army Nurse Poster (Reproduced with permission from Nursing Archive, Special Collections, Boston University Library.)

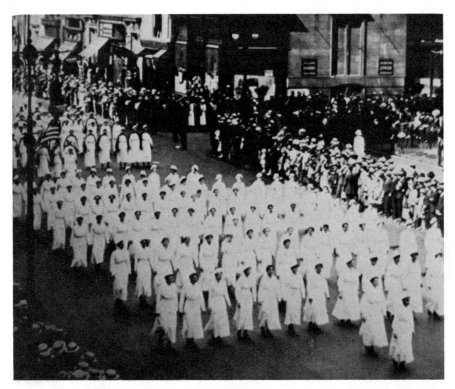

Figure 6.3. Nurses in uniform in a publicity picture. (Reproduced with permission from Nursing Archive, Special Collections, Boston University Library.)

The article covers many aspects of the long fight for official status and recognition. As the accompanying picture points out, nurses were used for publicity fund-raising appeals while at the same time having no secure position in the hierarchy.

This state of affairs led to the gradual gains which included establishment of an official uniform and the recognition within the chain of authority in hospitals and on army bases in general. The war ended with the problem still unresolved, but the nurses were committed to carry their work to its conclusion.

Some of the objections to nurses gaining rank were listed as follows:

· The bill would increase the cost of the Army at a time when the taxpayer was already overburdened.
· The alleged inferiority of some Army nurses made them unfit to become officers.

· It was feared that nurses, if given the privileges of rank, would lose their heads and become licentious.

The citing of letters, protests, legal maneuvers, and political pressures gives the struggle its former lifelike quality. It concludes in 1947 with the attainment of actual permanent rank.

The author highlights the importance of historical research in nursing by the following statement about his study:

> It is enlightening to look again at the debates and demonstrations that marked one of nursing's earlier active efforts in the political process. In this present atmosphere of concern over nursing's role in health care policy, it is well to remember that the tactics to be utilized in shaping political decisions that impinge upon the profession are not new.

Philip Kalisch: How army nurses became officers. Nursing Research 25, 3 (May–June 1976): 164–177.

The researcher conducting a historical study needs to carefully weigh the validity of the sources of information since they assume such a crucial role in the investigation. The sources of data are critically reviewed by means of a two-part process. EXTERNAL CRITICISM is utilized to appraise the genuineness and overall validity of the item. INTERNAL CRITICISM, the more frequently used of the two, is used to appraise the content of the data. This latter method assesses the accuracy of the statements and dates while determining the true meaning and value of the data. [4]

This "history" of the historical research in the nursing profession has been a consistent one of underutilization. This lack has been recognized by many leaders within the field and efforts have been instituted (such as the creation of Nursing Archives to preserve materials, and the existence of small grants to find historical projects) to stimulate the creative endeavors of nursing scholars.

Case Study Approach

Most nurses are familiar with the case study approach to collecting data about health-related information. The goal of a case study approach is to collect wide-ranging, in-depth data, to draw conclusions, and to make predictions based on that information. The medical sciences have long utilized this type of detailed analysis as a precursor of a more extensive research project.

Investigators in this type of study select their subject matter with a specific purpose in mind. The nurse may want to find out all the types of nursing problems encountered by a patient or a group of patients with a given medical problem. The focus of the information collected for the data base may start in the present, but often includes past events as well. Sociologists and anthropologists have traditionally used this approach to research in studying people, communities, institutions, and societies. The data are predominantly verbal, but may also include objects or artifacts. This is also true for health-related studies in which various objects such as x-ray films, still pictures, and drawings may become an integral part of the formal report of the research.

The investigator utilizing the case study approach should attempt to collect as many data as possible since the main benefit of this type of research is the in-depth level of insights that may result. This is particularly important in nursing where so much stress is placed on seeing the patient in a holistic light. Such a study would pave the way for the formulation of clinically viable hypotheses for use in later studies. Care should be exercised in selecting the objects for such a study since it would be important to note whether it would be more beneficial to find a subject who is most representative or most different from the group being studied. This is also important in light of the analysis of the findings. The applicability of results to different situations is an important consideration in any study, but particularly one in which th e subject matter is very limited in scope or number. The term IDIOGRAPHIC ANALYSIS is used when talking about the analysis of the one case under study. NOMOTHETIC ANALYSIS is the process of generalizing from the one case to a total group it is supposed to represent.[5]

Methodological Approach

Methodological research is undertaken for the specific purpose of developing ways of quantifying information. It deals with measurement in terms of mathematics, statistics, and various methods of obtaining and analyzing data. This approach includes a great deal of very needed work in nursing in the construction of instruments: scaling, the writing of items, and analysis of the usefulness of the items selected. Nursing lags behind other professions in this particular area, and it could be one of the major reasons for the small amount of completed research to date.

There are relatively few instruments available that can be used to collect information on or about nursing. Most of the available indices pertain to nursing education and the measurement of knowledge—predominantly in the theoretical sphere. Clinical tools for measuring or assessing nursing care or health promotion activities are a rarity. A psychologist who was planning a study that included the measurement of personality traits could look in one of the source books cataloguing psychological instruments and find information on numerous tests available for this very purpose.

Previous investigators in the psychosocial areas have laid the groundwork by developing, pretesting, and actually using the measurement devices in prior research work. This not only assists the investigator in economizing on time and money, but will also give them an idea about the degree of success in using the device. On the other hand, the nurse must conduct an extensive search for an instrument since nursing tools have not yet been developed and tested in sufficient quantities to permit the publication of such instrument resource books. In some instances the nurse can borrow and adapt previously devised measuring tools, but this process is not the most beneficial for quantifying aspects of the nursing care delivered to patients. Methodological research includes construction of interview schedules and the organization of observational techniques. Methods of selecting subjects can be included, as well as analysis of the results from the relatively straightforward, non-numerical process of content analysis, all the way up to the utilization of sophisticated statistical techniques.

Survey Approach

Survey research is the process of gathering current data from subjects so that new information can be obtained. Kerlinger notes that these studies are usually called *sample surveys* and states that "Survey research studies large and small populations (or universes) by selecting and studying samples chosen from the populations to discover the relative incidence, distribution, and interrelations of sociological and psychological variables."[6] Survey research is the label given to a number of distinctly different types of studies. The best feature of survey research is that it enables the investigators to collect current information about whatever it is that they wish to study. They have control over the form and the manner in which the information will be obtained. The survey is conducted expressly for the purpose the researcher indicates, unlike other approaches such as the historical in which the researcher has to make do with information that has been previously recorded. The word survey is appropriate in this instance since it implies that information is being collected from a variety of subjects who resemble the total group in the characteristic being studied. Although information on some facet of the subject's existence is being sought, this fact alone does not qualify the effort as research. A survey research study should not be confused with the taking of a census or the conduction of a public opinion poll. The research is set apart from polls since the researcher has set out in an attempt to add to existing theory or to extend the limits of what is known in a particular area. The main focus is then placed on the framework into which the new information is assimilated rather than on the information alone. Although authors differ on the classification of the types of survey research, most include aspects of the following.

EXPLORATORY
Studies are conducted to obtain more information on areas in which very little information is available. This type of survey might be conducted to determine the extent of nursing involvement in relation to a particular health problem or to identify possible hypotheses for further and more extensive study. An example of one study of this type would be an investigation of the nurse's role in caring for patients undergoing computerized axial tomographic procedures. The researcher in these types of studies moves forward with the expectation of charting new territory for research rather than with the goal of quantifying a particular variable.

DESCRIPTIVE
Surveys are carried out for the purpose of providing an accurate portrayal of a group of subjects with specific characteristics. Descriptive studies usually entail the precise measurement of phenomena as they currently exist within a single group. The example provided in Commentary 6.3 is a description of the attitudes of a group of nursing students about a health-related phenomenon. Descriptive studies are often utilized by researchers to determine the extent or directions of attitudes or behaviors. They are conducted many times as a prelude to the design of extensive and more precise projects. A volume entitled *Twenty Thousand Nurses Tell Their Story* was compiled in 1958 for the purpose of describing the then current state of the members of the nursing profession and the work in which they were engaged.[7]

Commentary 6.3
Want to Find Out About Nursing Student's Views About Contraceptives? Do A Survey!

Ruth Elder conducted a research project with a descriptive survey approach in order to obtain information on the attitudes of nursing students about providing contraceptive services. The sample consisted of 264 senior students who provided information about their attitudes by filling in a questionnaire. The students were generally permissive with regard to providing contraceptives to all groups except very young teenagers. One half considered that age 15 was the best time to educate teenagers in this area. Less than one-third of the group evidenced a permissive attitude when nonprofessional distribution (for instance, vending machines) of contraceptive devices was suggested. Those students holding a more permissive attitude were found to have more lenient attitudes toward premarital sex, more concern with population problems and more nontraditional views of the woman's role.

R. Elder: Orientation of senior nursing students toward access to contraceptives. Nursing Research 25, 5 (September–October 1976): 338–344.

EXPLANATORY

Surveys are conducted to provide causal explanations of phenomena or situations. According to Warwick and Lininger,[8] the following three conditions must be satisfied to establish a causal explanation: first, the cause and effect must be associated with each other. In other words, A must be present when B is present under specified conditions. Second, cause must precede the effect, and third, other possible explanations of the effect should be ruled out. This kind of survey is more specific than the two previously discussed types and requires a more sophisticated level of knowledge to enact. The investigators must familiarize themselves with previous studies and current literature in order to identify the causal relationships specific to the project. Explanatory surveys often involve hypothesis testing with an emphasis on the qualitative aspects of the data, as well as on the numbers collected. The study summarized in Commentary 6.4 is a typical explanatory survey.

Commentary 6.4
The "Rolling Stones" of Nursing

This exploratory study was conducted to study the rewards and incentives that influence the job turnover rate of staff nurses. Previous research in this topic indicated both key factors and some of the expected influences they might have in this situation. These rewards and incentives were grouped into the following categories: safety, social, and psychological. Seven different hypotheses were formulated to deal with personal characteristics of the nurse and specific factors that would affect her job longevity. Two of the specific hypotheses were presented like this:

   I.   Younger nurses leave jobs sooner than older nurses.
  VI. Among nurses, new graduates leave jobs sooner than older nurses.

Other hypotheses investigated the effect of such factors as marital status, salary of spouse, educational background, salary, and area of clinical specialization.

Ninety-four questionnaires were utilized in the study that surveyed nurses who had left their positions in metropolitan medical-surgical hospitals within the four months prior to the initiation of the survey.

The nurses in the sample were found to have less than the 70 percent turnover rate cited by previous work in this area. The findings concerning the two hypotheses listed above were as follows:

I.   Supported. Younger nurses left jobs sooner than older nurses.
VI. Supported. New graduates tended to leave the job in the first six months.

Other results indicated that overall rewards and incentives influenced job decisions in the following descending order of importance: psychological, safety, and social.

Joanne McCloskey: Influence of rewards on staff turnover rate. Nursing Research 23, 3 (May–June 1974): 239–247.

COMPARATIVE

Studies utilize set criteria to contrast two or more groups of designated variables. This popular type of survey has often been used by investigators to compare two distinct groups on the basis of such qualities as knowledge level, perceptions, or attitudes. The surveys are usually very broad comparisons as a result of the presence of a multitude of variables in the situation that are not under the control of the investigator. The usual procedure consists of choosing two groups that can be expected to vary according to a definite factor. When dealing with the complexities of human subjects, it is imperative to keep in mind the enormous lack of ability to screen out other factors and construct two groups equally comparable on a limited number of items. Comparative studies are characterized by carefully defined groups although the major effort is usually employed in selecting and refining the instruments used to measure the intergroup differences. The study summarized in Commentary 6.5 exemplifies a typical comparative study that was instituted to compare two groups of nurses on specific personality characteristics. The usefulness of comparative studies results from the relative ease, speed and accuracy with which they can be conducted by unexperienced researchers. This type of survey makes its biggest contribution to theory by generating feasible areas of further investigation and by suggesting future hypotheses for study under more controlled conditions.

Commentary 6.5
Personality Differences in Nurses

Lois Lukens conducted a study of graduate students to determine whether personality differences existed in nurses who choose two different areas of clinical specialization. She recognized this topic as an important area of study since satisfaction and retention within the field might be increased by better placement. Little is known about success in the field of clinical specialization, and the information available on nursing students does not generally extend to graduate level students. Counseling about placement within a clinical specialization could be based on research and facts if such information were available. Personality patterns of graduate nurses choosing a medical-surgical specialty were contrasted with those choosing psychiatric nursing. The sample consisted of 238 nurses who were enrolled as full-time graduate students in the two clinical specialties being contrasted.

The study results supported the major hypothesis: the personality patterns of nurses specializing in medical-surgical nursing differ from the personality patterns of nurses specializing in psychiatric nursing. Some of the major findings that differentiated the two groups were as follows:

MEDICAL-SURGICAL NURSES	PSYCHIATRIC NURSES
Higher needs for physical activity, organization, achievement, and intellectual development.	Higher needs for emotionality and reflectiveness.
More authoritarian with regard to social issues.	More psychologically minded.
Religious and humanitarian values higher than those of psychiatric nurses.	More willing to acknowledge socially undesirable feelings.
Higher value on background knowledge required in the field.	More value on the type of nurse-patient relationship developed.

Lois Lukens: Personality patterns and choice of clinical nursing specialization. Nursing Research 14, 3 (Summer 1965): p. 210–220.

EVALUATIVE

Surveys are being used more frequently today in conjunction with other data-gathering techniques to conduct evaluation research. This type of survey is defined by Warwick and Lininger as "the assessment of the process and for consequences of deliberate and planned interventions."[9] Evaluative surveys are appropriate in situations in which 1) a goal or objective has been identified, 2) a program has been instituted to meet the goal, and 3) the results of the program can be measured in terms of the degree in which the objective has been achieved.

The term evaluation implies that the worth or merit of something is being judged. Scriven[10] views the evaluation process as the assessment of both goals and results, and describes three distinct parts of the process. FORMATIVE evaluation is an internalized affair which is an ongoing part of the program development to improve it while it is being created and instituted. SUMMATIVE evaluation assesses the merit of the program after it has been developed and instituted. The summative evaluation is usually an external process reported outside of the agency developing the program and often conducted by an external evaluator. This type of evaluation is often used for comparison or for cost analysis. The last step is termed GOAL-FREE evaluation. This method is used to control bias by bringing in an evaluator who is unfamiliar with the objectives of the program and having him review the findings. This process is used to highlight unintended side effects of the program and is thought to present a consumer viewpoint.

Evaluative surveys will become more prominent in nursing as researchers strive to evaluate "nursing care" given to patients, discern whether programs are "cost effective," and to isolate critical variables and relationships that show promise for more extensive investigation.

Experimental Approach

The experimental approach to research is defined by Kerlinger as one in which "the investigator manipulates at least one independent variable."[11] Experimental research is considered to be the one and only true research approach by most investigators in the basic sciences. It is characterized by tight control over the variables and subjects. In fact, the researcher exerts so much control over facets of the study that less quibbling occurs over the results produced by such exactness. Experimental studies usually require more sophisticated knowledge of the problem, more in-depth planning, more expertise, and a greater expenditure of time than some of the other types of research. It often seems like many of the other types of studies are preliminary steps leading to "real experiments." This is very often the case since experimental studies can lead to clear-cut statements of cause and effect. These are the studies that many professionals regard as the "proving grounds" for theory development. There are two general types of experimental research—one is arranged and the other occurs in a natural environment. The arranged study is the laboratory experiment while the investigations occurring in their natural habitat are field experiments and field studies.

LABORATORY EXPERIMENTS

These types of studies have been utilized to the greatest degree in the social sciences by psychologists. A large number of the experiments are conducted with animals like rats and monkeys before being transferred to use with humans, and in this way parallel medical laboratory research. An experiment consists of arranging the conditions under which the planned treatment will take place. Silverman states that researchers utilizing this approach forsake the naturally occurring event in order to gain manipulation and control. He describes the scene of the research as follows:

> Though locations do vary, they have one consistent aspect: They are the habitat, in a phenomenological sense, of the experimenter and not the subject . . . Our manipulanda and measurements are not focused on normal life routines; rather, they constitute an exotic interruption of these.
>
> The advantages of conducting research in the experimenter's habitat are apparent. It affords a level of precision not readily attainable in the complex habitat of our human subjects.[12]

The laboratory research experiment has a great advantage in that many of the confounding variables can be screened out of a situation by secluding the interaction. The experimenter can plan a specific treatment, introduce it into the situation, and then measure the effects of the treatment. The treatment (independent variable) can be carefully arranged and applied without the intervention or interruption of factors that are not under the control of the investigator. The effect can then be clearly measured. The benefits of this type of study, however, are not accrued without the careful planning that is necessary to circumvent the problems that could arise.

Some scientists have questioned the extent to which laboratory findings fit into the real world since subjects in laboratory settings often display behavior that may be atypical. It has long been noted that the usual subject assumes a passive, subservient role in response to the experimenter's directions. The investigator needs to assure as much appropriateness to a natural situation as possible.

The response of the subjects to the experimenter's directions needs to be carefully evaluated. A response pattern set up for "social desirability" is one in which the individual seeks to deny unfavorable aspects of factors being measured, or, in other words, "fakes good." The opposite situation may occur in which the subject attempts to subtly undermine the study by a negative reaction. The latter often occurs when subjects are involuntarily "drafted" to participate.

A limited amount of nursing research has been conducted in laboratory settings to date. One example of a classical type of laboratory study was carried out by Beverly Raff, R.N. This nurse designed an experimental study to investigate prenatal conditions entitled, "The Relationship of Planned Prenatal Exercise to Postnatal Growth and Development in the Offspring of Albino Rats."[13]

FIELD EXPERIMENTS

Are very similar to laboratory experiments. The independent variable is manipulated by the investigator under carefully controlled conditions—but this time in a lifelike setting. Kerlinger notes the benefit of this type of study by noting that, "The more realistic the situation—the stronger the variable being studied."[14] This type of experimental study has been conducted by nurse researchers in the past few years in an effort to add to nursing's theory base. The experimenter exerts as much control over the situation as possible while preserving the natural atmosphere. This very lack of artificiality is the greatest benefit of field experiments since the subjects are usually more realistic and the findings are more directly applicable to a situation. This facet becomes even more important in clinical projects where a true-to-life flavor is imperative. Of course, these field experiments are subject to the same pitfalls of laboratory experiments and require planning and ingenuity to maintain adequate control. Commentary 6.6 describes a highly controlled field experiment in a medical-surgical setting.

Commentary 6.6
An Experimental Study on Nurses' Communication with Seriously Ill Patients

Ruth McCorkle designed and conducted an experimental study to determine the effects of touch as a means of communication with seriously ill patients. Sixty patients were assigned to experimental and control groups of 30 patients each. Experimental group patients were touched while talking with the nurse researcher, control patients were communicated with only through verbal channels. Four different instruments were used to measure the causal relationship between the touching behavior and the positive acceptance responses occurring in the patients. The hypothesis was:

Touching and verbally stimulating a seriously ill patient will produce an increase in the number of positive acceptance responses.

Positive acceptance responses were measured in three ways:

1. Observable reactions of the patient's pleasure or contentment to the researcher's touch as rated by two nurses who were watching the process.

2. Answers the patient gives to the questions of one of the observers after the researcher completes her interaction. (For example, How did the nurse show her interest in you?)
3. Heart rate and rhythm during the interaction as monitored by a cardiac tracing.

The following table displays a small portion of the results as recorded on the Behavior Interaction Worksheet by the nurse observers.

Table 1
Facial Expression Scores Recorded by Nurse Observers

	Experimental Group		Control Group	
Categories	Number of Patients (N = 30)	(%)	Number of Patients (N = 30)	(%)
Facial Expressions				
Total positive	29	(96.7)	24	(80.0)
Total neutral	7	(23.3)	9	(30.0)
Total negative	11	(36.6)	17	(56.7)

The hypothesis was supported by an increase in positive responses in the facial expression category and a separate rating of verbal interchanges. Some examples of the areas in which the hypothesis was not supported were "body movement, eye contact, and general response of the patient."

The results indicate that nurses can use touch to establish a positive relationship with seriously ill patients in a brief time span. Numerous implications are provided for other nurse researchers to utilize in developing their own communication studies with patients.

Ruth McCorkle: Effects of touch on seriously ill patients. Nursing Research 23, 2 (March–April 1974): 125–132.

FIELD STUDIES

Are the experimental studies that are closest to real life. Investigators seek to discover relationships between and interactions among variables in real social structures. Field studies do not usually have the independent variable that characterizes the more classical experimental studies. The researcher is often attempting to discern possible reasons for an occurrence after it takes place. Hence, much of this research is labeled EX POST FACTO since it denotes that the investigator is seeking answers to events that are occurring "after the fact" with regard to the variable being studied. Field studies are often called QUASI-EXPERIMENTAL or PARTIAL EXPERIMENTAL studies since they are not characterized by the rigor involved with the true experimental conditions. Katz[15] divides field studies into two classifications. EXPLORATORY field studies are instituted to discover variables and the relationships between them. They often lead to HYPOTHESIS-TESTING field studies that are instituted to test relationships among variables. Such studies can be utilized by nurses to build up the amount and quality of information available about nurses and the work they do. There are numerous follow-up studies of new baccalaureate graduates as they enter the work culture which could be classified as field studies. *In Reality Shock: Why Nurses Leave Nursing*, Marlene Kramer[16] reports the research she has conducted on neophyte nurses who have embarked on the beginning of their professional careers.

The main characteristics of the six research approaches are presented in Table 6.1 for a quick review of the main points.

RESEARCH DESIGN

The research design is the overall plan or blueprint the researchers select to carry out their study. According to Kerlinger, "the design has two basic purposes: 1) to provide answers to research questions and 2) to control variance."[17] Variance is controlled by planning the study in such a way as to rule out other hypotheses or other intervening variables as causes of the study outcome. The design entails all the steps in the research process from the definition of variables and formulation of hypotheses through the decision of how the data will be analyzed. The research design consists of the strategy used to find answers to the research question. This strategy, of course, is tailored by the objective of the study, the expertise of the researcher, the constraints placed on time and expenditures, the availability of subjects, and means to elicit information from them. The design must be both scientifically acceptable and practical enough to be manageable in the process of supplying useful information.

One aspect of the design is closely tied to the research approaches that are appropriate for use in studying the problem at hand. There are two overall classifications of design. The first classification is NONEXPERIMENTAL which consists of the bulk or research already completed in the nursing field. Studies falling under this heading are characterized by varying amounts of scientific precision and acceptable variability although none reach the amount of control and predictability of EXPERIMENTAL designs. This classification of research design is graphically presented in Figure 6.1.

Table 6.1
Characteristics of Various Research Approaches

	Philosophical	Historical	Case Study	Methodological	Survey	Experimental
Time frame	Present → past	Past	Present → past	Present	Present	Present → future
Researcher's objective	Trace development and/or present status of abstract ideas	Discover existing facts and combine to draw conclusions	In-depth analysis of subject; usually includes historical aspects	Develop instruments to measure variables; test statistical procedures for appropriateness	Discover new facts about subjects; make conclusions and interpretations	Prediction of events: discover cause and effect relationships under controlled conditions
Control over variables	None to minimal	None to minimal	Minimal	Moderate to extensive	Moderate	Extensive
Data collection source	Documents	Personal and public documents and records; artifacts; interviews in limited circumstances	Combination of data from subjects, documents, and artifacts	Subjects utilized for pretesting, retesting, reliability and validation of instruments	Subjects	Subjects
Type of research report	Narrative only	Narrative, sometimes includes objects or artifacts	Narrative with occasional numerical data; can include objects or artifacts	Numerical with accompanying narrative statements	Narrative that usually includes numerical data.	Narrative with great emphasis on numerical results

In addition to a decision about general amount of precision or control desired, the investigator must select an overall time reference for the conduction of the study. Some limitations may exist because of the research approach (historical studies cannot be conducted within a future-oriented time frame) chosen for the study. In many instances, the researchers have options available that may be greatly influenced by the kind of information they desire. Both the general time frame for carrying out the study and the time specified for the data collection must enter into this decision. CROSS-SECTIONAL studies are designed to be conducted with a focus of one particular point in time. They usually take place within a relatively short period in the present. Data are collected from subjects, analyzed, written-up, and that's it. A LONGITUDINAL study is one that is set up to follow a group of subjects over an extended period of time. During this extended period of study, data are usually collected at prescribed intervals. A PROSPECTIVE design entails locating a group of subjects and following them for a specified time in anticipation of effects that might result from some particular variable such as their health habits. RETROSPECTIVE studies are set up to start in the present while they delve into the past life of subjects for the remainder of the necessary information. Although this time frame of the past is frequently used, the investigator must be aware of the possible distortions of events that take place with the normal passing of time.

The research design is likewise concerned with the more specific issue of how the research question will be answered. The nonexperimental approaches are fairly straightforward in this regard since many contain just one group of subjects for data collection and there are usually no independent variables involved. The experimental designs are often more complex since they usually contain an independent variable resulting from the presence of the treatment that is applied by the investigator. Table 6.2 contains the set-up of a design for one group of subjects. In this structure, a "before and after" measurement is taken of the treatment instituted by the investigator.

The classical two-group design for experimental studies is contained in Table 6.3. The experimental and control groups are randomly selected before the initiation of the experiment to provide for equality. The treatment is applied to the experimental group only, followed by a measurement of differences between the two groups. An effective independent variable would produce a change in the experimental group and thus make it appear very different from the control group. This two-group design is illustrated with an example from a nursing study in Table 6.4. It is the plan of the researcher that differences between the two groups of patients will be related to the administration of nursing comfort measures. The differences here would be demonstrated by a difference in the average number of pain medication requests by the patients in the two separate groups.

Table 6.2
Structure of One Group (Before and After) Design

Group Classification	Assignment to Groups	Exposure to the Experimental Treatment (Independent Variable)	Measurement of Response to a Specified Factor (Dependent Variable)	Possible Comparisons as a Result of Experiment
Experimental group	Usually total group	yes	Two times (once "before" and once "after" treatment)	Differences *within* the one group; Comparison of the before and after state

Table 6.3
Structure of the Two Group Design

Group Classification	Assignment to Groups	Exposure to the Experimental Treatment (Independent Variable)	Measurement of Response to a Specified Factor (Dependent Variable)	Possible Comparisons as a Result of Experiment
Experimental group	Random	Yes	One time only (after the experimental treatment)	Differences *between* the two groups allows researcher to measure change resulting from the experimental treatment
Control group	Random	No	One time only	

Table 6.4
Two-group Design in a Study of Nursing Comfort Measures

Group Classification	Assignment to Groups	Exposure to Treatment (Independent Variable)	Measurement of Response (Dependent Variable)	Possible Comparisons
Experimental group	Random (from list composed of all patients on medical-surgical units)	Yes (Given treatment: specially designed nursing procedures consisting of pain relieving comfort measures)	Total number of pain medication requests at the end of 48 continuous hours of participation in the study	Differences *between* control and experimental group in total number of pain medication requests
Control group	SAME	No (routine nursing care)	SAME	

Table 6.5
Structure of the Matched Two Group Design

Group Classification	Assignment to Groups	Exposure to the Experimental Treatment (Independent Variable)	Measurement of Response to a Specified Factor (Dependent Variable)	Possible Comparison as a Result of Experiment
Experimental group	Random*	Yes	One time only (after the experimental treatment)	Differences *between* two groups populated by subjects with matching characteristics on preset criteria; permits a measure of change resulting from the experimental treatment
Control group	Random*	No	One time only	

* Random group assignment after matching subjects according to some preset criteria.

123

The structure of a two-group matched design is outlined in Table 6.5, and the resemblance to the classical two-group design is readily apparent. The structures can accommodate greater numbers of groups if the study called for them to be added.

SETTING OF THE RESEARCH STUDY

The investigators already have an idea of the setting by the time they determine the most appropriate approach and design. The locale of the research varies from highly controlled (laboratory experiments) to partially controlled (field experiments) to natural settings. The decision should take into account other factors, such as amount of artificiality desired, the overall number of subjects required (laboratory experiments have limited facilities), and the number of extraneous variables desired.

REFERENCES

1. T. Christy: The methodology of historical research: a brief introduction. Nursing Research 24, 3 (May–June, 1975): 189–192.

2. E. Durkheim: Suicide. Glencoe, Illinois: Free Press, 1951.

3. L. Montiero: Research into things past: tracking down one of Miss Nightingale's correspondents. Nursing Research 21, 5 (November–December, 1972): p. 526–529.

4. F. Kerlinger: Foundations of Behavioral Research. New York, Holt, Rinehart & Winston, 1973, p. 702.

5. H. Goldenberg, Contemporary Clinical Psychology. Monterey, California: Brooks/Cole Publishing Company, 1973, p. 11.

6. F. Kerlinger, Foundations of Behavioral Research, p. 410.

7. E. Hughes, H. Hughes, and I. Deutscher: Twenty Thousand Nurses Tell Their Story. Philadelphia, J. B. Lippincott Co., 1958.

8. D. Warwick and C. Lininger: The Sample Survey: Theory and Practice. New York, McGraw-Hill, 1975, p. 49–50.

9. D. Warwick and C. Lininger, The Sample Survey: Theory and Practice, p. 51.

10. W. Popham, (ed.): Evaluation in Education. Berkeley, McCutcham Publishing Co., 1974, p. 99.

11. F. Kerlinger, Foundations of Behavioral Research, p. 315.

12. I. Silverman: The Human Subject in the Psychological Laboratory. New York, Pergamon Press, 1977, p. 1–2.

13. F. Downs and M. Newman: A Source Book of Nursing Research. Philadelphia, F. A. Davis, 1977, p. 78–85.

14. F. Kerlinger, Foundations of Behavioral Research, p. 402.

15. L. Restinger and D. Katz: Research Methods in the Behaviorist Sciences. New York, Holt, Rinehart & Winston, 1953, p. 75–83.

16. M. Kramer, *Reality Shock* St. Louis: C. V. Mosby Co., 1974.

17. F. Kerlinger, Foundations of Behavioral Research, p. 300.

CHAPTER

7

Identifying Hypotheses and Selecting a Sample

Now that the general problem, the approach to its solution, and some of the guidelines for data collection have been outlined, it is time to turn the focus of attention to the specific aspects of the research methodology.

The methodology section of a research study provides the step-by-step guidelines the investigator followed in carrying out the research project. It generally includes the procedures for selecting a sample and an instrument and for collecting the information from the subjects, and it sometimes spells out the study design. The methodology relates in detail just how the research question in the particular study was answered. It is therefore the most important section to use as a pattern for repeating or replicating the study. It should provide a crystal clear picture of the procedures that were followed in the conduction of the project. At this stage decisions are made by the investigator about all of the kinds of questions that concern the neophyte researcher from the start: Who do I get answers from? How many people do I ask? How do I pick the people to ask? How do I know what to ask? Deliberate decisions are made, enacted, and recorded in written form. This must be explained in sufficient detail so that each part is self-explanatory. Other investigators should be able to follow these guidelines in order to be able to repeat the same study. This aspect of replication is essential since it makes it possible to confirm study findings in a variety of settings and situations. Replication and confirmation of findings will eventually help to build theory. Thus, the methodology section covers a variety of important areas that are a necessary aspect of a research study. This chapter will focus on the type of information desired, the people from whom it is sought, and the ways in which the subjects can be selected. The next two chapters will cover the types of tools or instruments that can be used to obtain data.

DEFINING KEY WORDS AND IDEAS

The researchers need to write out precise definitions of the important words they have been using all along during the development of the initial aspects of the study. This step is formally delayed until this middle phase of the research project to provide the investigators with an opportunity to read widely in the literature relating to the problem and to broaden their thinking about the factors they are investigating. Although the investigators may have jotted down a definition of a word or idea in some prior aspect of the research process, they must now pause to refine their definition to ensure that it is explicit, clearly phrased, and encompasses all aspects of the idea they wish to convey. It is also important that such definitions be meaningful and that they become integral parts of the study rather than terms copied from a dictionary. The time to make specific decisions about the practical aspects of the study is at hand, and it is necessary to define the important terms of the study first. There are a number of different types of words and ideas that will require definition, and they will be discussed in the following sections.

Table 7.1

Structure of the Two-Group Design for a Study of the Effects of a New Nursing Procedure on Premature Infants

Group Classification	Assignment to Groups	Exposure to Experimental Treatment (Independent Variable)	Measurement of Response to a Specified Factor (Dependent Variable)	Possible Comparisons as a Result of the Experiment
Experimental group (Has new nursing treatment)	Random (Random or chance placement in groups will lower the chance of putting babies who look like they would gain weight most rapidly into the experimental group)	Yes (Given the new nursing treatment during all shifts for the first three days after admission to the premature nursery)	One time only* (After experimental treatment. Weight measured exactly 72 hours after admission to premature nursery)	Differences be-*tween* the two groups. Allows researcher to measure change resulting from experimental treatment
Control group (Continues to be cared for with routine nursing procedures normally used in the unit)	Random	No (Routine care for all shifts for first three days after admission to premature nursery)	One time only* (Weight measured exactly 72 hours after admission to premature nursery)	Average weight gain or loss for each of the two groups is computed first. Then comparisons be-tween the experimental and control groups can be easily made

* Weight of each infant was recorded upon admission to the premature nursery before the study actually began so that the measurement of the dependent variable is a one-time-only measurement.

Variables

Variables are generally defined as the main factors that are being studied. They are the key elements that aroused the interest of the researcher in the first place. They derive their name from the very quality that draws investigators to initiate a study—they "vary." They change according to influencing conditions, can assume a variety of values, and thus create interest. There are numerous types of variables that influence the research process in a variety of ways, but it is essential to become aware of four types to be able to develop a beginning familiarity with research. The four types are independent, dependent, extraneous, and intervening variables.

Independent variables in a study are also known as causal, treatment, stimulus, or explanatory variables. The independent variable is a factor that is introduced into the situation or manipulated by the investigator to produce an effect. Therefore, independent variables are used in research studies only when the investigator wishes to study the effect or differences they produce. A descriptive study that is designed to form a picture of the role of the nurse in the premature nursery would not have an independent variable. The researcher conducting this study merely wishes to collect information that would describe the role of a particular group of subjects (nurses in the premature nursery.)

Independent variables are almost always found in experimental research since this type of design generally calls for some treatment or special condition (independent variable) to be applied to the experimental group of subjects so that its effects can be compared with those of the control group that did not receive the treatment. Supposing the researcher wanted to study the effects of a new nursing treatment designed to help premature infants gain weight. The new nursing treatment would be the independent variable. The best way to measure its effects would be to give the new nursing treatment to one group of premature infants while continuing with the established or routine nursing care for another group of premature infants. At the end of a specified time, the weight of both groups would be contrasted to measure whether the new nursing treatment had its expected effect. Note how the design of this study, presented in Table 7.1, closely resembles the two-group experimental design discussed in Chapter 6.

In order to get an idea of the way the researcher would answer the original question raised in the study, it is often most convenient to diagram the relationship of the independent variable to the subjects. Table 7.2 contains a simple skeleton table that would enable the researchers to show the results of the influence of their independent variable.

The need for defining the independent variable should become obvious after looking over the outline of the premature infant study. The new nursing

Table 7.2
Skeleton Table Designed to Show Results of the
Independent Variable

Experimental Group (New nursing treatment)	Control Group (Routine nursing care)
# (Average weight gain or loss for group)	# (Average weight gain or loss for group)

treatment is a strategic part of the experiment and as such, it is vital to define the variable in a way that would illuminate all the important aspects involved. The definition of the variable should be detailed enough to permit replication by readers who are located in another setting.

There are numerous types of independent variables, and some may seem more clear-cut than others. A condition that already exists may be used by the researcher as a type of independent variable in order to separate subjects into groups. For instance, the sex of the premature infants (although not caused or instituted by the researchers) may be used as a factor that separates them into groups. Thus, the previous study could have contained two independent variables that may have affected the subjects. The skeleton table for the premature infant study with two independent variables (sex of the baby and the new nursing treatment) is presented in Table 7.3. With this table the researcher can view the results in two ways—according to sex and according to treatment to find out the effect of either—and can also look at the effect of both variables working together.

Dependent variables are also known as effect or response variables. They constitute the factor that is being measured in a research study. There-

Table 7.3
Skeleton Table Designed to Show the Results of
Two Independent Variables

	Experimental Group (New nursing treatment)	Control Group (Routine nursing care)
Male Infants	# (Average weight gain or loss for the group)	# (Average weight gain or loss for the group)
Female Infants	# (Average weight gain or loss for the group)	# (Average weight gain or loss for the group)

fore, it is important to clearly define this factor. The dependent variable must have a commonsense relationship to the problem being studied and should imply some means of measurement. The dependent variable in the study of premature infants was the body weight that was to be measured at a specific time (72 hours after admission to the nursery). The dependent variable should not be mixed up with the instrument or tool being used to conduct the measurement of weight—which in this case would be a baby scale.

The dependent variable selected for use in a study must be used consistently with all the subjects who participate in the research. However, in an experimental study, the dependent variable is measured in both the treatment and control groups so that any differences can be noted.

It is not necessary to have an independent variable in order to measure some factor. Dependent variables can be measured in various types of survey studies in which no comparisons are possible. Take for instance the descriptive study about the role of the nurse in the premature nursery. Even though the descriptive study has no independent variable, the nurse's role can still be measured. The researcher could have designed an instrument to collect information about the nurse's role and could have asked a cross-section of nurses in that setting to fill in the tool. The dependent variable is the factor being measured—in this case the role of the nurse in the premature nursery. The instrument is the device used to record this measurement—in this case the questionnaire.

Some authors suggest various ways to organize, define, or categorize the dependent variable. Some label this explication of the dependent variable the criterion measures.[1] In the example of the dependent variable of role, the concept of role would be broken into its various components, parts, or criterion measures. For the concept or role, this could consist of components such as duties, functions, necessary skills or qualifications for that role. This idea of criterion measures is related to the validity or meaningfulness of the dependent variable. Its component parts should all relate directly and with relevance to the overall purpose of the investigation. In the study involving the nursing care of premature infants, the main purpose was to determine if the nursing treatment affected a gain in weight. Therefore, weight was a useful dependent variable for use in measurement in the study. The use of a measure such as the average number of ounces of formula consumed each day would not have been appropriate or meaningful in the study.

Extraneous variables is the term used to identify the many factors in a research study which may influence the outcome of the project even though they may not seem to have a direct influence on the results. The investigator may not be sure of their influence and may decide to identify them just in case. Or else, the researcher may wish to focus in on only one or two main variables while knowing full well that there could have been a number of other important influences that may have been affecting the situation (especially when dealing with human subjects). The important factors that are temporarily moved from the forefront of the situation are called extraneous variables. Extraneous variables may stem from a condition inherent in the individual subject (in which case they are called ORGANISMIC) or in the environment (termed ENVIRONMENTAL). The researcher has two choices with regard to the handling of extraneous variables: to control for them (set up the procedures to minimize their effects) or to keep tabulations on them. In the study involving the premature infants, the investigator could have decided that both types of extraneous variables were present in the situation. The investigator could have decided that weight gain could be influenced by factors other than the nursing treatment, such as the racial classification of the infant (organismic) and the type of isolette the infant is placed in (environmental). The researcher could "control for" the type of isolette by using only one model and excluding others, or by keeping track of the racial classification of the infants and looking at the data in light of this when analyzing the results. This would give a rough idea about the amount of influence of that one variable. Both extraneous variables could have been handled in the opposite fashion (by using subjects of only one racial classification and tabulating the type of isolette used for each infant.) There are numerous extraneous variables in all types of research studies, and the way in which they are handled will greatly influence the surety about study results, especially when determining cause-and-effect relationships. These variables need to be defined and then carefully evaluated for their influence in the study situation.

Intervening variables cannot be labeled or classified even though they may be influencing the outcome of the study. This terminology is used most often in describing psychological processes that are not directly observable in a research situation but which may be affecting the behavior of the subjects. The researcher should consider whether factors like motivation, hostility, or stress could possibly be influential in the conduction of the project. The researcher should note the presumed weight of such factors and plan the methodology to minimize their effect as much as possible.

The study described in Commentary 7.1 clearly demonstrates the manner in which the different types of variables need to be defined. Note the explicit features of the independent, dependent, and extraneous variables.

Hypotheses

The statement of relationship between two or more variables is known as a hypothesis. After the key variables of the study have been identified, it is important for the researcher to make a statement about how the variables appear to relate to each other. This statement, or hypothesis, gives a con-

Commentary 7.1
They've Tried Just About Everything, But—One More Time

It sometimes seems like every health care professional has his or her favorite treatment for decubitus ulcers or bedsores.

Suzanne Van Ort and Rose Gerber liked one in particular. They decided to run a small pilot study to see what results they would have in treating decubitus ulcers with insulin therapy. They carried out their experiment on fourteen patients in a nursing home. The seven in the control group received routine nursing care. The seven subjects randomly selected for the experimental group had treatment that consisted of the application of a small amount of insulin on the broken skin area twice a day. The size of the ulcer measured as a gauge of the rate of healing. After fifteen continuous days of treatment, the final measurements were taken and the groups contrasted. The group receiving insulin therapy had a rate of healing that significantly surpassed the routine care group. They caution that further studies should be carried out with larger numbers of patients to check the results. Why not use the study as a pattern and test out your own type of decubitus ulcer care?

S. Van Ort and R. Gerber: Topical application of insulin in the treatment of decubitus ulcers: a pilot study. Nursing Research 25, 1 (January–February, 1976): 9–12.

crete direction to the analysis of the findings. Often large-scale studies have a number of hypothese rather than just one. On the other hand, it is not necessary for each study to have a hypothesis. A descriptive study does not have an independent variable and would therefore not have a hypothesis. Sometimes studies without hypotheses have a "research question" stated to give some direction to the investigation. Kerlinger describes hypotheses as follows:

> Hypotheses are always in declarative sentence form, and they relate, either generally or specifically, variables to variables. There are two criteria for "good" hypotheses and hypotheses statements. One, hypotheses are statements about the relations between variables. Two, hypotheses carry clear implications for testing and stated relations.[2]

The hypothesis is often called an "educated guess" about the relationship between the independent and dependent variables. This estimation of the relationship or its direction usually comes from the expectations engendered by the literature and from similar studies that have been previously conducted. A straightforward or directional hypothesis in the study of the nursing care of the premature infants would be stated as follows:

> There will be a significant increase in the body weight of infants undergoing the new nursing treatment.

In the study presented in Commentary 7.1, the investigators were attempting to measure a definite relationship between the variables identified. The hypothesis was formulated as follows:

> There will be a significant increase in the rate of healing of the decubitus ulcers for subjects who receive the topical insulin therapy as evidenced by a decrease in the diameter of the ulcer.[3]

The two criteria specified by Kerlinger are present in the preceding hypothesis. The relationship between variables is spelled out as is the way of measuring its results. The final stages of the study will show whether or not the relationship has been supported by the evidence collected. The hypothesis is a concise statement of the cause-and-effect relationship being studied. If the data show that the relationship between variables was, in fact, in the predicted fashion, the hypothesis is said to be ACCEPTED.

The study summarized in Commentary 7.2 is a humorous example of the acceptance of a hypothesized relationship between the degree of revealing clothing and the amount of car rides offered.

If the data do not support the hypothesis, it is said to be REJECTED. In either event, the investigator has contributed to the amount of knowledge available about the problem by either advancing the position of a true relationship or by showing one to be unpredictable, unrelated, or spurious.

There are some instances in which it is not possible (due to lack of prior research or writing on the subject) to make a statement about the outcome of the relationship between the variables. In this case, a slightly different form

Commentary 7.2
Hypothesis Accepted . . . Ride Rejected

Two college girls in California came up with a rather unusual science project. Their study, they say, reveals conclusively that a girl who hitchhikes will get more rides if she wears revealing clothing. During the past several months, the two collegians thumbed rides dressed alternatively in baggy overalls and a blouse (a control costume) and in more revealing outfits (a test costume). Out of 425 motorists that passed by, 352 stopped to offer them a lift. The girls were wearing the test costume during 75% of the actual ride offers.

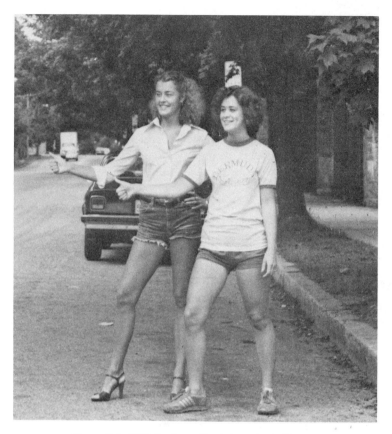

Figure 7.1. Will the hypothesis be rejected?

of hypothesis, termed a NULL HYPOTHESIS, is used. This means that the investigator formally states that no relationship exists between variables (even though it is hoped that one would turn up.) The null hypothesis is a declarative statement that begins with the words, "There is no relationship between . . ." and states the variables under consideration. If the researcher conducting the study of nursing care in the premature nursery wrote a null hypothesis, it would read as follows:

There is no relationship between the body weight of infants and the type of nursing treatment administered.

The researcher who is trying to demonstrate a relationship between the new nursing treatment and an increase in body weight wants to see the null hypothesis rejected. If the infants in the experimental group actually gained more weight and the null hypothesis was rejected, the finding would be stated as, "There is a relationship between body weight of infants and the type of nursing care administered." The acceptance of a straightforward relationship is often the same as the rejection of a null hypothesis. In the foregoing example, the acceptance of the straightforward and rejection of the null hypothesis would indicate the *presence of a relationship*. In summary, hypotheses are important elements in the world of scientific investigation because they serve the following important purposes:

Show how the problem is testable.
Help make theoretical ideas testable in the real world.
Serve as sources of generating new or slightly different hypotheses.
Show cause-and-effect relationships.
Lend objectivity to scientific investigation since they can be shown to be true or false.
Indicate a general direction for the researcher to follow in solving the research problem.
Condense the main point of the study.
Make the objective relationship available for further testing by other researchers.
Indicate ways to measure the problem.

Operational Definitions

Operational definitions are action-oriented definitions that spell out the exact meaning researchers are giving to any important terms (other than variables) they use in a study. The clear explication of terms provides future researchers with a means of duplicating a study as closely as possible. This means that investigators should explain the way they use the term in the study and not just include a standard definition copied from a dictionary. Individuals place a certain meaning on words as do dictionaries, but neither explanation may carry the same vital ingredients as an operational definition in a research project.

For instance, in a study designed to measure the effects of a patient-teaching program, the authors were concerned with length of hospitalization and operationally defined the term "length of hospital stay" as follows:

> The number of days the patient was hospitalized. Day of admission was counted as a day, day of discharge was not counted as a day. For subjects admitted for preoperative medical work-up, the first day counted was the day before surgery.[4]

Key terms need such attention, especially words in the statement of purpose and the hypothesis. The term "nurse" may be defined differently by researchers according to such criteria as educational background, length of professional employment, or area of clinical specialization. The precise meaning that is appropriate for the duration of the study must be spelled out in detail. There is no set rule about the placement of operational definions within the main body of a paper, so it is up to the researcher to find the most appropriate spot. They are most often located near the statement of the hypothesis or the definition of the variables.

THE SUBJECTS

Some of the most frequently asked questions of novice researchers concern the research subjects. The following section was designed to provide guidlines in this area. Who are they? The subjects of a research study are those people or objects from whom the information relevant to the study is collected. The selection of appropriate subjects is an important consideration since they will provide the data used to answer the research question or to support or reject the hypotheses. In short, the subjects need to be part of a group about which the investigator wants to draw conclusions as a result of the study. The findings can only be generalized or applied to a population from which the subjects were drawn. The selection of the TARGET POPULATION, or total group to whom the results can be generalized, is of extreme importance. The process of selecting the target population can be facilitated by answering the following questions before proceeding further:

1. What kind of population is required in this kind of study?
2. Is it necessary to exclude any parts of this group?
3. What are the feasible geographical boundaries for selecting subjects?
4. Are there any practical limitations?
5. Are there time limits that would affect the access to the subjects?
6. Does cost limit access to the subjects you wish to study?
7. How many people do you have available to help collect information from the subjects?
8. How convenient is it to contact the subjects?
9. Do you need to get information at more than one point in time?
10. Do you foresee any problem in gaining cooperation from subjects?
11. Are there any anticipated problems in acquiring information from subjects (such as language boundaries, physical handicaps, or developmental considerations, such as lack of reading or writing ability)?
12. Do you anticipate any difficulty in gaining agency permission to collect data from subjects (such as from hospitals or schools)?

Once investigators have identified a realistic target group to draw subjects from, they can then visualize a SAMPLING UNIT, or one of the typical subjects from whom they will gather information. It may be helpful to visualize this typical subject while thinking about the following areas.

HOW MANY DO I NEED?

The standard answer from most research textbooks would direct a student to use a sample as "large as possible." There is actually a purpose for the "bigger is better" idea when it comes to acquiring information from people. The more subjects there are in a group, the more representative the group will be of the population group from which it is drawn. The search for representativeness will lead to more valid conclusions about the group and thus more accurate answers to research questions. The whole point of gathering information from a group rather than from an individual or two is to decrease the error in the data.

Sometimes it is not possible to gather information from a large group of subjects because of constraints of time, money, or availability of cases. Take the example of a clinical study in which the patient population is limited because of the small number of available beds in a particular unit and a low turnover rate. Although the investigator may be limited to a maximum of 11 subjects in this case, the study can still be carried out. Researchers must be very careful in making generalizations about the findings and needs to keep reminding themselves that each person is almost 10 percent of the whole group. Of course, by adding seven or eight subjects to the group, the overall influence of any one of them is decreased to 5 percent of the total, yet this is not always possible to accomplish. Researchers should exercise common sense in making decisions about sample size. If there are three available cases of a fairly rare entity, use them all with a note of caution. If there are 5,000 subjects in the target population, then perhaps 200 or 300 would do.

Guidelines and formulas exist to aid in the selection of an adequate sample. Gay advises a minimum of 10 percent of a population for a descriptive study, (20 percent if it is a small group), a minimum of 30 subjects for statistical studies, and a minimum of 15 subjects for each group in experimental research.[5] Smaller sample sizes are generally more acceptable from homogeneous populations since the probability of selecting "typical" subjects is greater. A common rule of thumb which states that a minimum of 30 subjects should participate in each group for all types of studies has been cited by numerous authorities. This stems from the fact that statisticians have shown that sample means of groups of 30 or more approximate a normal distribution even if the attribute being measured is not normally distributed in the population.[6] A more in-depth treatment of the topic of sample size can be found in the following references:

D. Fox: The Research Process in Education. New York, Holt, Rinehart & Winston, 1969.

J. Cohen: Statistical Power Analysis for The Behavioral Sciences. New York, Academic Press, 1969.

J. Nunnally: Psychometric Theory. New York, McGraw-Hill, 1967.

WHAT SHOULD I TELL THEM ABOUT THE STUDY?

The investigator needs to give the subjects some information about the study in order to gain their consent to participate. The information should be truthful yet general. A detailed explanation of the purpose, rationale, or hypotheses of the study would most likely influence the subject's behavior. The subject should be made to feel comfortable about participating in the project, but not be made to feel that there are predetermined expectations about behavior or responses. Words need to be carefully chosen. A patient was once asked to participate in a study that was undertaken to determine patient's perceptions about nurses. The researcher asked the woman if she would fill in a form "To help find out if nurses ever treat you as you would like them to and whether you think they spend all their time giving medications and things like that." The researcher would most likely have received less biased replies if she had requested the woman to fill in a questionnaire "To help form a picture of the work nurses do." If the subjects ask questions that would require information that might affect the direction of their responses, it is best to tell them that you will be happy to answer such specific questions *after* they complete the questionnaire. You want to influence their answers or behavior as little as possible. Plan beforehand as much as possible what you will say to subjects and how you will say it. Remember that information can be transmitted through both verbal and nonverbal channels.

It is wise to plan to contact more than the minimum number of subjects that you decide you need to carry out the study. The average return rate for mailed questionnaires seems to hover somewhere around 50 percent. Even in the more actively controlled studies one should expect some drop-outs from the subject pool. The investigator should keep track of what happens to each subject who participates in the study in any way. The report should include a detailed description of the subjects, as well as the count of those not completing their participation much like the following:

> SAMPLE. The subjects were 168 registered nurses who were full-time employees of the two hospitals used as settings for the study. All had been working on the medical-surgical units for a minimum of one year. In the course of the data collection process, three nurses terminated employment resulting in a sample of 165 nurses.

The investigator should report something about the difficulty rate in getting subjects to participate, if this was an important factor. A recent clinical study was conducted in a gynecology clinic of a municipal hospital. The number of subjects participating in the study was reported as 22. The investigators noted that approximately 60 women were asked to participate and almost two out of three declined. Although this information is not sufficient cause to invalidate the findings, it certainly enables us to view the results in the proper perspective.

HOW CAN I GAIN THE SUBJECTS' COOPERATION?

The best way of gaining the cooperation of subjects is to make the participation voluntary. An atmosphere tinged with subtle coercion or demands may produce anything from half-hearted responses to out-and-out sabotage. Various aspects of the researcher's expectations about subjects should be reviewed: the amount of time required, the convenience of the testing circumstances, the nature of the behavior expected, and the subject's familiarity with the circumstances under study. Many subjects will willingly volunteer to take part in a study once they have been given baseline information about the reason for the study and the basic expectations regarding their participation. It is not unusual today to find studies that obtain subjects' cooperation by offering a token payment or service to the participants.

The many ethical and legal concerns regarding subjects will be covered in detail in the next chapter. It is important to note here that most subjects will be concerned with the confidentiality of their responses. Researchers need to take steps to protect the identity of participants if they have made this bargain with subjects. It may entail spending extra time coding subjects' answer sheets to keep the replies anonymous during data analysis, but it is an important issue that should not be overlooked. The written report of the study should be presented in such a way that none of the subjects could be identified by the information provided. This also holds for agencies and other types of institutions. A hospital should be described in a study in global terms (500-bed private urban hospital used by several medical schools) unless specific permission has been obtained to identify it in the report. The next question at this point should be: *How do I find the subjects?* This will be explained in the following section.

SAMPLING

One very important aspect of any research study is the process used to select or choose the subjects. The manner in which the subjects are gathered will have a great influence on the overall accuracy of the results. It will also affect the extent to which the investigators can generalize the findings of the study or view them as "typical" results. Thus, the quality of the results and the applicability to the entire population of possible subjects will be directly related to the process by which they are selected. SAMPLING is the term used to identify this process the researcher utilizes to pick out study subjects. Sometimes it is possible to contact many or all of the individuals in a group the researcher is interested in studying. However, it is more often the case that the goal in selecting a SAMPLE or group of subjects is to establish a small group that is a microcosm of the larger group. A researcher who wished to study the attitudes of registered nurses in the United States would simply be unable to survey each and every one of them. Constraints of time, energy, and cost would make this an impossible task. It would also be an unnecessary task if the researcher could select a small group of nurses who would be completely representative; there are ways of sampling that provide more surety of accomplishing this result. There are two broad classifications or sampling procedures that can be employed. Random sampling (also known as probability sampling) is the type utilized when a truly representative sample is required. The second classification consists of nonrandom sampling methods (also known as nonprobability sampling) which, although useful in many circumstances, provide less chance of obtaining a representative cross-section of a population.

Random sampling is a process of selection in which each individual has an equal chance of being chosen. Randomness implies that in so far as everyone is familiar with the concept of a selection by lottery or with drawing names out of a hat. This time-honored way of choosing people from a group evolved because the probability of being selected should be identical for each of the names stuck in the hat. Thus, every name had an equal chance of being picked. Researchers have modernized the hat technique and have developed more sophisticated means of selecting samples according to the same principle of random selection. The following steps are a general outline of the random sampling process:

1. Make a master list that includes the names of all subjects in the population.
2. Assign consecutive numbers to each subject on the list. (Be sure to use equal digit numbers, such as 01 to 99 for less than 100 subjects, 001 to 999 for less than 1,000 subjects, and so on.)
3. Utilize a table of random numbers to obtain as many subjects as you need from your master list. A table of random numbers is a lengthy list of digits that have been placed together in no discernible pattern. (Most statistics textbooks contain tables with a complete list of random numbers.)

A brief example of the actual steps of the process will demonstrate that it is simple to enact. Suppose an investigator wanted to select six nurses at random from a total group of 40. The numbered list would look like the one in Figure 7.2. In order to select the six subjects at random, the investigator would use a table of random numbers similar to the excerpt in Figure 7.3.

Before entering the table, the researcher must decide the order in which to take numbers from the table. This may be done by either going across the rows or by going up and down the columns. This researcher decided to take numbers by going across rows. The next step entails the designation of a starting point in the table. Without looking at the actual numbers, the researcher puts a pencil down on the table of random numbers and records the two digits closest to this point. The first number selected in this way was 39, and it has been circled for demonstration purposes in Figure 7.3. This number designates the first subject to be selected from the master list in Figure 7.2. As the researcher moves horizontally across the row, the second number circled is 88, which is larger than any of the numbers assigned to subjects on the list and is therefore discarded. The third number circled is 03 which designates the second subject to be selected. Inspection of the master list shows that Mary Wieners (39) and Penny Burgess (03) have been selected as subjects thus far. This process is continued until all six

---

Master List of Possible Subjects

01 Grace Andrews	21 Ronna Krozy
02 Jill Bloom	22 Karen LaFare
03 Penny Burgess	23 Jalma Marcus
04 Diane Carser	24 Marcia McPhee
05 Barbara Connolly	25 Karen Noonan
06 Edward Connolly	26 Rita Olivieri
07 Mary Ann Corcoran	27 Marguerite O'Malley
08 Shawn Crossett	28 Mary Pekarski
09 Robert Davis	29 Marian Reed
10 Cynthia Doctoroff	30 Pauline Sampson
11 Mary Ellen Doona	32 Helen Saxe
12 Joyce Dwyer	33 Rachel Spector
13 Ellen Freeman	34 Agnes Sweeney
14 Mary Ann Garrigan	35 Marcella Tierney
15 Marjory Gordon	36 Phyllis Vitti
16 Carol Hartman	37 Miriam-Gayle Wardle
17 Marion Heath	38 Ronetta Watrous
18 Barbara Hedstrom	39 Mary Weiners
19 Elizabeth Hickey	40 Patricia Wood
20 Jean Ikegami	

Figure 7.2

```
EXCERPT FROM A TABLE OF RANDOM NUMBERS
  62898    93582    04186    19640    87056
  21387    76105    10863    97453    90581
  55870    56974    37428    93507    94271
  86707    12973    17169    88116    42187
  85659    36081    50884    14070    74950

  55189    00745    65253    11822    15804
  41889    25439    88036    24038    67192
  85418    68829    06652    41982    49159
  16835    58653    71590    16159    14676
  28195    27279    47152    35683    47280
```

Figure 7.3

subjects have been designated. If there had been 175 individuals on the list, the numbering system would commence with 001, and the researcher would be selected three-digit numbers from the table. The preceding example would in this case have resulted in the selection of the following three-digit numbers: 398,803,624, and so on, until six subjects were identified.

This random process results in a minimal amount of bias in the selection of subjects. If the six subjects were tested in some kind of experiment and then sent back to their places in the original list of 40, the selection of a second set of six subjects would theoretically be just as representative of the entire group as the first six. The system of using a table of random numbers can be time-consuming, particularly in situations in which large populations of potential subjects are involved. This process has been greatly accelerated with the advent of computerized random selection.

The selection process just described is the basis of probability sampling. This classification has been subdivided into several different categories that have distinct features.

1. *Simple random* sampling is the process of selecting a group of subjects from a population in which each member has an equal chance of being chosen. It basically involves the process previously described.
2. *Stratified random* sampling is a variation of simple random sampling that has been devised to ensure representation of subgroups. It is used when it is necessary to subdivide a population according to some characteristic in order to obtain true representativeness in the final sample. Suppose that a researcher wanted to obtain a sample of workers in a particular type of hospital. The first step would entail finding out the varied types of

workers and their relative numbers in relation to the total staff. The breakdown in one such institution was as follows:

Nurses	50%
Administrators	10%
Physicians	10%
Physical therapists	05%
Occupational therapists	03%
Dietitians	05%
Nursing assistants	10%
Housekeeping	05%
Maintenance	02%
	100%

The researcher wants to select a sample containing representation from the various groups of workers that is proportionate to the share of the total population they hold. After determining the number of subjects necessary for the study, the researcher would assemble separate master lists for each sub-group. A table of random numbers would be used to select subjects from each list that is proportionate to the make-up of the population. If 100 hospital workers were required for the sample, 50 subjects would be selected from the master list of nursing names, ten from the list of administrators, ten from the list of physicians, and so on.

3. *Cluster* sampling involves the random selection of groups rather than individuals. This is a necessary variation of simple random sampling when it is not possible to obtain master lists of subjects or when the setting does not allow for dealing with individuals rather than groups. Clusters may include such things as classrooms, hospitals, or schools. Suppose a researcher wanted a sample of professional workers in state supported mental health clinics in a particular geographical location. After obtaining some background information, the researcher learns that there are ten clinics fitting the criteria which employ an average of 12 workers each. The researcher could then randomly select the required number of clusters (clinics) that would provide a sufficient sample. If a minimum sample of 30 was needed, the researcher could select three clinics from all of the staff in each one. This method would provide for economy in obtaining data by saving time, travel, and expense. The biggest drawback may be lack of representativeness since the subjects are not chosen completely at random.

4. *Systematic* sampling is a process of selecting a sample according to a system of choosing subjects at fixed intervals. This would involve such procedures as selecting every tenth, or seventh name on a list. It could include selecting patients assigned to even numbered rooms in a clinical setting. This type presupposes that the researcher has compiled a list in

random order or has no predetermined reason for selecting even- or odd-numbered rooms.

Each sample has been moving further away from the true definition of random selection. The next section clearly moves away from any attempt at randomization even though some attempt is always made to seek a somewhat representative sample. Although the nonprobability methods of selecting a sample back the statistical soundness of a random selection, they are frequently used in social science research for a variety of reasons. Some of the main types of nonprobability sampling are as follows:

1. *Purposive* sampling involves the selection of particular subgroups because of the presence of some desired characteristic. Researchers go out of their way to pick the group by exercising their own judgment about what would be a typical or representative group. An example would be the purposive selection of nurses working in orthopedic clinics in several urban hospitals. Researchers may need a group with selected skills and experiences and may gather data from as many of these individuals as they can.

2. *Expert* sampling is closely related to purposive sampling and is characterized by greater selectivity. A group of experts may provide a type of data unlike that which could be obtained from a cross-section of a particular field. They may generate hypotheses and provide fascinating information relevant to case studies. The usefulness of this method is demonstrated in the example of sample selection in Commentary 7.3.

Commentary 7.3
Is There a Scientific Way to Get Nurses to Agree With One Another?

Carol Lindeman wanted to find out the most pressing problems in patient care settings in order to draw up a prioritized list of areas for clinical nursing research. She wanted to obtain in-depth opinions of a divergent group of nursing experts. She used the Delphi Technique to gather and combine these opinions and used a series of four questionnaires to produce group consensus about the problems. Her efforts resulted in the compilation of a large mass of data from 341 respondents. The top three areas of research identified by a subgroup of nurse administrators were:

1. Determine valid and reliable indicators of quality nursing care.
2. Determine and evaluate interventions by nurses that are most effective in reducing psychological stress of patients.

3. Determine effective means of communicating, evaluating, and implementing change in practice.

C. Lindeman: Nursing research priorities. *Journal of Nursing Administration* V, 6 (July–August, 1975): 20–21.

3. *Quota* sampling involves setting goals for a predetermined number of cases in the categories being studied and seeking subjects who fit the criteria for inclusion in each category. For example, a group of researchers may wish to compare a group of patients who have attended natural childbirth classes with a group who have not attended such classes. The research could set a goal of 50 subjects for each group and could then keep collecting data until the full quota had been filled for both groups. This method is frequently used when there is little opportunity to gather names for a master list and to select patients at random. A researcher may find that she can easily fill a quota of 50 expectant mothers in a municipal hospital setting who have not attended natural childbirth classes. She would automatically stop looking for subjects in that category once the quota was met, but would continue to look for expectant mothers who had completed natural childbirth instruction for as long as it took to reach 50.

4. *Convenience, haphazard*, or *accidental* sampling consists of gathering just about any kinds of subjects who will take part in the study. Although planning must take into consideration the likelihood of finding viable subjects in a particular location, any subject who gives consent to participate will be included. For instance, a group of nursing students wanted to collect information from local citizens about their attitutde toward mandatory licensure for nurses. They selected a large supermarket as a site for data collection (rather than an exclusive store) since it would ensure the largest cross-section of the local citizenry. They ask all of the store patrons to fill in a questionnaire before entering the shopping area. Two separate half-days of data collection by this convenience method resulted in the completion of 140 questionnaires.

5. The use of *volunteers* is a frequently used method of obtaining subjects. Signs, posters, and newspaper advertisements are utilized to attract subjects who are willing to take part in research projects. There are a variety of factors that may set the volunteer apart from the "typical" subject one would ideally like to test, and the subject's motivation for taking part in the study (to get a grade, to make money, to help pass the time, for the experience of doing something different) may influence the results.

The researcher using any of the nonprobability methods of obtaining a sample must keep one point in mind when talking about the results. The findings may not be generalized to larger populations of individuals since the subjects were not randomly selected. Whatever the findings are, and no matter how fascinating they seem, the results of studies using nonprobability sampling are applicable only to the specific subjects who participated in the study itself.

The next chapter covers the information needed to answer the next logical question the beginning researcher might ask. Now that the subjects have been identified and chosen, the investigator must focus on ways of obtaining information from subjects. It is about this time that the beginning researcher wonders, "What is the best way to get the information from the subjects that I have chosen?"

REFERENCES

1. F. Abdellah: Criterion measures in nursing. Nursing Research 10, 1 (Winter, 1961): 21–25.

2. F. Kerlinger: Foundations of Behavioral Research. New York, Holt, Rinehart & Winston, 1973, p. 18.

3. S. Van Ort and R. Gerber: Topical application of insulin in the treatment of decubitus ulcers: a pilot study. Nursing Research 25, 1 (January–February, 1976): 10.

4. C. Lindeman and B. Van Aernam: Nursing intervention with the presurgical patient-the effects of structured and unstructured preoperative teaching. Nursing Research 20, 4 (July–August, 1971): 319–332.

5. L. Gay: Educational Research: Competencies for Analysis and Application. Columbus, Ohio, Charles E. Merrill, 1976), p. 77.

6. D. Warwick and C. Lininger: The Sample Survey: Theory and Practice. New York, McGraw-Hill, 1975, p. 83.

PART

III

Gathering Information

One of the most important decisions that researchers need to make centers around the information they require about the subjects under study. This section begins with Chapter 9, which presents general topics such as legal and ethical constraints, and covers varied strategies that should be considered in planning the data collection activities. While the various techniques for accessing information are covered in Chapter 8, the following two chapters cover specific steps in obtaining and assessing instruments. Chapter 9 discusses available instruments while Chapter 10 provides guidelines for designing data collection devices. The latter chapter covers the preliminary steps that researchers should take with the instruments as soon as they have been completed by the subjects.

CHAPTER

8

Collecting Data: Plans and Procedures

ETHICAL AND LEGAL CONSIDERATIONS IN DATA COLLECTION

The first step in data gathering should consist of a review of the ethical and legal concerns involved in this process. The investigator must be cognizant of the varied aspects of these codes as they relate to the conduction of research. Purposeful decisions about data collection should be enacted only after the researcher scrutinizes the ethical and legal ramifications of each action.

Nurses are currently involved in research in two distinct ways. First, as researchers, nurses either conduct studies or work as members of research teams in carrying out investigations. Second, nurses give clinical care to patients who are subjects in a research endeavor (such as a medical study to evaluate an experimental therapy). In both instances, the nurse would be expected to be knowledgeable about the research project and to follow professional guidelines for its conduction.

Ethics is a branch of philosophy that deals with human behavior. Since human behavior is such a multifaceted entity, it is not possible to draw up lists of all-inclusive rules to govern action, but only to sketch out guidelines that can be used as rough indices. As Juanita Fleming has stated:

> It is important that we recognize and bear in mind that, in many cases, there are no sharp lines that divide what is ethical and what is unethical. It is not likely that there is ever 100 percent ethical behavior or 100 percent non-ethical behavior. There is a point at which a large number of small alternations becomes an important difference. It is those little things that add up to make big differences. It is necessary that scientists be cognizant of *that essential point* at which just a small amount more will make more than a little difference[1]

The basic element of the nurse-patient relationship is trust. Modern scientific and technological advances have made it all the more important for the nurse to assume the role of advocate, protector, and collaborator, as well as caregiver. Each profession must establish its special code or rules to govern the behavior of members so that it may be objectively evaluated. The medical profession has devised a series of safeguards for providing ethical guidelines for patient research. Since nurses are often involved in providing direct care to subjects of medical research, it would be important to know the recommendations that guide doctors with respect to patient consent for participation in research. The Declaration of Helsinki reads as follows:

> In the treatment of the sick person, the doctor must be free to use a new therapeutic measure if, in his judgment, it offers hope of saving life, re-establishing health, or alleviating suffering.
>
> If at all possible, consistent with patient psychology, the doctor should obtain the patient's freely given consent after the patient has been given a full explanation. In case of legal incapacity, consent should also be procured from the legal guardian; in case of physical incapacity, the permission of the legal guardian replaces that of the patient.
>
> The doctor can combine clinical research with professional care, the objective being the acquisition of new medi-

cal knowledge, only to the extent that clinical research is justified by its therapeutic value for the patient.

In the purely scientific application of clinical research carried out on a human being, it is the duty of the doctor to remain the protector of the life and health of that person on whom clinical research is being carried out.

The nature, the purpose, and the risk of clinical research must be explained to the subject by the doctor.

Clinical research on a human being cannot be undertaken without his free consent, after he has been fully informed; if he is legally incompetent, the consent of the legal guardian should be procured.

The subject of clinical research should be in such a mental, physical, and legal state as to be able to exercise fully his power of choice.

Consent should, as a rule, be obtained in writing. However, the responsibility for clinical research always remains with the research worker; it never falls on the subject even after consent is obtained.

The investigator must respect the right of each individual to safeguard his personal integrity, especially if the subject is in a dependent relationship to the investigator.

At any time during the course of clinical research, the subject or his guardian should be free to withdraw permission for research to be continued. The investigator or the investigating team should discontinue the research if, in his or their judgment it may, if continued, be harmful to the individual.[2]

The International Council of Nurses has not yet taken a formal stand on ethics in research, but includes ethical values in a code for proper conduct in the practice of any type of nursing. The code states that in providing care, the nurse must "promote an environment in which the values, customs, and spiritual beliefs of the individual are respected."[3] The Commission on Nursing Research of the American Nurses' Association has prepared a paper on human rights guidelines in response to the rapid changes taking place in nursing practice. The document produced by this group entails two kinds of rights as follows:

One set is concerned with the rights of qualified nurses (those with research preparation) to engage in research and to have access to resources necessary for implementing scientific investigations. The other deals with the human rights of all persons who are recipients of health care services or are participants in research performed by investigators whose studies impinge on the patient care provided by nurses.[4]

The first right paves the way for benefits to the whole of society through individual support of research projects. The number of qualified nurse researchers is growing. Members of the profession should muster support and cooperation for studies while providing collaboration through the reading, critiquing, and utilization of research findings.

The second set of guidelines deals with the subjects of the study. There are two general areas of consideration with this framework. The initial set deals with the manner in which the researcher obtains her facts; the second set is concerned with what she does with the facts after she gets them.

For researchers who wish to obtain further information in this area, the Commission on Ethics of the American Nurses' Association has a brief 1980 publication entitled, "Ethics in Nursing: References and Resources that is available on request.

Guidelines for Obtaining Facts

INSTITUTIONAL PROCEDURES

The researcher must obtain permission to collect data for the study from the institution or agency in which the subjects are located. In many hospitals, some kind of research review board will meet to review the research proposal and then recommend whether or not permission to conduct the research should be granted. Specific procedures vary from agency to agency; so, it is an important step in the organization of a study to determine the exact policies of the facility in which the target population can be found. It is best to obtain some form of written permission from an agency before collecting any data from subjects. The permission form can be drawn up by the researchers if the agency does not have a standard version. The agreement form in Figure 8.1 is a facsimile of a form granting permission to a group of students to conduct their study in a hospital setting. The form contains the necessary basic information: dates of period during which permission is requested to conduct the research, summary of proposed study, details of data collection procedures including a copy of the instrument, names and titles of individuals signing the agreement, and the date of the agreement. Hershey and Miller have prepared a guide for investigators and administrators that reviews legal aspects of gaining permission for conducting studies with human subjects.[5] It is important for nurses to become aware of the existence of institutional review boards and to become knowledgeable about the policies and procedures that are in effect in the health care agencies with which they are in contact. Eileen Hodgman has outlined the evaluation criteria used by the administration in one metropolitan teaching hospital that provide valuable information for those who may wish to investigate institutional review procedures in more detail.[6] Many agencies that support research through funding require additional proof of the enactment of research safeguards. For instance, the U.S. Department of Health, Education and Welfare requires written assurance of the protection of human subjects in any research study as a part of all grant applications.

Example of Agency Permission Form For Conducting Research

AGREEMENT BETWEEN COMMUNITY AGENCY AND BOS-
TON COLLEGE

It is agreed that the Boston College Senior Nursing Students listed below may utilize the facilities of _____ in order to engage in a nursing care study. The students expect to be in the agency between _____ and _____ , 19_____ , and request permission to employ the following areas as the setting for their project:

_____ .

The study proposal is as follows:

The students agree to submit a report of the study to the Director of Nursing Service.

Signature of Students: _____

_____

_____

Signature of Community
Agency Representative: _____
Title: _____
Signature of Boston
College Faculty: _____

_____

Figure 8.1

CONSENT

All research guidelines include sections on gaining subjects' informed consent for participation in an experiment. The "informed" part signifies that the subject is appraised of sufficient information about the study so that he can make a valid decision about his obligations as a participant. He needs to be informed about his rights as a subject. This is of particular importance in clinically oriented studies in which the patient should not be coerced or subjected to a lesser quality of care as a result of his decision. Commentary 8.1 is a fine illustration of the process of "informed consent" from its minimal

Commentary 8.1
Insuring Privacy by Obtaining a Truly Informed Consent

Catherine Rosen is a psychologist who conducted a study about patient authorization of the release of personal information. The project was conducted in a state supported mental health facility which provides care for approximately 4,600 low-income clients a year. The crux of the study involved the issue of the patient's understanding of what consequences would result from his action in signing or not signing the information release form. This is a step beyond the usual action taken in mental health agencies which entails telling the patient why information is needed and where it is going to go. Rosen went beyond ensuring mere comprehension of the written consent form, and intended to see what would happen if patients felt that the services offered to them would not be jeopardized by refusal to sign the consent form.

	Control Phase	Experimental Phase		
		No option	Option	
			Presented by clerk	Presented by therapist
Percentage who signed form	100	100	41	20
Percentage who refused to sign form	0	0	59	80

Over 1,000 patients were participants in the 14-month study. The patients studied in the control phase were presented with a standard type of legal consent form authorizing the state to release personal information to appropriate agencies. All signed.

The experimental phase included two different types of consent forms. The "no option" variety was essentially a simplified version of the legal consent form. All signed. The "option" version included insertion of the following statement:

> If you do not sign this paper, this identifying information will not be sent into the state offices in the Capitol and will be kept only locally. The services you get will not depend on your choice. In other words, if you don't sign you will get the same services from us as if you did sign.

In this "no option" setting one group of patients was presented with the consent form by a clerk and another group had the form presented by a professional therapist. The number of patients who signed the information release form, after being assured that they truly had a free choice of whether or not to do so, dropped dramatically.

The researcher concludes that professionals in the mental health field have the responsibility to see that neither the content of the consent form or the manner in which it is presented pressure the patients into signing their names. It is very important to ensure that such personal data are released as a result of a free choice.

C. Rosen: Signing away. Civil Liberties Review III, 4 (October–November, 1976).

to optimal level of enactment. It can clearly be seen that implied messages can be transmitted by the manner in which a subject's consent or permission is obtained.

The area of informed consent extends beyond the scope of giving intelligent subjects a full explanation of the many options available to them. There are a number of complicating conditions that pose consent problems to all types of medical researchers since they are often collecting data in situations affected by extraordinary circumstances. Ramsey asks searching questions such as, "Who consents to fetal research?" and provides guidelines for dealing with issues of permission for research on unusual types of patients, such as the unborn, condemned, dying, and unconscious patients.[7]

PRIVACY

The individual's right to privacy and dignity should remain intact despite agreement to participate in research. The investigator assumes responsibility for study conditions and must safeguard the confidentiality of material and anonymity of subjects during data collection phases and in the communication of study results. Subjects must be treated with dignity at all times.

FREEDOM FROM RISK

The study subjects, whether human or animal, must be protected from undue physical or emotional risk during participation in a research project. The possibility of risk needs to be specified by the director of the study so that the subjects can be briefed on as many of the possible consequences of research participation as possible. Research procedures have been classified into five categories of increasing risk by Reynolds as follows:

1. No positive or negative effect on the subject.
2. Temporary discomfort such as tension, temporary anxiety, or physical pain. The discomfort is no more than encountered in day-to-day living, and ceases with the termination of the experiment.
3. Unusual levels of temporary discomfort. The normal state is usually attained within a brief period after cessation of the experiment, but intervention such as postexperimental treatment or debriefing may be required.
4. Risk of permanent damage.
5. Expectation of permanent damage as a result of experimentation.[8]

With regard to the legal issues surrounding risk or bodily harm to subjects, Creighton and Armington state:

> The majority of legal and ethical problems concerning human research have occurred not in the formal research but in connection with the malpractice of doctors, nurses, and other health workers accused of experimenting during the ordinary treatment of patients. While people have been used extensively in experimental situations, there is not an impressive set of legal precedents to indicate proper procedures in carrying out research on human beings.[9]

DECEPTION

It is a common practice for psychologists to conduct studies on subjects who are not aware of the variables being studied. In order to conduct such experiments, the investigator gains the consent and cooperation of the subject by emphasizing a part of the experiment that is not really being studied at all. This is often necessary since an awareness of the true goals of the study might considerably alter the subject's behavior while in the situation. The study described in Commentary 8.2 utilized deception in the methodology.

Commentary 8.2
Love a ("Highly Attractive") Nurse P.R.N.

Two female undergraduate students at Yale carried out a research project to identify factors that influence a male's choice of a romantic partner. Previous studies had shown that people become the most interested in partners of the opposite sex who are extremely physically attractive. This attraction to the physical appeal of the opposite sex was found to be present in both physically attractive and physically unattractive people. This tendency to seek a partner of objectively higher attractiveness has been attributed to the fact that people do overevaluate themselves in many types of situations. One factor that is known to influence an individual's opinion of himself is his level of self-esteem. The researchers thought that males with a high level of self-esteem would actively seek out attractive females since they would either inflate their own physical attributes or feel that other factors (such as intelligence or personality) made up for their lack of physical attractiveness. The researchers felt that feelings of low self-esteem would influence the active selection of a partner in a converse way. They reasoned that males with low self-esteem would see a highly attractive partner as "hard to get" and would choose someone less desirable (and thus more congruent with the low opinion they held of themselves as well). The study hypothesis was as follows:

> The lower the self-esteem, the lower would be the attractiveness of a chosen romantic partner.

The 37 male subjects chosen for the study were mostly undergraduate and graduate students. The study was planned so that two levels of self-esteem, high and low, would be present in a group of males. This differentiation of self-esteem was achieved by setting up a testing situation in which the males were led to believe that they were either doing very well or very poorly on an intelligence test. It was assumed that those who were told they were doing very well on the test would experience a temporary high level of self-esteem and thus overevaluation of self, while those who fared poorly on the test would experience a temporary low level of self-esteem and no overevaluation of self. Observations were set up to measure each subject's romantic behavior toward two kinds of females—a very attractive group and a moderately attractive group.

The subjects were ostensibly recruited for the study to take a one-hour intelligence test. A male experimenter told the subjects that he was establishing norms and that the test had already been given to hundreds of students. He emphasized the fact that the test was accurate and reliable and that it predicted "success in life." To reduce variance in subject performance, the test was made extremely difficult so that the experimenter could easily create a high or low self-esteem condition for the subjects by conveying that their performances were either very good or inferior. During a break from the test, he took a subject to a cafeteria for a cup of coffee, introduced him to one of the female confederates, and excused himself from the scene.

The two female confederates appeared randomly in either a "high" or "moderate" level of attractiveness. In the "moderate" attractiveness condition, each confederate wore her hair pulled straight back, no makeup, heavy glasses, and sloppy clothes which clashed. During the period of interaction with a subject, the confederate was directed to act the same way (accepting, interested) each time. In order to decrease bias, she was not aware of the level of self-esteem of the subject. The experiment lasted for the first half hour of the time the subject and confederate were together in the cafeteria, and observations of his behavior in certain categories of romantic behavior were recorded. Some of the types of romantic behavior exhibited during these interactions are presented in the chart below. The hypothesis was supported. This lends credence to the belief that self-esteem will affect the type of romantic partner chosen. The authors interpret the results to mean that self-esteem affects what the person thinks is a realistic or practical choice. Changes in the perceptions of the self will in turn affect perceptions of the chance for probable success or "payoff."

Percent of Subjects Displaying Romantic Behaviors

ROMANTIC BEHAVIOR	EXPERIMENTAL CONDITION			
	High Self-Esteem		Low Self-Esteem	
	Moderately Attractive Confederate	Highly Attractive Confederate	Moderately Attractive Confederate	Highly Attractive Confederate
Asked for date	10	19	27	13
Offered to buy coffee, etc.	0	25	18	25
Expressed compliments	0	25	18	0

At the end of the experimental session, the confederate "debriefed" the subject and took pains to emphasize the real nature of the intelligence test.

S. Kiesler and R. Baral: The search for a romantic partner: the effects of self-esteem and physical attractiveness on romantic behavior. In K. Gergen and D. Marlowe (eds.): Personality and Social Behavior. Reading, Mass., Addison-Wesley, 1970.

Subjects were led to believe that "intelligence" was being studied when the experiment was actually designed to create different levels of self-esteem and to see how the self-esteem affected romantic behavior.

Although deception is a useful adjunct to some study designs, it should be used cautiously, and only when necessary. Silverman has written extensively on the role of the subject and the subject-experimenter relationship. He subscribes to a decline in the use of deception by researchers as he writes:

> The demise of introspectionism began with the functional schools of the early 1900's and, for all purposes, was completed with the advent of Watsonian behaviorism in the second decade. Then the concept of subject underwent a marked transition from "collaborator-observer" to "object." From that point, psychological experimentation required that the subject be untrained and uninformed about the investigator's intentions. Rather than observer . . . he was regarded as a passive entity . . . and gave off measurable responses.
>
> History has a way of reappearing, and, as we come to this understanding, there is a faint, but unmistakable call for a return of sorts to introspectionist methods.[10]

If deception of any sort is used, the experimenter must build a formalized "debriefing" session into the postexperimental phase of the study so that subjects will be cognizant of the true goals of the study. This debriefing is utilized to remove any misconceptions about the study and to reestablish a feeling of trust between the researchers and the subjects who are likewise potential consumers of the findings.

Guidelines for Utilizing Facts

CONFIDENTIALITY

The investigator is obligated to protect the identity of individual subjects who participate in a study. The types of subjects and their location is described in general terms in the descriptions of the target population and sample, but specific subjects are not named. In a large study in which numerous people have access to the data, a coding system is developed by the experimenter to keep exact identities a secret. In studies utilizing an interview or observation for data collection, the subjects are obviously not completely anonymous since they are seen by one or more raters. The raters in this type of study would be pretrained by the investigator to respect the confidentiality issue. The identities of hospitals, schools, or other types of institutions should be kept confidential unless the researcher has specific permission to acknowledge them.

WITHHOLDING OR MISREPRESENTING FACTS

Researchers are ethically obligated to report findings in an accurate and unbiased manner. They should not purposely misrepresent or disregard study findings if they don't coincide with the framework or thrust of the study.

Many facets of the ethical and legal implications must be kept in mind during all of the stages of a research project, but most notably in the planning of data collection. The subject may be a patient who is directly benefitting from the treatment or may be a patient or volunteer who is gaining no personal benefit while contributing to the advancement of knowledge. Each case must be approached with equal care. Figure 8.2 contains a brief checklist of some of the ethical guidelines that should be considered by nurses when they encounter patients in their care who are participants in research projects.

**Checklist for Assessing Adherence to
Ethical Guidelines in Research Projects**

1. Art participants adequately protected from:
    ____ Physical stress
    ____ Mental stress
    ____ Serious risks
    ____ Invasion of privacy
2. Have the researchers made provision for:
    ____ Procedures for screening out high-risk participants?
    ____ Safety precautions?
    ____ Monitoring for unintended stresses or risks?
    ____ Respectful treatment of participants?
    ____ Removal of any misconceptions at the end of the study?
3. Has adequate communication been carried out between:
    A. Researchers and subjects in regard to:
    ____ Informed consent (clear and fair agreement between experimenters and subjects) regarding participation?
    ____ Adequate knowledge about the provision of services if they refuse to participate in a study?
    B. Researchers and nursing staff in regard to:
    ____ Role and responsibilities of the nurse in relation to the study?
    ____ Identity of the investigator and any research assistants?
    ____ Means of contacting them or an appropriate resource person in the institution in regard to questions, concerns, or important observations which should be made known?

Figure 8.2

METHODS OF COLLECTING DATA

There are three general methods of data collection investigators may utilize in conducting their study. Often the researcher uses a combination of methods in order to collect the most meaningful information. Each method is composed of various techniques that provide a wide variety of creative approaches to gathering facts about a problem.

EXISTING DATA is the classification used for information that has been accrued for purposes which are not usually related to research but which can be used in a meaningful way in a research context. There are all kinds of official documents that provide useful information for statistical (government census) and content (medical records) analysis. These official documents can provide a wealth of information to scientists who are looking at similar areas from different vantage points. Commentary 8.3 summarizes a study that used existing data to gain answers to the research question posed. The grant proposals utilized in that study were located in the appropriate agencies and, although not collected expressly for the purpose of conducting this study, were able to provide all the required information. One drawback of using existing data results from the fact that it was not collected purposefully for the study and often does not provide specific or sufficient answers to the research question.

Unofficial documents, such as letters, diaries, and unpublished papers, can often be used as raw data. Historical researchers often use these types of documents in their quest for building up information about an individual or

Commentary 8.3
Factors Affecting the Success of Nursing Grant Proposals

The funding of research proposals becomes a very important consideration to nurses attempting to set up sizeable research projects. In an effort to shed light on the variables that are most strategic in this grant-seeking process, Jeanne Berthold investigated the responses of two national granting agencies to proposals submitted for nursing studies.

> The purpose of the current study was to compare approved and disapproved proposals on all dimensions available through a review of the records consistently kept by the National Institutes of Health (NIH) Division of Nursing and American Nurses' Foundation.

The final sample consisted of 328 proposals of which 136 had been approved and 192 had been disapproved. The results showed that funding was influenced by:

· Significance of the problem area
· Background development
· Design
· Quantification of the variables
· Operational procedures
· Population or sample
· Data analysis
· Budget
· Institutional setting
· Competency of the investigative team (independent of investigator background variables such as sex or academic degree.)

J. Berthold. Nursing research grant proposals. Nursing Research 22, 4 (July–August, 1973): 292–299.

event. Such documents may be found in archives, special collections, or private collections.

An added development in this area has brought modern technology into the picture. The day has arrived when people write relatively few letters while relying more on media to transmit messages. This has led to the use of magnetic tape devices to capture information about people and events of the present and near past. These ORAL HISTORIES are, in fact, interviews that are conducted to be preserved on tape for use by future researchers. This form of data is utilized to provide original data and to improve the record for future scholars. Many aspects of this technique of gathering information have been explained by Safier and, although relatively new, should not be overlooked in the quest for existing material.

In a similar vein, researchers have utilized artifacts in a number of different ways. Investigators use objects in conducting historical research (the Nursing Archives at Boston University contain Nightingale lamps and early nursing uniforms), in reporting field studies (anthropologists utilize cultural objects d'art), or in developing case studies (many patient-related case studies contain still pictures, x-ray films, or specimens). Such items, if properly utilized, may lend authenticity, color, and a nonverbal dimension to a study report.

OBSERVATION is a popular means for collecting data for research purposes. There are basically two varieties of observation: that in which the researcher is directly involved in the action (PARTICIPANT OBSERVATION), and that in which he or she is uninvolved or distinctly apart from the action

(NONPARTICIPANT OBSERVATION). In using either type of method, the nurse researcher is at a particular advantage. Many facets of nursing involve observations—of patients, of situations, of signs and symptoms. Most nurses have keenly developed power of observation that can be readily captured for use in a research study. This is particularly important in the development of clinically oriented research studies. Observations can be made concurrently with the administration of patient care. Nurses spend so many hours of their work day in close conjunction with patients that the use of observation as a method of data collection has a variety of uses. Nurses collect all kinds of information this way, but it needs to become a better organized routine to become meaningful. The two main types of observation have different characteristics that can be noted as follows.

Participant Observation is the technique used to collect data that is characterized by a direct interaction between the observer and subjects. The degree of awareness that the subject has about the research endeavor may vary greatly according to the objectives of the study. The data in each instance pass through the observer and are then recorded for use in the study. An interview is a popular technique employed by researchers to collect data. The subject's cooperation is obtained and questions are posed that can vary from a very formalized or "structured" set of questions to an informal, nondirective interview. The questions are verbally presented to the subject either face-to-face or by transmission over media such as the telephone. This type of data-collecting technique has a great advantage in that it provides the opportunity to gather in-depth information on a subject since there is leeway for follow-up or pursuit of an important topic. The use of interviews as a means of collecting information from subjects has a long history in the annals of medicine as can be seen in Commentary 8.4.

Formalized nursing interactions may be utilized to record information gathered from a patient by the interview technique. The recording of a nursing history interview and assessment may take place in a more overt fashion than a psychiatric interview that is later documented by means of a process-recording technique.

Field studies are commonly carried out by having the observer participate in the activities of the group being observed. Anthropologists and sociologists have long utilized this technique. William F. Whyte pioneered the perfecting of this type of data collecting, and provided a well-rounded picture of group activities in his well-known *Street Corner Society*. Two senior nursing students once designed a participant-observer study of the "culture" of a coronary care unit for an anthropology course project. Both felt they had a definite advantage in collecting data in this way since they were legitimate members of such a culture and knew the "language" and "mores." They soon discovered that many facets of the culture were second nature to

Commentary 8.4
The First Participant-Observers in the Field of Medicine

No doctor shortage here

Medicine was not practiced in ancient Babylon by individual "professors of medicine." However, according to historians of the time, those who suffered from disease were carried to a public square where they could be interrogated by passers-by concerning the nature of their afflictions. Any passer-by who had been afflicted with a similar disease was thus able to communicate the process by which his own recovery had been effected. It was unlawful in Babylon for anyone to pass by a diseased person in a public square without inquiring into the nature of his complaint.

Courtesy of *The Boston Globe.*

them and were taken for granted. They had to "sensitize" their powers of observation as if they were visiting a foreign land.

Nonparticipant observation is a technique utilized by researchers to collect data by having an objective observer rate behavior or other types of observations in which she takes no active part. The classic type of nonparticipant observer is physically removed from the room where she can collect information without the subject's awareness. The covert type of arrangement for nonparticipant observation can be carried out by utilizing a two-way mirror or any type of mechanical recording device that screens the observer from the subject. The purpose of separating the action from the observations is to gain more realistic behavior from subjects while limiting the amount of interference in executing the observations.

Overt nonparticipant observations are made by individuals who are present during interactions yet somehow set apart from the action itself. In the early stages of hospital research, many "time and motion" studies were conducted. An observer would arrive on a hospital unit wearing street clothes and carrying a clipboard. The job of this nonparticipant observer was to write down the activities and whereabouts of the nursing staff at specific time intervals. He took no active part in the activities of the staff since even a brief, innocuous conversation would influence the "time and motion" of the subjects. A number of nonparticipant observer studies were carried out in hospitals using sociologists as observers. Nurses have traditionally had the most difficulty being observers of this sort since they have been reluctant to simply record rather than interact in situations. Unable to let an IV run dry or to make an uncomfortable patient wait for a bedpan, nurses have been more prone to leave the on-the-spot nonparticipant observation to others. However, studies utilizing recording devices (such as videotapes) to capture the action for later scrutiny by nurse raters have been much more successful.

DIRECT MEASUREMENT of data is a method utilized to collect information directly from the subjects in a situation. This data collection method eliminates the interference of a second party (observer) and eliminates the necessity of "making do" with information previously recorded. Direct collection of data is probably the most widely used means of gathering the information the researcher deems necessary. There are three general sources of direct information, and the techniques to collect this information are as follows.

Questionnaires are the most widely used technique for collecting information from subjects. This paper-and-pencil device is used to collect beliefs, opinions, characteristics, perceptions, and attitudes of subjects on an infinite variety of topics. They may be constructed in an overt manner in which straightforward information is sought, or may be covert in the sense of having a fairly obvious purpose while collecting the sough-after information in a less obvious fashion. There can hardly be a nursing student in existence who has not filled in at least one questionnaire.

Tests are another technique for collecting information in which facts are solicited and then evaluated for the degree of appropriateness to the situation. Objective tests are classified into two broad groups. Inferential tests take the subject's answers and match them against a predetermined set of response patterns. Personality and vocational interest inventories are structured so that a new individual's responses to sets of questions are compared to the responses from a large group of subjects who have previously taken the test. In this way, the subject's responses can often be pictured in a graph or profile that shows how he matches up with individuals who have already completed the test. On the other hand, noninferential tests rate the subject's success rate in displaying the information he possesses about a particular subject. Knowledge tests fit into this category. National League for Nursing achievement tests are examples of this data-gathering technique.

Projective tests collect information directly from subjects but often change the form of the data before making use of them. A psychologist may use drawing or story-eliciting cards to coax individuals into giving information they are not consciously aware of transmitting. Projective devices are stimuli that encourage the subject to create his own type of responses. They are particularly useful in obtaining thoughts or feelings that the subject could not consciously articulate. Although many projective devices require expertise in scoring and interpreting results, a wide range of creative possibilities exist for use from the novice to the expert psychometrician.

Mechanical devices are available in every size, shape, and form since they are used in conjunction with all phases of health care. Nurses are extremely fortunate to have so many mechanical devices available in their everyday clinical milieu. Mechanical devices provide a certain amount of accuracy in the data collection routine and, what's more, provide numeric indices of whatever they are measuring. Just take a look around the clinical setting and visualize the variety from the everyday thermometers and sphygmomanometers to the intricate monitors of sophisticated settings.

It is customary for investigators to conduct the data collection phase of the study by utilizing COMBINED methods. This is especially true when it is

Table 8.1
Summarization of Data Collection Methods and Techniques

Methods	Existing Data	Observation	Direct Measurement
Techniques	1. Official records (such as medical records or government census documents) a. Statistical analysis b. Content analysis	1. Participant a. Interview b. Formalized nursing interactions (such as process recordings or nursing histories c. Field studies	1. Questionnaires (such as devices used to gather information on attitudes or opinions)
	2. Unofficial documents (letters, diaries, or unpublished documents	2. Nonparticipant a. Covert 1. Direct observation (two-way mirror) 2. Recording devices (audio and videotapes) b. Overt	2. Tests a. Objective 1. Inferential (personality and interest inventories) 2. Noninferential (knowledge tests) b. Projective (sentence completion and human figure drawings)
	3. Artifacts (uniforms, equipment, x-ray films, and specimens)		3. Mechanical deviances (sphygmomanometers and thermometers)

important to approach the measurement of a variable from several different directions simultaneously. The combination of different methods can serve as a double-check on each other, can lead to a more in-depth or sophisticated treatment of the problem, or can be a necessity for gathering the required information on a topic since some kinds of data are gathered more appropriately by one mode rather than another. The main methods and techniques of data collection are summarized in Table 8.1.

TYPES OF DATA

In selecting an appropriate technique for collecting data, the researcher needs to determine the type or the form of the information she needs. This is a prelude to selecting a method of data analysis as well. There are two main types of data that researchers collect from the great variety of techniques available: words and numbers. They are subdivided into two classes each and are commonly referred to as MEASUREMENT SCALES. They are defined as follows.

Nominal scales consist of equally weighted word categories and are the simplest way of classifying information. There are two requirements for setting up a nominal scale: each must be mutually exclusive (each piece of data would appropriately fit into only one category) and together they must be all-inclusive (categories must be available for all possible pieces of data).

Ordinal scales consist of word categories that have an implied order or hierarchy. Ordinal categories go from large to small in varying degrees according to the entity being measured. Figure 8.3 shows an example of both a nominal and ordinal scale for the variable of occupation.

Interval scales are a step beyond ordinal scales in that they consist of a hierarchy in which there is an equal distance between each category. Interval scales are measured in numbers—a thermometer is a prime example of a commonly utilized interval scale.

Ratio scales are numerical scales that contain an absolute zero point. This means that mathematically any point on a ratio scale can be reported as a multiple of any other. It has become quite common to combine numerical scales when referring to them in studies. Numerical scales are more desirable in many instances since they are more precise than word scales. The contrast between the ordinal scale and interval-ratio scale for the variable of body temperature in Figure 8.3 is readily apparent. The choice or word of numeri-

---

Examples of Different Types of Rating Scales for Measuring Each Variable

1. Variable = occupation

   NOMINAL
   SCALE   nurse   photographer   biologist   secretary   other

   ORDINAL
   SCALE   unskilled   semi-skilled   clerical   semi-professional   professional

2. Variable = body temperature
   ORDINAL SCALE   cold   tepid   warm   hot   sizzling

   INTERVAL-RATIO
   SCALE   96.2–97.1   97.2–98.1   98.2–99.1   99.2–100.1   100.2–101.1

Figure 8.3

cal types of scales to categorize data will have long-range effects on the type of analysis and statistical procedures that can be performed on the data collected.

THREATS TO ACCURACY OF DATA

This last section on the process of data collection concerns an important issue in the enactment of any type of research study. The amount of confidence with which an investigator can view his results will have a direct relationship to the amount of error that played a part in the overall data collection and handling process. There are four general types of error that must be kept under a watchful eye.

Sampling error is a type of error that occurs when the sample used in the study is atypical and leads to results that are different from those of the study of the whole target population. Figuring out the sampling error involves using mathematical formulas and varies according to the summary measures or statistical procedures which are utilized in the study.

Observer error involves mistakes made by the observers or raters in the process of recording the information. Random errors are accidental slipups. Systematic errors occur routinely as a result of inadequate training of observers or of some bias that is influencing their observations. Observer error must be carefully guarded against since it can greatly influence the accuracy of the data.

Response error occurs when subjects err in responding to questions. Care should be taken to construct self-explanatory questions to give adequate directions, and to elicit complete replies from respondents in order to prevent accidental errors.

Processing errors are inaccuracies that result from mistakes in handling the data once they have been collected. Technical mistakes of varying degree and quality affect the accuracy during the analysis. Transcription errors, the incorrect categorization of open-ended questions, and improper application of statistical procedures all add up to processing errors.

The investigator must take steps to prevent errors from damaging the precision of the data at each step of the process. Careful planning, wise selection, and attention to detail help to keep the data as correct as possible.

The next chapter will cover the tools or instruments the researcher can utilize to record and collect the data. Now that the varied considerations of the data collection process have been covered, investigators can make a more insightful decision about the specific type of instrument required for the conduction of their study.

REFERENCES

1. J. Fleming: Human rights and ethical concerns of scientists. Issues in Research: Social, Professional, and Methodological. Kansas City, American Nurses' Association, 1974, p. 37.

2. Declaration of Helsinki: Recommendations Guiding Doctors in Clinical Research. Adopted by the 18th World Medical Assembly, Helsinki, Finland, 1964.

3. Code of ethics. International Nursing Review 20, 6 (1973): 116.

4. Human Rights Guidelines for Nurses in Clinical and Other Research. Kansas City, American Nurses' Association, 1975, p. 1.

5. N. Hershey and R. Miller: Human Experimentation and the Law. Germantown, Md., Aspen Systems Corp., 1976.

6. E. Hodgman: Student research in service agencies. Nursing Outlook 26, 9 (1978): 558–565.

7. P. Ramsey: The Ethics of Fetal Research. New Haven, Yale University Press, 1975.

8. P. Reynolds: On the protection of human subjects and social science. International Social Science Journal 24, 4 (1972): 694–695.

9. H. Creighton and C. Armington: Legal concerns of research and nurse researchers. Issues in Research: Social, Professional, and Methodological. Kansas City, American Nurses' Association, 1974, p. 21.

10. I. Silverman: The Human Subject in the Psychological Laboratory. New York, Pergamon Press, 1977, p. 5.

CHAPTER

9

Selecting and Using Existing Instruments

INTRODUCTION

The INSTRUMENT is the device or tool used by the researcher to collect and record the data that are obtained from the subjects. The instrument is probably the most well-known aspect of the entire research process. This process of capturing information is a vital part of all types of studies since the results and data are used to answer the original questions posed by the researchers. As mentioned in Chapter 8, the ways in which the information is collected from subjects can differ greatly. Data can be collected by means of direct contact, such as personal interviews, or by indirect methods, such as the observations made by behind-the-scenes observers. However, care should be taken to avoid confusing this process (the general ways to collect data) with the instrument. The instrument is the actual contrivance used to gather, record, and store information about the subjects being studied. Although most people immediately think of a questionnaire when the word instrument is mentioned, there are numerous other kinds of devices available. The instrument plays an important role in any research study and should be selected and used with care. There are three main categories of instruments available for use by researchers that coincide with the three methods of data collection: utilization of existing data, observation, and direct measurement. The two types that will be covered in this chapter are observation and direct measurement. These two classifications are the most frequently used. The instruments used to collect existing data are fairly uncomplicated and usually designed specifically for a particular study. This chapter will cover the kinds of instruments that have already been devised and are available for research purposes. The next chapter will cover the steps that are necessary in constructing an instrument of your own in the event that the existing ones are not suitable for your particular project.

DIRECT MEASUREMENT INSTRUMENTS

DIRECT MEASUREMENT INSTRUMENTS is a rough classification for tools that have one common feature: the information or data are in the form of verbal reports supplied directly by the subject. This means that the researcher can expect to end up with the actual written words, thoughts, or reported feelings of the subjects being questioned. These answers are not interpreted by observers or middlemen, and are not dependent on machines or other equipment for their transmission. These direct types of instruments are found in a variety of different forms as can be seen by the following examples.

Questionnaires

The questionnaire is by far the most widely used instrument in the research information-gathering process. The questionnaire consists of a series of preset questions to which the subject responds by providing written answers. The range of subject matter that can be covered by a questionnaire is vast. Attitudes, feelings, opinions, ideas, experiences, and perceptions may be investigated by using questionnaires to poll the respondents selected for a study. The degree of specificity of the answers will depend on the way in which the questionnaire is designed. Some are highly structured and offer the subject a "forced choice" of responses from which to select an answer. Others are semistructured in which case the subject is allowed some leeway to provide a more personalized response to a preset list of questions. The third type, an unstructured design, presents a stimulus situation or poses a leading question and leaves the type of response completely up to the subject. This variation in structure affects the kind of response that can be expected from the subject, as well as the depth of the information obtained. The variation will likewise produce different needs as far as the scoring procedures are concerned. The structured questionnaires are relatively easy and quick to score from an answer key. The semistructured responses pose serious problems in terms of categorization and interpretation of the wide range of answers that are usually given to open-ended questions. There are advantages and disadvantages in utilizing all three structures when asking for information from subjects. The depth of information desired, the conscious availability of answers from the subject (many people are not able to clearly articulate some of their attitudes), and the expertise of the researcher in interpreting data are some of the important factors to weigh in deciding which kind of tool to use. In order to demonstrate the structured differences in questionnaires, the three types of structures are contrasted in Figure 9.1. Questionnaires are often used to gather information that will be used to describe characteristics of the subjects. DEMOGRAPHIC DATA or background information on subjects, such as age, sex, area of residence, educational level, national origin and socioeconomic level, is often obtained through asking the subject to fill in a questionnaire. The sizable differences among structured, semistructured, and unstructured styles should become apparent after visualizing the types of responses one could expect from each of the three styles. Note that the researcher gradually loses control over the nature of the information gathered as the question becomes less structured.

Questionnaires are most often used to get information on topics for which there are no "right or wrong" answers. They provide a relatively easy way of collecting information that can be used to describe individuals. For instance, questionnaires have been constructed to determine attitudes of individuals so that the opinions of large numbers of individuals can be summarized to describe the overall attitude of a group on a certain topic. Questionnaires can also be used to identify certain subgroups within a larger group. For example, in a study in which the subjects were asked to complete two instruments, the questionnaire results were used to separate the sample into two groups—one with a positive attitude toward some attribute and the

Example of Structural Variation in Questions Designed to Obtain Demographic Data

Structured Questions	Semi-Structured Questions	Unstructured Questions
1. Please circle the category which describes your occupational group:	1. Please circle the term which most closely describes your occupational group:	1. What is your occupational group? (please specify:) _____

registered nurse	attendant	professional
doctor	licensed practical nurse	skilled
social worker	psychologist	semi-skilled
recreational therapist	dietitian	unskilled
occupational therapist	laboratory technician	
physical therapist	x-ray technician	
respiratory therapist	ward clerk	

other (please specify): _____

Figure 9.1

other with a negative attitude toward the same attribute. The researcher was then able to see if one group scored higher than the other on a second instrument—a knowledge test.

Questionnaires differ greatly in the degree of directness they use in communicating with subjects. Some are obvious in setting forth information on the variables the researcher is trying to measure, while others have a more covert approach. The descriptions that follow are of the overt type.

RATING SCALES

Rating scales are used to extract definite ratings on obvious factors. The subjects are fully aware of the entity being evaluated and are asked to make judgments about the strength or the amount of varied factors from their point of view. The rating scale is not normally constructed for the purpose of finding "hidden" or semiconscious information. The value of the scale comes from the explicitness or directness with which the rater can use the tool to assess the factor being investigated. The rating scale in Figure 9.2 is a self-assessment type of instrument. The subjects are asked to rate their ability to communicate with patients from two viewpoints. They were asked to designate a rating that corresponds with the way others (instructors) have judged them, and to indicate their own rating as well.

Note how the subjects have the opportunity to rate different aspects of communication in varying degrees from a high of A+ to a low of F. The numbers 1 to 11 were substituted for the letters to obtain a total score for the scale or find an average score for certain items on a subscale. The subjects were asked to rate their ability to communicate in a clear-cut, overt fashion.

An Example of a Rating Scale

These questions were designed to have you evaluate your ability to communicate with patients and health team members in your role as a professional nurse. Circle only one value for each question. The scale allows you to designate varying degrees of ability from a high of A+ to a low of F.

1. In regard to *verbal communication* with patients, my nursing instructors have rated me overall as:

    A+ A   A− B+ B   B− C+ C   C− D   F

2. In regard to *nonverbal communication* with patients, my nursing instructors have rated me overall as:

    A+ A   A− B+ B   B− C+ C   C− D   F

3. In regard to *verbal communication* with patients, I would rate myself as:

    A+ A   A− B+ B   B− C+ C   C− D   F

4. In regard to *nonverbal communication* with patients, I would rate myself as:

    A+ A   A− B+ B   B− C+ C   C− D   F

5. In all aspects of communication with patients, I would rate myself as:

    A+ A   A− B+ B   B− C+ C   C− D   F

6. In overall aspects of communication with all members of the health care team, I would rate myself as:

    A+ A   A− B+ B   B− C+ C   C− D   F

Figure 9.2

CHECKLISTS

The checklist is a simple list of factors that the subjects are asked to check or mark off. The checklist in Figure 9.3 is an example of an instrument used to determine the subjects' image of nurse researchers. A variety of factors that have been found to make up different images people have of them are enumerated, and the subjects are instructed to check the items that coincide with their views on this matter. The checklist differs from the rating scale in that the degree, or strength, of opinion cannot be designated since there is no scale incorporated into the questionnaire. Only the presence or absence of an item can be denoted by the response to the checklist.

Psychological and Sociological Measures

There are a great variety of instruments that attempt to quantify the feelings, attitudes, or opinions individuals hold on a particular concept. The attempts at measuring these vague and often hidden (even to the subject) thoughts extend from the use of simple attitude scales to the employment of sophisticated projective devices. This section will touch upon some of those most often used.

Example of A Checklist

The following characteristics are commonly attributed to researchers. Read through the list and check off any items which correspond with *your picture of nurse researchers*.

__ Scientifically oriented   __ High achievers

__ Innovators   __ Creative

__ Low technical skills   __ Impractical

__ Ivory tower thinkers   __ Highly intelligent

__ Critical thinkers   __ Independent professionals

__ Highly respected   __ Statistically competent

Figure 9.3

Examples of Items on an Attitudinal Scale

QUESTIONNAIRE

Directions: Please read each of the following statements and circle one
response. Please be sure to answer all questions.

1. I rather like the idea of being the first to try a new nursing procedure
   Strongly Agree   Agree   Disagree   Strongly Disagree

2. I dislike doing anything just on the spur of the moment.
   Strongly Agree   Agree   Slightly Agree

3. Few things are more upsetting than a sudden unexpected change of
   work routine.
   Strongly Agree   Agree   Disagree   Strongly Disagree

4. In whatever one does, the old and established procedures are always
   the best.
   Strongly Agree   Agree   Disagree   Strongly Disagree

5. I never start anything I can't finish.
   Strongly Agree   Agree   Disagree   Strongly Disagree

Figure 9.4

ATTITUDE SCALES

Many researchers use questionnaires to elicit the subjects' attitudes on a
variety of topics. It may be expected that the subjects would differ in the
strength of their opinions on a certain topic, so the researcher isn't necessarily scoring one answer as correct and a differing opinion as incorrect. The
questions presented in Figure 9.4 are excerpted from a questionnaire that
was constructed to measure attitudes of individuals toward everyday life
situations. These attitudinal questions are fairly obvious, in that the subjects
are asked to give their opinions on each item, and it is not too difficult to
figure out that the investigator wants to find out how flexible the subjects may

Example of An Item Extracted from An Attitudinal Scale Concerning Nursing Actions

It is a hospital policy that all patients must be discharged in a wheel-chair, accompanied by a member of the hospital staff. Mr. Smith, recovering from a stroke, has had a long and difficult period of rehabilitation and is now ready to go home. He has finally learned to walk with the aid of two canes and is proud of this accomplishment and wants to show his daughter how well he is doing when she picks him up at the hospital entrance. He objects to having to ride in a wheelchair to the hospital entrance. You, as the nurse, judge that Mr. Smith is quite capable of walking the distance required and that forcing him to ride in the wheelchair will threaten his slowly developing self-confidence. However, it is a hospital rule.

Indicate the extent to which you would choose each of the listed behaviors.

	Strongly Agree	Agree	Undecided	Disagree	Strongly Disagree
A. Let Mr. Smith walk down to the hospital entrance since it is very important not to threaten his slowly developing self-confidence by making him ride when he feels he is capable of walking.	___	___	___	___	___
B. Explain to Mr. Smith that he may become weak and tired and that it would be unsafe for him to walk that far. Have him use the wheelchair.	___	___	___	___	___
C. Have Mr. Smith ride to the hospital entrance in a wheelchair, explaining to him that it is a hospital rule made for the benefit of all patients.	___	___	___	___	___
D. Call the physician and ask him if it is all right for Mr. Smith to walk to the hospital entrance.	___	___	___	___	___
E. Call your supervisor and ask her if you might break the hospital rule so that Mr. Smith might walk to the entrance.	___	___	___	___	___
F. Let Mr. Smith walk to the hospital entrance, accompanied by an orderly wheeling an empty wheelchair in case Mr. Smith gets tired and wants to ride.	___	___	___	___	___

Figure 9.5

be. Note that these questions are worded in such a way that the subjects can react in a characteristic manner. They have been worded to make it seem as if the readers are talking so that they can recognize familiar statements, and react to a statement that does not agree with their known attitudes. The subjects are allowed to respond according to the strength of their agreement or disagreement rather than simply a clear-cut agree or disagree. Note that there are four choices to make in response to a statement. This is called a four-point scale. This type of instrument is probably one of the most common. The investigator could have added a "slightly" agree and disagree category and ended up with a six-point scale. Notice that the neutral category is missing from the tool. The neutral choices (undecided, neither agree or disagree) may be present on a number of instruments, but should be used with caution. It is often easier to remain neutral or "on the fence" with regard to an attitude or opinion, and the very presence of an easy way out may keep some subjects from expressing a true opinion.

Attitudinal scales may take many shapes and forms. The question in Figure 9.5 was one item on a scale constructed to pick up varying attitudes of newly graduated nurses (toward such things as enforcing bureaucratic rules and utilizing their own clinical judgment).

SEMANTIC DIFFERENTIAL SCALES

Attitudes and perceptions of concepts are often hard to explain verbally. Often, the subjects are truly unaware of their attitudes or feelings, and at other times questions, such as those required in attitude scales, are cumbersome and awkward. One device often utilized by researchers to uncover this information in a more covert manner is the semantic differential scale. This scale consists of bipolar sets of adjectives that are selected by the researcher and used throughout the instrument. Each set is rated according to its overall positive or negative relationship to the concept being evaluated. The subjects would be requested to fill in the response set for a number of different concepts in order to construct a composite feeling about each one. The example in Figure 9.6 would elicit both the overt and covert feelings of the subjects about the concept "nurse."

PERSONALITY AND INTEREST INVENTORIES

Much of the educationally oriented research of the past has centered on measuring the personality characteristics of subjects. Psychologists have devised a great many instruments of this type that are in widespread use. Some of the more popular of these tests that you may come across in reading reports are *The Minnesota Multiphasic Personality Inventory* (MMPI), *The California Psychological Inventory* (CPI), *The Omnibus Personality Inventory* (OPI), and *The Edwards Personal Preference Schedule* (EPPS). Most of

---

Example of An Item Extracted from a Semantic Differential Scale

Directions:

In the following section, there are a series of adjectives which might be used to describe something or someone. The adjectives are grouped in pairs with the two adjectives in each pair referring to more or less opposite characteristics (e.g. Positive/negative). Check (√) the line on the scale which you feel comes closest to describing the keyword listed above the sets of adjectives. *Work as quickly as possible, trusting your first impression.*

Example:

MOTHER

positive	___ ___ ___ _√_ ___ ___	negative
strong	___ _√_ ___ ___ ___ ___	weak
valuable	___ ___ _√_ ___ ___ ___	worthless

1.   NURSE

positive	___ ___ ___ ___ ___ ___ ___ ___	negative
strong	___ ___ ___ ___ ___ ___ ___ ___	weak
valuable	___ ___ ___ ___ ___ ___ ___ ___	worthless
good	___ ___ ___ ___ ___ ___ ___ ___	bad
progressive	___ ___ ___ ___ ___ ___ ___ ___	traditional
peaceful	___ ___ ___ ___ ___ ___ ___ ___	ferocious
right	___ ___ ___ ___ ___ ___ ___ ___	wrong
sensitive	___ ___ ___ ___ ___ ___ ___ ___	insensitive

Figure 9.6

these measurement devices have specific directions for administration and are highly standardized. Most break up the subjects' responses into subscales of various personality characteristics (such as autonomy, deference, or flexibility) and are usually machine scored at special centers. Interest inventories, such as the *Strong Vocational Interest Inventory* (SVII) and *The Kuder Preference Test*, have also been widely used in studies of the characteristics of nursing students and nursing personnel. They are primarily used to classify interests related to vocational endeavors, but can be utilized for other purposes. The researcher can even order computerized interpretations of the results of some of these devices (such as the MMPI and the SVII). Most of these inventories have special profile sheets that enable the tester to place the subjects' scores on a preprinted scale and thus make comparisons of different subscores within the individual profile, as well as in relation to the "norm" or average group.

PROJECTIVE DEVICES

This type of instrument presents a stimulus to the subject with the aim of obtaining less obvious, hidden, or partially unconscious information. The researcher records the reactions or responses of the subjects and analyzes the information by going through a set of procedures designed to classify the responses as objectively as possible. The most commonly known projective instruments have been set up to quantify underlying personality constructs. The famous Rorschach Inkblot Test and the Thematic Apperception Test (TAT) have been used in numerous studies. The administration of such devices is fairly easy and often more interesting and challenging for subjects. One word of caution should be mentioned, however. Projective tests and closely related projective drawings should only be used by researchers who are properly trained in the scoring of projective techniques.

The difficulties encountered most often by beginning researchers, when seeking information on attitudes, are in scoring or classifying the responses, since many are relatively easy to process.

Stories told in response to situational pictures can be evaluated for major themes or topics. The investigator of the study summarized in Commentary 9.1 devised a projective device for her study that was basically similar to standard psychological tests such as the Rosenzweig Picture Frustration Study.

Commentary 9.1
One Way to Draw Upon Your Research
Background . . .

One researcher wanted to assess nurse-patient role perceptions and expectations. In choosing an instrument for measuring this type of information, she had to keep in mind that the literature suggests that such perceptions are not always readily available for the asking. Often times such thoughts are at a low level of awareness and are more openly conveyed to others through story telling, picture drawing or humorous anecdotes. Thus, a projective device is required to delve into the area. A unique instrument was devised for collecting data from patients and nurses in this study. The nurses and patients were given sets of cartoons that were constructed to elicit certain kinds of perceptions. The subjects were given four frame cartoon strips. The first three frames set up the theme of the story. The last frame showed a patient or nurse with a blank area where the words should appear. The subjects were instructed to "put words into the nurses (or patients) mouth." The words, of course, would be based on their own perception of the situation. The great advantage of using a projective technique is the variety of answers which can be produced since the creativity of the subject is stimulated. The first 3 sets of cartoons on p. 186 are like the ones used in the study. Why not try your skill with the fourth set of cartoons? Go ahead and put the words in the student's mouth about the research course.

Do the words you wrote in frame four convey your perception of the role of research in nursing?

The responses of the patients and nurses who took part in the "cartoon" study had to be rated by judges to introduce as much objectivity as possible in the analysis. The patients had some very interesting things to say about the nurses, and vice versa . . .

L. Copp. A projective cartoon investigation of nurse-patient psychodramatic role perception and expectation. *Nursing Research* 20, 2 (March–April 1971): 110–112.

Tests

VERBAL TESTS

The purpose of a test is to measure the amount of some specific factor or characteristic that an individual possesses. The use of intelligence, aptitude, and achievement tests is widespread throughout our entire educational system. The subject can be evaluated either by comparison to a set numerical scale (for example, a passing grade for a course may be set at 70) or by comparison to the "norm" or average group of those previously taking the test (for instance, the "average" score on the College Entrance Examination may be calculated at 500). The use of knowledge tests is widespread throughout nursing research literature. Scores on tests devised to measure accuracy of such factors as knowledge of diabetes and venereal disease can be readily interpreted by most students.

PERFORMANCE TESTS

Some tests have been devised to measure the ease with which subjects perform certain tasks. The tasks are most often devised to measure factors that can be scored in relation to the individual's achievement in motor skills. These tasks can measure such things as manual dexterity, muscle coordination, and creative problem solving. The investigator who set up the study described in Commentary 9.2 used a well-known performance test as one of the measures of the dependent variables in her study.

Commentary 9.2
Using the Fruits of Other's Work

One nurse wanted to study the relationship between pica (the ingestion of non-edible substances) and the developmental level of a group of two-year-old children. The information about the child's pica practices was acquired by interviewing the mother. The researcher however, had to make an important determination about the developmental level of the child, and needed an instrument she could rely on to get the rating. She selected the Denver Developmental Screening Test (DDST). This is a well-known device which is used to detect the developmental delays in young children. The delays can be detected in four categories:

gross motor   language
fine motor-adaptive   personal-social

In this instance, it was important to secure a tool that had been developed and pre-tested by experts in the field. As a result of testing 90 children, this researcher found that children who practiced pica and exhibited other consistent hand-mouth behavior were lagging behind in certain developmental areas assessed by the DDST. She was then able to give some suggestions for nursing actions that were related to her results.

P. Robischon. Pica practice and other hand-mouth behavior and children's developmental level. *Nursing Research* 20, 1 (January–February, 1971): pp. 4–16.

Mechanical Devices or Instruments

Health-related research studies often utilize mechanical instruments to collect data from subjects. The large variety of such devices add both interest and precision to research studies. Instruments, such as thermometers, sphygmomanometers, and all kinds of sophisticated monitoring devices, are readily available to nurses in clinical settings. Such instruments provide for objective and precise readings or scores. The exact reading 98.6° for a body temperature provides an unbiased and fairly exact reading that can be com-

Examples of Projective Devices Used to Collect Information About Underlying Attitudes

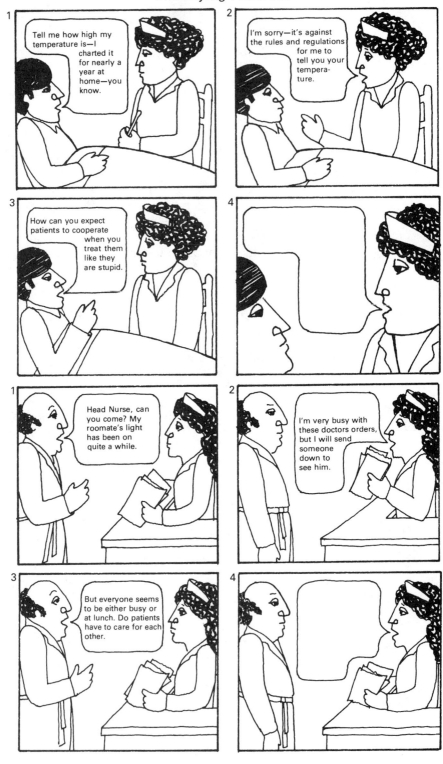

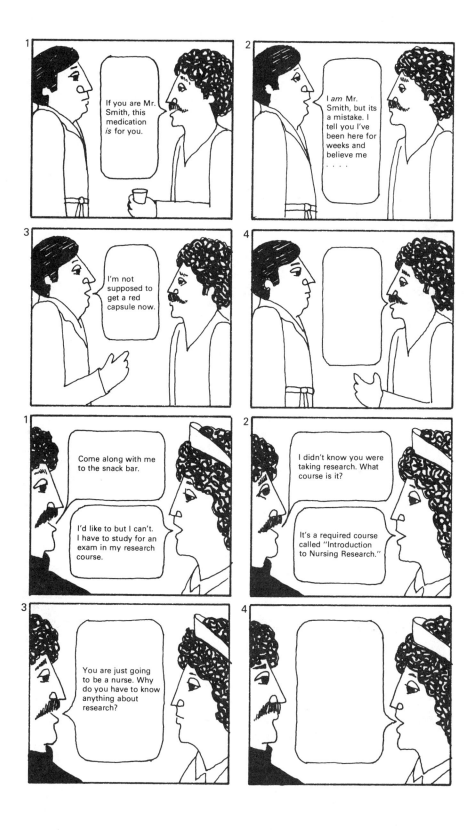

pared with a later reading. The numbers or scores supplied by these devices allow for the application of more sophisticated statistical analysis of the results.

INSTRUMENTS UTILIZED TO COLLECT INFORMATION IN AN INDIRECT MANNER

Throughout nursing research literature there are many examples of the indirect method of collecting data. This means that the responses from the subject are transmitted through some other agent before being recorded. This method necessarily reduces the amount of anonymity that can be guaranteed to the subjects. However, indirect data collection may be the preferred or even the only plausible way to get certain information.

Interviews

There are two basic types of interviews: structured and unstructured (with lots of room for variation in between). The classification depends mainly on the amount of organization and standardization that is done during the interaction between researcher and subjects. Interviews provide the researcher with the opportunity to gain more in-depth information and provides an opportunity to explore and clarify issues that could be missed on a questionnaire or from an existing record. The interaction allows the investigator to get a more personal feeling about the subjects. This is obviously more time-consuming than some other means, but may be well worth the investment.

UNSTRUCTURED INTERVIEWS
Are generally pretty freewheeling data-gathering conversations. The researcher knows the general type of information she would like to obtain, but usually "plays it by ear" and pursues the topics that come up in the conversation. This type of interview is most often used by researchers who are trying to pin down a vague topic or who are very experienced.

STRUCTURED INTERVIEWS
Are planned in detail in an attempt to standardize them as much as possible. This means that several interviewers can approach a number of subjects and gather fairly consistent data. Such details as the wording of

individual questions and the order in which the questions are posed to each subject are planned out well in advance. Sometimes interviewers have schedules or written guidelines they can follow directly during the interaction. An example of a previously utilized structured interview schedule can be seen in Figure 9.7. The utilization of an interview involves the same kind

---

Sample Instrument for a Structured Interview

Patient's Initials_____

Admission Date_____   Assessment Date_____

Introduction:

Mr., Mrs. or Miss_____, I am_____

I would like you to answer some questions in order that we may plan your care better while you are here in the hospital.

  I. Do you have any problems with your

    Hearing?
    Sight?
    Passing urine?
    Bowels?
    Menstrual periods (if female)?
    Teeth-Mouth?

  II. There are some questions I need to ask you about the things you do daily.

    Some people go to sleep early in the evening and wake up early in the morning. What do you usually do?

    Some people eat their meals at about the same time each day. Do you?

    In your opinion do you eat a lot at meals?

    Do you snack between meals?

    Some people like to bathe in the morning. Others in the evening. When do you prefer to bathe?

    Would you rather take a bath or a shower?

    What time of the day do you seem to have the most energy?

(Continued)

Figure 9.7

Do you have some time for leisure activities?

Do you have any hobbies? (If yes) Tell me about them?

Some people prefer being alone. Others would rather be with groups. Which do you prefer?

Some people like quiet activities such as reading, sewing, and playing cards. Other people like active pastimes such as dancing, swimming, or tennis. What things do you enjoy doing?

Some people feel lonely, even in a crowd. Others seldom feel lonely. How would you describe yourself?

Some people get angry very easily. Other people rarely seem to let things bother them. Which sounds more like you?

Some people fear being alone, in high places, or closed areas. Others fear situations they are placed in with people. How would you describe your fears?

Some people feel tense and nervous a lot of the time. Other people feel relaxed most of the time. Which one sounds most like you?

Some people read, take a walk, or work in the garden when they are lonely or upset. What do you usually do?

Some people see themselves as overweight while others think they are underweight. How do you see yourself?

Some people think others see them as shy. Others think people see them as outgoing. What way do you think others see you?

Some people jump at the slightest noise while others barely notice it. How do you usually respond?

Some people cry when they are sad. Others cry when they are happy. What are you most prone to do?

What grade were you in when you left school?

Do you see yourself as being dependent or independent?

Do you have any allergies to medications, food, pollen, feathers, dust, etc.?

How do you feel about having people visiting you while you are here?

Are there any people you would prefer not to have visit you?

Are there any problems you feel I need to know?

Are there any things that you didn't get finished before you came to the hospital that I could help you take care of?

III. (Directions to nurse: Observe in the following areas and record while with the patient)

Figure 9.7 (cont.)

General Appearance: *Cue Guide*
                       Personal hygiene
                       Nails, Hair
                       Skin condition
                       Body odor, etc.

Communication Patterns: Quiet
                           Talkative
                           Comfortable
                           Anxious

Body Language: Posture
                  Gestures
                  Eye contact
                  Mannerisms

Nurse_____Time Spent_____

Figure 9.7 (cont.)

of planning effort as does the construction of a written instrument. The investigator needs to consider the following points:

1. The length of time for the interview
2. The interview setting
3. The manner of recording the information (by committing statements to memory, writing responses, audio- or videotape, etc.)
4. The appearance and demeanor of the interviewer
5. The manner of approaching the subjects and gaining their cooperation
6. The use of probing questions to gain further clarification of issues
7. The wording and order of questions
8. The types and kinds of observations that will be made about subjects

Observation

At times, researchers employ raters or judges to make decisions about some type of behavior displayed by the subjects. Usually, several raters are used to add more weight to the decisions by ensuring group consensus on the phenomenon. The raters undergo training sessions to sharpen their skills in this area and to learn how to use the instrument involved in the project. It is important that all the raters are in agreement (called inter-rater reliability) if the outcome is to be meaningful. There are numerous types of rating scales, and it is quite important for the scale to be comprehensive yet simple to use since the rater is often being asked to make judgments about fast-paced interactions and behavior. Figure 9.8 is an example of a scale used by an individual to rate the performance of another person. Note that the rating

---

Sample of a Performance Rating Scale
Dry Sterile Dressing Procedure

Nurse being rated: _____ Rater: _____

		Yes	No
1.	Performs handwashing procedure before donning gloves.	☐	☐
2.	Dons gloves while maintaining sterile condition.	☐	☐
3.	Uses proper procedure to clean wound.	☐	☐
4.	Maintains sterility of sterile field.	☐	☐
5.	Positions patient in a safe, comfortable position.	☐	☐
6.	Explains procedure to patient.	☐	☐
7.	Disposes of soiled equipment according to prescribed procedures.	☐	☐

Figure 9.8

scale asks for specific judgments to be made about a limited number of factors in a particular situation The rater is able to designate a place on a scale (from a small to a large amount) to show the degree of presence or absence of the factor being considered. The training of observers takes on added importance when you are relying on their judgement and when you consider how quickly an activity can take place. The rater must be able to record the decisions quickly and with little chance of error if the observation is to be worthwhile.

The form in Figure 9.9 is an example of the types of observational ratings made by nurses about mothers and babies in a high-risk population group. The observational ratings are filled in after home-visit interviews are completed by the public health nurse. The layout and coding of this instrument was set up specifically to facilitate computerization of the data. A more complete description of this instrument and its use can be found in *Nursing Information Systems* by H. Werley and M. Grier.

GASTON COUNTY HEALTH DEPARTMENT
High-Priorty Infant Identification Form

BABY'S NAME _____

| Last (1-34) | First | Middle | Sex (35) |

IDENTIFICATION NUMBER ___ ___ ___ ___ ___   (To be assigned by clerk.)   COHORT NUMBER ☐ 79
36 37 38 39 40 (First two digits = year of birth.)

FORM NUMBER ☐ 80

	For Clerical Purposes	High-priorty factors on birth Certificate	For Clerical Purposes
	41 42		Yes No
Month of birth		Mother's age under 18	☐ 50 ☐
Day of birth	43 44	Mother's age over 35	☐ 51 ☐
Race of mother	45	Parity above 4	☐ 52 ☐
Month of pregnancy prenatal care began	46	*previous live-born now dead	☐ 53 ☐
Total number of prenatal visits (coded)	47	APGAR 6 or less at 5 min	☐ 54 ☐
0 = none		Mother's education below 9th grade	☐ 55 ☐
1 = one thru three visits 2 = four thru nine visits 3 = ten or more visits 9 = unknown		*No prenatal care or care began in 8th or 9th month.	☐ 56 ☐
Expected source of health care	48	*Birth weight under 2,500 gms.	☐ 57 ☐
		Out of wedlock birth	☐ 58 ☐
Visited in hospital by PHN or office nurse Yes ☐ 49 No ☐		Total number of high-priorty factors from birth certificate (Cols. 50-58)	59

Maternal Characteristics Identified By Nurses and Indicative of Infant High-Priorty Status:	
*Poor coping ability with a previous baby or with this baby.	☐ 60 ☐
Feels powerless or lacking in control over her life	☐ 61 ☐
*Seems emotionally unstable	☐ 62 ☐
Expresses hostility toward baby	☐ 63 ☐
Illiterate or of apparently low intelligence	☐ 64 ☐
Very poor housing or other indication of extreme poverty	☐ 65 ☐
*Baby ill before discharge from hospital	☐ 66 ☐
*Low maternal-child attachment noted in hospital or at early home visit	☐ 67 ☐
Total number of nurse-identified high priority factors (Cols. 60-67)	68
(0 = none, 1 thru 7 = one thru seven, 8 = eight or more) Total of all high-priorty factors (Col. 59 + 68) (use actual number)	69
Baby assigned to high-priorty follow-up.	☐ 70 ☐
Baby's age at time of assignment to high-priorty follow-up (coded data-see code sheet)	71
Private M.D. notified of baby's possible high-priorty status.	☐ 72 ☐

*Presence of any one of above starred factors should result in automatic assignment.

73 Deceased

Mother's Name: _____
First   Middle   Last
Address: _____
Street or Rural Route

City or Town   County   State
Phone: _____

MIH—1 GCHD, Aug. '76

Baby's expected residence during first 3 months:
(If different from mother's address-include hospital or other institution.)

Street or Rural Route
_____

City or Town   County   State
Name of expected
Caretaker _____
First   Middle   Last
Relationship of
Caretaker to baby: _____

(Continued)

Figure 9.9

Sample of an instrument used to record observational ratings made by nurses.

Date _____   **GASTON COUNTY HEALTH DEPARTMENT**   5/24/77

                              High-priority Infant Follow-up Form   Revision

CHILD'S NAME _____   _____
(Please print) Last (1-34)   First   Middle   35
                                                                      Care Status of Private Pediatrician
IDENTIFICATION NUMBER _____   Babies
                      36 37 38 39 40

            (See code for use in completing this form)

____ (41) Age of Period of Child   HEALTH STATUS INDICATORS
____ (42) Present Location of Child in Relation to Need for
____   Follow-up Care   ____ (60) Immunization   DPT
____ (43) Primary Caretaker   ____ (51)   Status: Polio
____ (44) Daycare   ____ (62)   Measles
____ (45) Current Member of WIC Program
                                                      ____ (63) Hemoglobin Level
        NUMBER OF SICK-CARE VISITS: ____ (64) Development Level
           (since last age period)   ____ (65) Weight-height Centile
                                                      ____ (66) Congenital Anomalies
____ (46) hospitalizations
____ (47) to emergency room   ____ (67) Maternal-child Attachment
____ (48) to private M.D.   ____ (68) Maternal Emotional Stability
____ (49) to H.D. clinic   ____ (69)*Maltreatment (abuse or neglect)
____ (50) to other sources of sick-care   ____ (70)*Physical Problems (exclude all coded above)
____ (51) total outpatient sick-care visits   ____ (71) Estimate of Severity of Most Important Health
                                                               Problem (60-70)
        WELL-CHILD CARE: ____ (72) Estimate of Intensity of Need for Special Service
        (since last age period)
                                                      ____ To be completed only at 3-month age period:
____ (52) primary responsibility for well-child care
____ (53) change in primary source of well-child care ____ (73) Initial prenatal home assessment
____   since last age period   ____ (74)*Failure to regain birthweight by first clinic visit
____ (54) number of well-child visits to primary source ____ (75)*Mother had postpartum check
____ (55) number of broken appointments at primary source
                                                      ____Number of Prenatal Group Education Sessions:
        HOME VISITS (since last age period)
                                                      ____ (76) with nutritionist
____ (56) for initial home assessment   ____ (77) with PHN
____ (57) other home visit   ____ (78) with health educator regarding Family planning

____ NUMBER OF GROUP EDUCATION SESSIONS: ____ (79) COHORT NUMBER
        (since last age period)   ____ (80) FORM NUMBER

____ (58) with nutritionist   *Single identification factors warrenting
____ (59) with PHN   high-priority follow-up; for physical problems
                                                        this results only if illness occurs before two
                                                        months of age.

                         HEALTH STATUS INDICATORS

Column
Numbers   Immunization Status:

    60   DPT - Total number of shots received to date:
            0. None
            1. One
            2. Two
            3. Three
            4. Four or more
            9. Unknown

                        (Continued)

                   Figure 9.9 (cont.)

Column
Numbers

61   Polio - Total number of doses of oral vaccine received to date:
(Use same code as for DPT in Column 60.)

62   Measles (rubeola)

0.   None
1.   Measles (rubeola) alone
2.   Measles and rubella M-R
3.   Measles + Rubella + Mumps M-M-R
4.   Measles vaccine of unknown kind
9.   Unknown

63   Hemoglobin Level

1.   11 or above
2.   10 to 10.9
3.   8.5 to 9.9
4.   Below 8.5
9.   Unknown

64   Developmental Level   0.   Unknown

1.   Apparently normal - no information to nurse (Do not use this code if child has ever received Codes 2 thru 8)

Assessment   (2.   Question of deviation - Nurse alerted on lab slip
incomplete   (3.   Probable deviation - referred for pediatric assessment which is not yet complete

(4.   Previously questioned deviation (Code 2) now thought to be resolved.
Re-assessed as O.K. (5.   Diagnosed by pediatrician or D.E.C. as no deviation

Assessment   (6.   D.E.C. or pediatrician diagnosed deficiency - special follow-up in progress — no
completed.   (change noted.
Follow-up   (7.   D.E.C. or pediatrician diagnosed deficiency - special follow-up in
in progress   (progress — diagnosed improvement

Follow-up   (8.   D.E.C. or pediatrician diagnosed deficiency - special follow-up not in progress
action needed   (9.   Assessment or re-assessment indicated and not done.

65   Weight-Height Centile

1.   5th centile or less — definitely underweight
2.   6th or 10th centile — question of underweight
3.   11th to 25th centile
4.   26th to 74th centile
5.   75th to 89th centile
6.   90th to 94th centile — question of overweight
7.   95th centile or greater — definitely overweight
9.   Not recorded

66   Congenital Anomalies

0.   None
1.   Suspected — diagnosis in progress
2.   Diagnosed — no action needed at present
3.   Diagnosed — recommendations for action just made
4.   Diagnosed — approriate action currently in progress
5.   Diagnosed — approriate action completed
6.   Diagnosed — recommended action not being taken
9.   Diagnosed — action unknown

67   Maternal-child Attachment (Or other primary caretaker)

1.   Apparently satisfactory
2.   Apparently unsatisfactory — receiving PHN follow-up only
3.   Apparently unsatisfactory — receiving follow-up from outside agency
4.   Apparently unsatisfactory — no follow-up
9.   Unknown — little or no contact with mother

(Continued)

Figure 9.9 (cont.)

68   Maternal Emotional Stability (Or other primary caretaker)
       1. Apparently stable
       2. Apparently unstable — receiving PHN follow-up only
       3. Apparently unstable — receiving specialized mental health care
       4. Apparently unstable — no follow-up
       9. Stability unknown — little or no contact with mother

69   Maltreatment (Abuse or neglect)
       0. No reason to expect or suspect
       1. Not suspected but high potential believed present (i.e., due to previous maltreatment or other known
           predisposing factors)
       2. Current maltreatment suspected but not diagnosed — supportive action being taken.
       3. Current maltreatment suspected but not diagnosed — no action being taken
       4. Recent maltreatment officially reported to DSS and program being implemented
       9. Unknown — no contact with caretakers

70   Physical Problems (Code follow-up status for most important physical problem not coded elsewhere; e.g. under
       hemoglobin or anomalies. Include injuries resulting from maltreatment.)
       0. Examined and none found (Do not use this code if code 5 or 6 could be used for follow-up of a prior acute
           problem.)
       1. Assessed chronic - apprpiate treatment or supervision in progress
       2. Assessed chronic - appropiate treatment or supervision not in progress
       3. Assessed chronic - treatment or supervision no longer needed
       4. Assessed acute — appropiate treatment or supervision in progress
       5. Assessed acute — treatment or supervision completed — problem resolved
       6. Assessed acute — no action taken — problem resolved
       7. Assessed acute — no action taken — problem not resolved
       8. Follow-up of assessed problem unknown
       9. Not examined — problem status unknown

Figure 9.9 (cont.)

Combinations of Instruments

Sometimes investigators utilize several types of instruments in collecting data from subjects. The researcher must consider the practicalities of the situation (time, expertise, funds, and the type of information required) and then relate these to the optimum way of collecting data. The following description of the data collection in a study of nonverbal communication illustrates the use of multiple instruments within a single project. The researchers in this specific study attended to the following:

> Observation of the patient-investigator interaction by two observers (both nurses), a questionnaire administered by one of the observers at the end of the interaction, a tape recording of the verbal interaction, and electrocardiographic tracings of the patients on cardiac monitors.[1]

SELECTING INSTRUMENTS

The investigator must take great care in this phase of the project since the instrument can greatly affect the meaningfulness of the entire project. The following general points should be reviewed:

Criteria for Selection

1. Does the instrument require special talents or experience in administration or scoring? It should be noted that as a general rule of thumb, it is best to administer the test according to the instructions provided. The standardization of the instrument and its comparability with other results from the same instrument are based on this point. Likewise, using one subscale (of say 25 items) from a standardized test (of say 399 items) is altering the potential test results to an unknown degree.
2. How expensive are the instrument, answer sheets, and machine scoring if required?
3. Is specialized equipment needed?
4. How many subjects can be tested at any given time? Are the test booklets reusable?
5. How much time does it take to administer the instrument?
6. Is more than one instrument appropriate and available? If so, gather information on each (from literature, test reviews, and consultation).
7. Is a test manual available? If so, review it for other pertinent information.
8. The possible familiarity of the subjects with the instrument may affect the selection of a particular instrument.
9. There are several well-known indices that influence the selection of instruments. The reliability, validity, and sensitivity of the devices are commonly reviewed in the test selection process. These important factors can be applied as follows:

RELIABILITY

A reliable instrument is a consistent one. This means that the device will yield the same type of response in a variety of situations. A reliable thermometer will read 98.6° each time it is utilized to measure the temperature of subjects who are at the designated normal point. A reliable test is one that results in consistent responses from the subjects. Two of the most common ways of determining the reliability are as follows:

Test-Re-Test. In this instance, the researcher gives the test to a group of subjects and then repeats the administration of the test at a later time. This retest normally occurs from several weeks to six months after the original testing. The responses to the questions are compared to see if the subject has given a similar response both times.

Statistical Computations. The use of statistical formulas, such as the Kuder-Richardson 20 and the Spearman Brown formula, eliminate the retest (as well as avoid chance reasons for a fluctuating performance, such as the subject's health status). Some of the formulas compare each item of the test with every possible combination. This is a feat that would otherwise take an incredible amount of time per instrument.

VALIDITY

This relates to the meaningfulness or relevancy of the test to the variable being measured. There are several ways to ensure validity. The previously designed instrument will often be accompanied by information on validity. Face validity is present when the test looks realistic, legitimate, and related to the factor being studied. Other types of validity (content, construct) pertain more to the content of the device. Is it related to major knowledge in the field, is it comprehensive, and does it yield the same results as similar instruments?

SENSITIVITY

This generally means the degree of accuracy with which the instrument can measure the variable being studied. A word scale is generally not as sensitive as the score on a mechanical instrument. Researchers need to determine the approximate level of sensitivity that they need for their particular study.

LOCATING INSTRUMENTS

There are several means of locating existing instruments.

1. Look through published research reports that cover your general area of interest. Most describe the instruments that have been utilized in the study in detail. Some include a facsimile of the instrument for visual inspection by the reader.
2. If the instrument looks like it may be useful in your project, write to the author of the article to ask for a complete copy, for further information on reliability and validity, and for permission to utilize the instrument in your investigation.
3. Investigate standard sources for instruments in social sciences like the following:
   O. Buros, (ed.): Tests in Print II. New Jersey, The Gryphon Press, 1974. (Descriptive bibliography of 2,467 commercially available tests).
   O. Buros, (ed.): The Eighth Mental Measurements Yearbook. New Jersey, The Gryphon Press, 1978.
   (Descriptions of 1,184 tests; test reviews by specialists; bibliography of books on testing).

4. A compilation of specific nursing research instruments is available from the following source:

    M. Ward and M. Fetler: *Instruments for Use in Nursing Research.* Boulder, Colorado, Western Interstate Commission for Higher Education, 1979.

It might be wise to start a card file on the nursing and clinically related instruments you come across when reading studies.

5. *Dissertation Abstracts International* contains the abstracts of many doctoral dissertations. Look under the subject since most abstracts include mention of the instruments utilized in the study.
6. Utilize a previously published instrument (or some of the basic ideas from a test protocol) to adapt one for your particular needs. The next chapter deals with specific suggestions on designing your own tool.

PRETESTING INSTRUMENTS

The instrument you have selected should always be pretested on a small number of individuals who are similar to the subjects you later wish to study. The pretest is like a practice session for the investigator and a "dry-run" of the instrument. This need not be an elaborate step in a small project, but is a very important measure in assuring that the data collected in the actual study are meaningful. The data collection instrument cannot be altered once the study is underway. (How could you describe the results of the first instrument *and* the revised form all in one study?) Use a neat, official-looking copy of the proposed instrument with the accompanying equipment, answer sheets, #2 pencils, and whatever else you plan to use in the actual experiment. Note the following points about the pretesting:

1. The time it takes the subjects to complete the task.
2. The difficulty of the items. (Is the wording understandable to all? Are the questions ambiguous or too easy?)
3. Can you flag problem items or questions? (For instance, are people leaving one particular item blank or giving evasive answers?) Are the directions clear?
4. Are the test results sufficient to answer the questions you posed when beginning the study?
5. Are there problems that need to be solved with equipment, procedures, or perhaps the setting?

6. Seek the reactions of the pretest subjects immediately after the testing. Did they feel rushed? Did they encounter any small problems they may not have asked the administrator about? Was there any further information they wanted to have added to the questions?
7. Revise the instrument as needed and pretest again if substantial revisions have been incorporated.

This chapter has discussed the procedures for selecting and using existing data collection instruments. In particular, discussion focused on direct measurement instruments. You may wish to review your understanding of these instruments by referring to the following outline:

DIRECT MEASUREMENT INSTRUMENTS

A. Questionnaires
   1. Rating scales
   2. Checklists
B. Psychological and Sociological Measure
   1. Attitude scales
   2. Semantic differential scales
   3. Personality interest inventories
   4. Projective devices
C. Tests
   1. Verbal tests
   2. Performance tests
D. Mechanical Devices or Instruments
   1. Indirect data collection
      a. Interviews
         1. Unstructured
         2. Structured
      b. Observation
E. Combination of Instruments

REFERENCES

1. K. Chun, S. Cobb, and J. French: Measures for Psychological Assessments: A Guide to 3,000 Original Sources and Their Application. Ann Arbor, Michigan, Institute for Social Research, 1975.

2. D. Lake, M. Miles, and R. Earle: Measuring Human Behavior. New York, Teachers College Press, 1973.

3. J. Robinson and P. Shaver: Measure of Social Psychological Attitudes. Ann Arbor, Michigan, Institute for Social Research, 1973.

4. M. Shaw and J. Wright: Scales for the Measurement of Attitudes. New York, McGraw-Hill, 1967.

5. J. Snider and C. Osgood: The Semantic Differential: A Sourcebook. Chicago, Aldine Press, 1968.

6. H. Werley and M. Grier (Eds.): Nursing Information Systems. New York, Springer, 1980.

7. Reprinted with permission from Reality Shock: Why Nurses Leave Nursing by M. Kramer. Copyright 1974 by the C. V. Mosby Co.[7]

8. Cartoons in Sets 1, 2, and 3 were adapted from: L. Copp. A Projective Cartoon Investigation of Nurse-Patient Psychodramatic Role Perception and Expectation. *Nursing Research* 20, 2 (March–April 1971): 100–112. Copyrighted material was reprinted with permission of the American Journal of Nursing Company.[8]

9. Copyrighted material reprinted by permission of American Journal of Nursing Company. From: Marshall, G. and Feeney, S. Structured Versus Intuitive Intake Interview. *Nursing Research* 21, 3 (May–June, 1972), p. 270.[9]

10. The system was developed by Marion E. Highriter in conjunction with Mrs. Edith Rogers, Health Director and Mrs. Hilda Newton, Nursing Director of Gaston County Health Department in Gastonia, N.C. as a part of the technical assistance program of the University of North Carolina School of Public Health. Copyrighted material reproduced with permission of Springer Publishing Co., 1980.[10]

CHAPTER

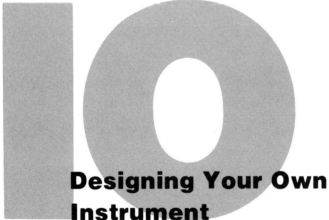

10

Designing Your Own Instrument

INTRODUCTION

Very often it is necessary for researchers to design their own data collection instrument. This situation arises when there isn't a suitable instrument available or when the uniqueness of the particular situation necessitates the design of a special instrument. Since there are few nursing-related tools available, nursing students often choose to adapt an existing instrument into a workable device, or to design a simple instrument from scratch for use in their first research project. See Figure 10.1 for an example of a student-designed questionnaire. Therefore, we feel that a discussion of the steps involved in creating one's own data collection instrument is most appropriate. Since the questionnaire is one of the most frequently used methods of collecting data, this chapter will concentrate on the steps involved in designing this type of instrument and will conclude with some guidelines for observational devices.

One very useful technique to use before beginning the formal design of a questionnaire is to spend some time designing what your results will look like. This does not mean that you should anticipate what the answers will be, but rather the way in which they will be presented. In fact, if you can actually design the tables that you wish to include in your final report, so much the

---

SAMPLE ITEMS ON A QUESTIONNAIRE DESIGNED BY NURSING STUDENTS TO DISCOVER ATTITUDES OF NURSES TOWARD INSTITUTING A NEW NURSING PROCEDURE

1. I prefer to vary basic procedures rather than get into a routine.
    TRUE   FALSE
2. I would be willing to try a drastically different new bath procedure if I were confident that it would be safe for my patients.
    TRUE   FALSE
3. I have often thought that the manner in which nurses give baths to patients could be modernized.
    TRUE   FALSE
4. I would enjoy learning to give a patient a bath in a new and different way, but I would have to think about it awhile before actually trying it out.
    TRUE   FALSE
5. I don't forsee any problems in introducing a radically different procedure to a patient.
    TRUE   FALSE
6. I would only consider trying out a new bath procedure on a patient who was newly admitted since he wouldn't really know that I was doing anything in a different way.
    TRUE   FALSE
7. I think my patients would enjoy experiencing a new procedure and then giving me their reactions to it.
    TRUE   FALSE

Courtesy of J. Tellier, M. Guay and N. Tomlinson.

Figure 10.1

better. By going through this exercise in detail, the researcher is in a far better position to know what questions must be asked in order to get the data to fill in those tables. All too often, beginning researchers "design the output" while the data are being gathered and recorded on the instrument. As a result, they often find that they "forgot to ask" this or that particular question or asked it in the wrong way. We have found this "mapping out of results first" approach most helpful in ensuring that all the data necessary for later analysis are, in fact, gathered.

ASKING QUESTIONS ABOUT THE RESPONDENT

Questionnaires have four general aspects: the directions, the demographic section about the respondents, the research questions, and the answering system.

Generally, the first section of a questionnaire seeks objective personal information about the respondent. There is usually a tendency to ask for every bit of information possible about the person filling out the form. One is often worried that once the respondent leaves, the "one piece of information you wish you had" will be lost forever. While this is true, the designer should be careful to select only questions that will be necessary for the eventual analysis of data. The following is a fairly exhaustive list of the information that might be obtained from objective questions.

Age	Current licensure
Sex	Income
Marital status	Basic educational program
Number of children	Highest degree obtained
Ethnic background	Major field of study
Occupation	Religion
Place of employment	City
Full-time or part-time status	State
Membership in professional	Country
organizations	Political affiliation

The selection of items that contain information of some importance to the study is up to the discretion of the researcher. For example, if inferences are going to be made about the difference between the way males and females respond to a set of questions, then obviously, the sex of the respondent needs to be recorded. On the other hand, information about the city or state of the respondent may be totally irrelevant.

OPEN-ENDED AND CLOSED-ENDED QUESTIONS

When asking questions, the designer has two basic options. The questions may be "open-ended" where the respondents must supply their own answers (like a fill-in-the-blanks or essay-type response). Asking for the occupation of a respondent could be done via an open-ended question.

On the other hand, with closed-ended questions, respondents must select their answers from a list provided by the researcher. For example, a question seeking information on a respondent's marital status might be as follows:

1. Please indicate your current marital status:
    single   ____
    married   ____
    divorced   ____
    separated   ____
    widowed   ____

Once again, the choice of whether or not a particular question is open- or closed-ended is up to the researcher. In most cases, there is some choice. For example, the researcher may be interested in the respondent's actual age and thus ask an open-ended question. Or, the researcher may only be interested in the range of the age (teenager, middle aged, elderly) and ask a closed-ended question.

Both types of questions have advantages and disadvantages. Open-ended questions will need to be coded prior to the analysis of data. Thus, if an open-ended question were used to solicit a respondent's occupation, all the different occupations would have to be listed (after reviewing the collected data) and assigned a numeric code. Thus, processing can proceed only after this intermediate step. Many researchers feel very comfortable with closed-ended questions since they can be sure of getting some uniformity in the responses they receive. In addition, these types of questions are often easily coded right on the questionnaire and thus are simpler to process.

However, some caution must be exercised in creating closed-ended questions. There are two terms that describe some important factors to consider. They are taken from probability theory: collectively exhaustive and mutually exclusive. The choices in a closed-ended question must be collectively exhaustive. This means that all of the possible answers that might be anticipated are provided. Consider, for example, the following sample question:

1. Please indicate your religion by checking the appropriate blank.
   a) Catholic   ____
   b) Protestant   ____

How would a person of the Jewish faith answer this question? What about the athiest's response? Clearly, this question is not collectively exhaustive. All the possible responses have not been included. Some designers include a "catch all" response such as Other____ to get around this problem. It is usually beneficial to put a blank line next to the "other" category and request that the subject specify the reason for designating the other category. While using this technique is certainly okay, the researcher should be careful to include as exhaustive a list of responses as seems relevant to the study.

The term mutually exclusive means that only *one* response from the set of responses can be selected as the answer. Consider the following question:

1. Which topic should be covered in the nursing curriculum?
   a. Computers in health care   ( )
   b. Diagnosis by nurses   ( )
   c. The role of the nurse practitioner   ( )

If respondents wished to indicate that they felt the first *and* third topics should be covered, they might check two boxes in response to this question. The choices are not mutually exclusive. (They could have been made so by rephrasing the question, for example, Choose the *one* topic that you would like to have discussed . . .)

After a little practice, the researcher can easily develop an adequate question with a set of feasible alternatives for possible answers. The best way to go about it is to write out the item as it will appear on the questionnaire and pretend you are one of the subjects who will be filling in the tool. Are all the likely answers provided for? The next step is to ask a fellow student or colleague to look over a set of items. An objective reader may pick up very simplistic errors that the researcher easily could have overlooked by being too close to the work. After a number of questions have been laid out, place the items on a "dummy" or preliminary questionnaire and ask several people who are similar to the intended subjects to respond to the questions. This type of assistance is quite helpful since these individuals can offer both unbiased and constructive suggestions.

One way to develop feasible alternatives for closed-ended items is to ask a few people to give responses to an open-ended question. The range and variety of answers could be assessed prior to designing the entire instrument.

ASKING QUESTIONS ABOUT YOUR RESEARCH TOPIC

Certainly, open-ended and closed-ended questions could be used throughout your questionnaire (not just in the section that seeks information about the respondent). However, the most frequently used question is one that is named after the social researcher, Rensis Likert. These questions are said to have a "Likert scale" that uses standardized response categories. Most of you will recognize these scales immediately after an example or two.

Examples are:

1. A nurse should be required to have a college education in order to become registered.

        SA   A   U   D   SD

(The instructions would have indicated that SA = strongly agree, A = agree, U = uncertain, D = disagree, and SD = strongly disagree. The respondent would circle the appropriate answer.) Another example:

1. A nurse evaluates how well a pain medication is working.

        A   D   DK

(Again, the respondent would have been informed that A = agree, D = disagree, and DK = don't know.)

The researcher should be certain to allow for a "don't know or "uncertain" response when it is appropriate to a question. This often provides valuable information. Without this option, respondents may circle a response that is their guess, or they may simply leave the question blank (however, do not assume that this is equivalent to a "don't know" response.)

As an example of the variety of scales that might appear on a questionnaire, look at the following:

In each of the questions that follow, SA = strongly agree, A = agree, DK = don't know, D = disagree, and SD = strongly disagree.

1. It would be a good thing if the government were to provide health care to all its citizens.   SA A DK D SD
2. Nurses should perform more fundamental research.   SA A DK D SD
3. Which of the following courses should be required of all nursing students prior to graduation? (Check yes or no as appropriate.)

	Yes	No	Don't Know
a) Statistics	( )	( )	( )
b) Computer Science	( )	( )	( )
c) On Death and Dying	( )	( )	( )
d) Introduction to Management	( )	( )	( )

GENERAL HINTS FOR CONSTRUCTING QUESTIONS

Regardless of the type of question or scale that is used, the questions themselves must be carefully constructed.

1. Questions should be clear and easy to understand.

This is perhaps the most important point to be made about constructing a question. If the respondent does not understand what you are asking because the question is ambiguous (unclear) or the language being used is not easily understood, there is very little likelihood that any meaningful data will be gathered concerning that question. Choosing the proper wording for a question is not always an easy task. The researcher must follow that fine line between being too technical and being too patronizing. In fact, some care must be exercised in selecting particular words if the questionnaire is to be filled out by people from different parts of the country. For example, consider the different usage of the word "tonic" in New York (something for your hair) and in Massachusetts (a soft drink). There are, to be sure, certain words that are tipoffs to the researcher that a question may be ambiguous and in need of clarification. A list of some of the "key words" that should be avoided is provided below:

| many | often | usually |
| occasionally | any | fairly |

2. Do not ask for one answer to a combination of questions. This is often referred to as asking a "double-barreled" question. An example might be:

"Do you plan to leave your nursing job and look for another one in the current year?"

Consider the possible dilemmas facing a respondent. Perhaps she is planning to leave her nursing job but *not* look for another one in the current year. Perhaps she already has a new job. What about the person who is leaving her nursing job to look for a non-nursing job in the current year? How should she respond? The watchful researcher can keep a sharp lookout for double-barreled questions by, once again, looking for tipoffs. The key word to watch for in this case is the word "and." Questions containing this word are candidates and should be carefully reviewed before being included in the questionnaire.

3. Avoid the use of leading questions, or emotional words.

A leading question is one that "leads" or directs the respondent toward a particular answer. For example, a question that begins with "Don't you agree that . . ." is a perfect candidate for being a leading question.

The researcher would also do well to maintain a list of key words that are emotional rather than descriptive and refer to this list as questions are being constructed. Some of the words that would almost certainly be found on everyone's list would be:

fascists	black leaders
reds	communist
radical students	imperialist
big business	people on welfare

4. Questions should be short and to the point.

After all the questions have been developed, it is often a good idea for the researcher to reread each of them with the objective of shortening questions whenever possible. Many times this process, by itself, reduces ambiguity in a questionnaire. Furthermore, a respondent should be able to read a question quickly and provide an answer without difficulty.

5. Some questions may not have to be completed by all the respondents.

In some questionnaires, certain questions are relevant to one class of respondents and not relevant to others. For example, you may wish a certain set of the questions on a questionnaire to be answered only be registered nurse respondents who attended a three-year diploma program. Questions of this type are called CONTINGENCY questions (whether they are to be answered or not is contingent upon the respondent's response to an initial question.)

6. The order of the questions is important.

The order in which the questions are answered can affect the respondent's answers. For example, if the first several questions dealt with the positive aspects of a nurse/patient relationship, it is likely that the response will have been influenced by those prior questions.

The opening questions should be interesting and provide some motivation for the respondent to want to continue. In light of this, most researchers will leave the routine objective or demographic questions about the respondent until the end of the questionnaire. In this way, the questionnaire is not perceived as simply another routine form.

Sometimes the researcher will attempt to minimize the effect of the order of the questions by randomly placing them within the questionnaire. Unfortunately, this can at times confuse the respondent and add to the difficulty with which a questionnaire can be completed. The best advice is to be sensitive to the fact that the order of the questions can influence the results and design the instrument with this in mind.

THE FORMAT OF THE RESPONSE

There are many ways in which responses may be recorded on a questionnaire. This section will illustrate some of the more common methods.

A. Technique: Check the Appropriate Answer.

Example:
1. How often have you visited a patient in the hospital during the last 12 months?
   ( ) Not at all
   ( ) Once
   ( ) Two to five times
   ( ) Six to ten times
   ( ) More than ten times

This method has the advantage of being easy for the respondent to complete and easy for the designer to prepare (most typewriters have brackets and/or parentheses).

B. Technique: Circle the Appropriate Answer.

Example:
1. What is your opinion about the quality of patient care in the hospital in which you work? (Circle one)
   a. Excellent
   b. Good
   c. Fair
   d. Poor

One of the major advantages of this method is that the responses are quite easy to prepare for later processing. Since the answers do not have to be coded (See Section 10.7), tabulation of keypunching can begin immediately.

C. Technique: Frequency responses.

Example:
1. What percentage of your time on the job is spent on each of the following activities?

____% spent on direct patient care
____% spent on administrative paper work
____% spent on preparing nurse's notes
____% spent with patient's family
____% spent on miscellaneous items
Total % = 100

D. Technique: Open-ended response.

Example:
1. What is your present occupation? _____

2. What do your see as the three most pressing areas of concern for the staff nurse?

Other techniques are more unique. For example, the "story identification" technique presents two stories, with characters, about a particular situation and asks the respondent to identify the character that they feel is most representative of themselves.

E. Technique: Scaling responses.

There are, of course, many other forms that the response choices on a questionnaire may take. Some of them are consistent with the above examples. The Likert scale questions, for example, could be constructed using either the checking or the circling technique. Consider the following two versions of the same question.

1. Registered nurses should be required to pass a periodic comprehensive examination before having their licenses renewed.
   (Circle one)   SD   D   U   A   SA
2. Registered nurses should be required to pass a periodic comprehensive examination before having their license renewed.
   (Check one)   ( )   ( )   ( )   ( )

The "semantic differential" method makes use of a scale with two end points. The respondent is asked to locate where on the scale their response would fall. For example:
1. Most nurses are:

Conservative   ____ ____ ____ ____ ____ Liberal
Intellectual   ____ ____ ____ ____ ____ Non-intellectual

Warm						Cold
Feminine						Masculine

F. Technique: Contingency responses.

Contingency questions have a format all their own. At the very least, these questions must be easy to follow. That is, if a respondent is to continue to answer some additional questions (because of a prior response), the instructions on what to do next must be clear. One very useful technique is to place the additional questions in a special box that highlights when questions should be answered. Consider the following example:

1. Have you ever heard of the proposed requirement for continuing education credits for nurses?   ( ) yes   ( ) no
   If yes:
   a. Do you generally agree or disagree with that requirement?
      ( ) Agree
      ( ) Disagree
      ( ) Uncertain
   b. Have you received any continuing education credits during the last 12 months?
      ( ) Yes
      ( ) No
   Continue with Question 2.

G. Technique: Ranking responses.

Finally, some responses need to be ranked by the respondent. Once again, the instructions need to be clear to the person filling out the questionnaire.

1. Please rank the following in terms of their importance in evaluating the potential effectiveness of a nurse.
   (1 = most important, 5 = least important, etc.)
   Rank
   ( ) nursing school attended
   ( ) years of nursing experience
   ( ) age of nurse
   ( ) sex of nurse
   ( ) years of nursing education completed

See Figure 10.2 for another example of a question where ranking is used.

ITEM FROM A QUESTIONNAIRE DEVISED BY NURSING
STUDENTS TO DETERMINE THE RANK ORDER OF
RESPONSES

Please read each of the following situations carefully. Following
each two preference lists can be found. In the section labeled *PERSON-
ALITY TRAITS* select five groups of qualities which you would like to see
in the leader of the given situation. Label each in the order of preference
1–5.

Ms. C. is head nurse on a thirty bed medical-surgical unit. She
is working over the extended Christmas weekend. There are twelve
patients on her floor during this time period. It will be Ms. C's responsibility to make this time as pleasant and joyous as possible for those under
her care.

PERSONALITY TRAITS (Select 5. Label in order of preference 1–5).

____ a.   Demanding, Firm, Challenging
____ b.   Receptive, Supportive, Approachable
____ c.   Direct, Structured, Expectations understood
____ d.   Creative, Original, Innovative
____ e.   Clinical expertise, Technical mastery
____ f.   Faith, High ethical, moral and value formation
____ g.   Direction, Purpose, Motivation, Consistency
____ h.   Intelligence, Problem solving ability, Decisiveness
____ i.   Flexible, Open-minded, Adaptible
____ j.   Integrity, Trustworthy, Credibility
____ k.   Enthusiasm, Sense of humor, Optimism
____ l.   Self discipline, Solitude, Commitment
____m.   Organization, Executive ability

Courtesy of E. Kelly, C. McCarthy, and E. Burke.

Figure 10.2.

Before leaving the subject of the format of responses on a questionnaire, one additional technique that is often overlooked deserves mention.
All of us have, at one time or another, taken a test (using that old favorite, the
#2 pencil) that was to be machine scored. The forms that are used for these
tests can also be used for recording the responses to a questionnaire. In fact,
most suppliers will design (at a minimal charge) a specific form to meet the
researcher's needs. Many institutions have computer programs available that
will not only tabulate the results for the researcher, but also provide an
analysis of each item on the questionnaire. In addition, the information on
these forms can be automatically punched onto cards and used as input for
more sophisticated analyses of the data.

Two disadvantages of this particular format are (1) these response sheets are somewhat more difficult for the respondent to fill out, and (2) there is a greater error rate in the recording of answers.

INSTRUCTIONS FOR FILLING OUT THE QUESTIONNAIRE

A questionnaire must contain clear instructions as to what is expected of the respondent. Generally, a questionnaire would begin with a few brief introductory comments concerning the intent and objectives of the study (if appropriate). Next, any general instructions would be provided. For example, respondents might be told "to place an x in the box beside their selected answer" or "SA = strongly agree, A = agree, U = uncertain, D = disagree, and SD = strongly disagree."

Some questions may require specific instructions. Ranking questions, contingency questions, and some open-ended questions are examples.

In any case, instructions are intended to guide the reader more easily through the questionnaire. They should therefore be brief, informative, and clear.

PRECODING THE QUESTIONNAIRE

When designing the questionnaire, the researcher should have begun with a detailed plan of what tables and charts would be used to display the results of the analysis of the data. At the same time, some consideration must be given to the way in which the data will be analyzed. That is, how will they be processed? Will the tabulations and statistical tests be done by hand? Will a computer be used? Are special forms required?

To facilitate the processing of the data on the questionnaires, some coding is often necessary. The reason for this is that some questions may have been Likert-type questions, some may simply be check marks or circled items. To make the processing easier, it is common practice to assign a numeric code to each answer (*e.g.*, a YES is a 1, and a NO is a 2).

To illustrate the techniques of coding a questionnaire, we shall examine two sample questionnaires. (1) A questionnaire on which the data will be processed by hand, and, (2) A questionnaire on which the data will be processed by computer.

The concept of "scoring" a questionnaire is different from the concept of coding and will be discussed at the end of this section.

Figure 10.3 shows a questionnaire that will have its data processed manually. This is often feasible when questionnaires are relatively short and few in number. If this is not the case, the researcher should give serious consideration to having the data prepared for processing by the computer.

In the case of the questionnaire in Figure 10.3, the information can, in fact, be processed without any coding being necessary (this will not always be the case). Many times a researcher must add up the responses to several questions to obtain a score for the questionnaire. This almost always necessitates some form of coding.

In this case, however, the data processing can be effectively accomplished by using a set of tally sheets to accumulate the summary information that is necessary for the analyses being performed. Figure 10.4 shows some of these tally sheets. Note that the researcher need only place a check in the appropriate column of the tally sheet for each question on the questionnaire. After having gone through the entire set of questionnaires, the researcher will only need to add up the check marks for each category in order to prepare some tables containing the frequency of each response to each question (See Figure 10.5).

It is more common to have the data on the questionnaires prepared for processing by computer. This means that there should be a numeric code to

---

A Questionnaire that will have its data processed manually.

SAMPLE QUESTIONNAIRE

1. Please enter your age (in years) ....☐

2. Your sex (circle one)   MALE   FEMALE

3. Should nurse practitioners assume tasks now performed by doctors in providing primary patient care? (circle one)
STRONGLY   DISAGREE   AGREE   STRONGLY
DISAGREE   AGREE

4. Should the B.S. in Nursing be a requirement for licensure?
STRONGLY   DISAGREE   AGREE   STRONGLY
DISAGREE   AGREE

5. How many times have you been admitted to the hospital as a patient in the last 10 years? ....☐

Figure 10.3

AGE	FREQ	SEX	FREQ	QUESTION	Q3 FREQ	Q4 FREQ	Q5 FREQ
UNDER 20		MALE	//	STRONGLY DISAGREE	//		
20 to 40	///	FEMALE	/	DISAGREE			/
40 to 60				AGREE	/		/
over 60				STRONGLY AGREE		///	/

Figure 10.4. A tally sheet for the questionnaire in Figure 10.3.

represent the responses to each question. While alphabetic information can, of course, be processed by computer, it is more cumbersome to prepare (by a keypuncher) and takes longer to process (by a computer). The intent here, then, is to present the data in a form that will lend itself to being easily keypunched onto cards for later processing by computer.

The questionnaire in Figure 10.6 was designed with this in mind. Note that all questions have a numeric code associated with them. If the answer itself is numeric, then no code is necessary (see Question 5). The easiest way to prepare the data for keypunching (either by the student or by a profes-

---

The frequency tables (Assume 300 respondents)

SEX	NO.	%
MALE	100	33
FEMALE	200	67

AGE	NO.	%
UNDER 20	30	10
20 TO 40	30	10
40 TO 60	180	60
OVER 60	60	20

QUESTION #3	NO.	%
STRONGLY DISAGREE	0	0
DISAGREE	60	20
AGREE	210	70
STRONGLY AGREE	30	10

Figure 10.5

SAMPLE QUESTIONNAIRE

1. Please enter your age (in years) .... ☐

2. Your sex (circle one) .... MALE   FEMALE ☐
                                                           1   2

3. Should nurse practitioners assume tasks now performed by doctors in providing
    primary patient care? (circle one)

    STRONGLY   DISAGREE   AGREE   STRONGLY   ☐
    DISAGREE   AGREE
       1   2   3   4

4. Should the B. S. in Nursing be a requirement for licensure?

    STRONGLY   DISAGREE   AGREE   STRONGLY   ☐
    DISAGREE   AGREE
       1   2   3   4

5. How many times have you been admitted to the hospital as a patient in the
    last 10 years? .... ☐

Figure 10.6. Questionnaire prepared for processing by computer.

sional keypunching service) is to create a coding form that is constructed to represent how the information is to be punched onto a card (i.e., what columns of the card are to be used.) See Figure 10.7 for an illustration of such a coding form.

Certainly, it is necessary to have some idea of what options are available for processing the data on a computer. The student will be introduced to all of these options in the computer section of this textbook. For now, it is sufficient to know that the coding of a questionnaire into a numeric format will greatly facilitate the processing of the data by computer *whether you write the programs yourself, hire someone else to do it, or use your data with your computer center's existing programs.*

Actually, the questionnaire in Figure 10.6 is clear enough that it could have been sent directly to the keypuncher for processing. The instruction sheet in Figure 10.8 would ensure that the data were properly prepared. Note that the instructions tell the keypuncher what to do if there are blanks on the questionnaires. These instructions need to be very specific.

When having data keypunched by a professional keypunching service, it is quite common to also request that the data be verified. This essentially means that the punched cards are fed through a second time and "re-punched" to check for errors. This extra step is designed to minimize the number of errors in the data deck that you finally receive.

A Coding Form with Instructions

RESPONDENT	AGE	SEX	Q3	Q4	Q5
CC 1–3	CC 5–6	CC 8	CC 10	CC 12	CC 14–16
001	25	1	3	3	003
002	55	1	2	4	000
003	16	2	1	2	010
004	67	1	3	3	007
.	.	.	.	.	.
.	.	.	.	.	.
.	.	.	.	.	.

(CC stands for Card Column. Thus, the age of the respondent should be punched in columns 5 and 6. Note that leading zeros have been punched.)

Figure 10.7

Some questionnaires are quite detailed and actually include punching instructions right on the form (see Figure 10.9). When this method is used, the instructions should explain that the respondent should disregard these numbers as they are only there to facilitate later processing of data.

The advantages of having the data prepared directly from the questionnaire itself rather than having to go through the process of copying them

Instructions to the keypuncher

To the keypuncher:
1. There are 300 cards to be punched.
2. There should be one punched card for each questionnaire.
3. There is no alphabetic data.
4. The columns to be used when punching the data are given directly on the coding forms.
5. All leading zeros should be punched.
6. Type missing data as zeros.
7. Keypunch and verify all data.
8. If any questions arise, please contact:
   Ms. Joanne Foley
   33 Wander Rd.
   Woburn, Ill. 02212
   Telephone: 729-9878

Figure 10.8

onto coding sheets cannot be overemphasized. The time savings to the researcher often outweigh the costs of properly preparing the questionnaire at the start. One of the biggest mistakes made by the beginning researcher is that of failing to consider how the data will be processed once they have been collected. By being careful to consider the alternatives early in the design process, the researcher will save much wasted time and anguish later on.

Sometimes, it is necessary to "score" a questionnaire. That is, the responses to a particular set of questions need to be totaled and recorded. One method, of course, is to leave the totaling to the computer and simply proceed to have the data prepared according to the techniques described above. However, to have the computer do the totaling for specific questions would usually require the writing of a special program. While this is not as difficult as you may initially guess, it does involve an additional step in the processing cycle.

Suppose, for illustrative purposes, we decide to score the questionnaire in Figure 10.9 and have this number as part of our coding sheet (Figure

---

1. Please enter your age (in years)..................................☐ CC 1–2

2. Please enter your weight (in pounds)...........................☐ CC 10–12

3. Please enter highest year of education completed.   ☐ CC 15–16

4. Your sex (circle one)   Male (1)   Female (2) ☐ CC 20

5. Overweight people like to eat out at restaurants.................☐ CC 31
        1   2   3   4   5

6. Overweight people always have desserts.........................☐ CC 41
        1   2   3   4   5

7. Overweight people are always jovial and happy..................☐ CC 51
        5   4   3   2   1

8. Overweight people eat more than 3 meals a day..................☐ CC 61
        1   2   3   4   5

(Respondents would have been informed in the instructions for the questionnaire that for questions 5 to 8 a (1) means **strongly disagree** and a 5 means **strongly agree** etc.)

Figure 10.9. Keypunch instructions coded on the form itself.

10.10). The score for a respondent is obtained by adding up the responses to questions 5, 6, 7, and 8. Question 7 is a reversed scale item and therefore must be adjusted before this total is obtained. Note that the process of keeping coding sheets for the questionnaire is easily amended to include this new data.

One final comment on coding is appropriate. Many researchers prefer to place an identification number on the top of each questionnaire and to have the identification number punched right along with the data for that questionnaire. This facilitates the identification of a questionnaire with a particular punched card should this becomes necessary later on in the processing cycle. For example, suppose that the analysis of data indicated that a respondent answered with a number 2 to a question about his age. When the punched card containing this "2" is located, the identification number on the punched card can be used to find the original questionnaire and correct the data.

DATA GATHERING OPTIONS

There are many ways in which the data for your research study can be gathered. The four most common ways are (1) the personal interview, (2) the telephone survey, (3) the mailing out of your questionnaire and (4) the completion of the questionnaire by small groups or individuals while you are present.

Scoring a questionnaire
CODING SHEET

Respondent	Age	Weight	Education	Sex	Q5	Q6	Q7*	Q8	Total
001	25	175	14	1	5	2	2	3	12
002	56	202	9	1	1	1	2	1	5
003	45	185	17	2	3	4	5	4	16
.	.	.	.	.	.	.	.	.	.
.	.	.	.	.	.	.	.	.	.
.	.	.	.	.	.	.	.	.	.

* Note that question 7 has a reversed scale. Enter reversed value in table before adding up questions 5, 6, 7, and 8 to obtain the respondent's total score.

Figure 10.10

The personal interview is a very powerful method of gathering data, particularly with a well-trained interviewer. There is often a much stronger motivation on the part of respondents when they are face-to-face with the interviewer. Because of this, response rates are usually quite high, sometimes in excess of 80 percent. This is also true of the telephone survey. In addition, both of these methods allow the interviewer to clear up ambiguous answers and explain any questions that are not clear to the respondents.

Despite the high response rates of these two techniques, the most frequently used method is the mailed questionnaire. This is due in part to its low cost and its attractiveness in reaching a broader audience. The typical procedure that is followed is to include a self-addressed, stamped envelope along with the questionnaire when it is sent out. Response rates to mailed questionnaires are, however, usually quite low. Some researchers have found that the following factors can favorably influence the rate of return:

1.   Sending the questionnaires via first-class mail.
2.   Using colorful stamps rather than prestamped envelopes.
3.   Including a personally typed letter.
4.   Follow-up phone calls (if appropriate).
5.   Follow-up postcards.
6.   Avoiding lengthy, complex questions (and questionnaires).

In some cases, the data can be gathered by distributing the questionnaire to small groups of individuals. An example of this might be distributing them to a class of students or setting up a table at the local shopping center. While this technique would seem to include many of the advantages of the other methods, the researcher must recognize its limitations. First, the sample may not be as representative as the researcher would like. For example, the shopping center chosen may reflect a certain economic or social class of respondents. The students, by the very fact that they are in a class together, may represent a biased sample.

Whatever method is selected, the researcher must consider (1) how representative a sample is desired (2) how expensive the data-gathering effort will be, and (3) what response rate is required. Table 10.1 presents a comparison of the techniques described in this section.

WHAT TO DO WHEN THE QUESTIONNAIRES ARE COMPLETED

The major steps that must be taken once the questionnaires have been completed are editing and coding them before processing begins. Editing is an important means of ensuring the quality of the data that have been obtained.

Table 10.1
Comparison of Data Gathering Methods

Method	Possible Length of Ques- tionnaire	Level of Difficulty of Ques- tionnaire	Possible Expenses	Average Response Rate
Personal interview	Short to moderate	Simple to complex	Interview travel, salary	80%+
Telephone interview	Short	Simple to complex	Telephone expenses; in- terviewer time	80%+
Mailed ques- tionnaire	Short to moderate	Simple to moderate	Envelopes; stamps; follow-up cards	30%
Small groups	Short to moderate	Simple to complex	Administrator's time; travel	50%+

The edit checks that are made are:

1. Checking for incomplete questionnaires.
2. Checking for inconsistencies.
3. Checking legibility.
4. Checking for improbable responses.
5. Handling missing values.

If a questionnaire has substantial omissions, it must either be discarded or sent back (if possible) to be completed properly. Incomplete questionnaires should not be used in later analysis.

Occasionally, the person doing the editing will detect some inconsistencies in a questionnaire. For example, a respondent may have checked MALE for sex and WIFE elsewhere. Sometimes, other items on the questionnaire can resolve the inconsistency. If an inconsistency cannot be resolved, it is either left alone, or the questionnaire is discarded according to the wishes of the researcher.

Since the data must at some point be coded, it is important to ensure that the information is legible and clear. There must be no doubt as to what answer or response was intended.

The editor should also check each questionnaire for any improbable responses. For example, in a list of 50 true-false questions, it is unlikely that someone who checked "true" 50 times was sincere in responding. Of course, the questions themselves may show inconsistencies that support this. In these cases, the researcher is usually well advised to discard that questionnaire. Caution should of course be exercised since the researcher, through careless editing, can significantly alter the results that will be obtained later on.

The most difficult problem that faces the researcher is what to do with a "missing value." This may simply be a blank response because the question was not understood, an illegible response, a blank response through an oversight, or the failure of the respondent to follow instructions. Whatever the reason, something must be done to account for the missing value. Care must be taken not to "infer" what the respondent meant by leaving the response blank. Rather, missing values should be treated as a category and analyzed along with the other data. It may be found, for example, that those leaving a particular question blank are primarily males. This may have some important implications for the study. One mistake that is often made is to assume that a blank response is equivalent to a response of "Don't Know."

The second part of the data preparation process is that of coding the information. This is done primarily to facilitate the processing of the data. While the coding of questionnaires has been covered earlier in this chapter, it is appropriate here to list several comments concerning the final coding of a questionnaire.

1. What code will be used for missing values?

It is best to use a numeric code (perhaps a 0 or a 9). There are two important factors to consider in selecting this particular code. First, the code for a missing value should be the same throughout the questionnaire. It should not be a 0 for questions 1 through 12 and a 9 for questions 13 through 15. Second, the number selected for this code should not be among the set of potential answers. For example, using a code of 9 to denote a missing value may cause some difficulty with a question asking for a respondent's age (a nine-year-old may have been the respondent).

2. Are there any open-ended questions that need to be coded? For example, the question "What is your occupation?" is likely to generate a wide variety of responses. Usually, the researcher can scan some of the questionnaires and develop a coding list for each occupation. That is, a registered nurse may be coded as a 1, a teacher as a 2, and so forth. In large studies, this can be a tedious chore, and the researcher may have been better advised to list several general categories on the questionnaire from the start.

3. Will any part of the questionnaire need to be "scored?"

Very often, a set of responses on a particular questionnaire are added up or accumulated in some way to obtain a "score" for that respondent. This may be part of the coding process. If, however, the data analysis is to be done by computer, the researcher is advised to leave the scoring to the computer. Computer program "packages" usually have the option of combining several variables together to create a new variable. Even if the computer program is being designed specifically for your application, it is easier to have the program prepared to do any scoring that is necessary.

4. Do any of the variables in your questionnaire need to be "recoded?" For example, the questionnaire may have asked for raw income data, but in your analysis you want to refer to income groupings (under $10,000; between $10,000 and $15,000, and so on). If this is the case, those particular data will

have to be recoded. If the researcher is interested in both forms of the data, the information must either be coded twice or the analysis done by computer. Once again, the computer analysis programs that are now widely available can "regroup" raw data quite easily into whatever groupings the researcher wishes.

5.   Have you used any "reversed scales" for any of the questions in the questionnaire? If reversed scales have been used anywhere, those particular questions must be scored differently than the rest of the questionnaire. At the risk of being redundant, the computer program used for analysis can "re-score" these questions.

6.   Does each questionnaire have its own unique identification number? It is quite useful to assign a number to each questionnaire and to have this number coded along with all of the related data. By doing this, it is easier to trace back to a questionnaire that may contain an error or some unusual data. Also, should your coded deck of cards be dropped, it is much easier to reorder them if there is a unique identification number on each card.

7.   Are the coding forms well organized, unambiguous, and easy to complete? Spending a little time designing the form that will contain the coded data from the questionnaires can greatly facilitate both the successful encoding of the information by the coders and the later analysis of the data. These forms should be well-labeled with instructions, when appropriate, for filling them out correctly. Plenty of room should be allowed for the data so as to make the data-processing phase easier for either the keypuncher who will prepare the data for computer processing or for the researcher who will be analyzing the data.

8.   Have the coders been trained?

If the data are to be prepared properly, some training of those who will be doing the coding is an absolute necessity. The researcher should prepare a set of "test" questionnaires that contain many of the exceptions that are likely to occur. For example, the test questionnaires may contain some missing values, multiple answers to a single question, reversed scale questions, and so forth. Only by actually going through the coding process can the coders become thoroughly familiar with the coding conventions for your particular questionnaires.

Several times during the previous discussion, we have mentioned the ease with which the computer can be used to process data. Chapters 14 through 17 will present a thorough and quite useful orientation to this very powerful tool.

For now, it is sufficient to say that it is unlikely that the researcher of today can afford not to use the computer. Certainly, with any substantial collection of data, processing and analyzing by hand is exhausting. In addition, preprogrammed packages for performing quite complex analyses are available and quite easy to use (*i.e.*, one does not have to be a "computer expert"). This additional resource allows the researcher to spend more time on the interpretation of the results rather than on the processing of the data.

PROJECTIVE DEVICES AND OBSERVATIONAL RATING SHEETS

There are numerous sources of information about constructing objective tests and questionnaires if one looks for them. The design of more loosely structured instruments such as projective devices and observational rating sheets is usually left to the imagination of the researcher. The creativity, originality, and talent of the experimenter can often be utilized in this

	a		b		c		
	Start	Stop	Start	Stop	Start	Stop	Bed No. 1
Age:	____	____	____	____	____	____	
Sex:	____	____	____	____	____	____	
Diagnosis or type of surgery:	____	____	____	____	____	____	
Yes No	a		b		c		
	Start	Stop	Start	Stop	Start	Stop	Bed No. 2
Age:	____	____	____	____	____	____	
Sex:	____	____	____	____	____	____	
Diagnosis or type of surgery:	____	____	____	____	____	____	
Yes No	a		b		c		
	Start	Stop	Start	Stop	Start	Stop	Bed No. 3
Age:	____	____	____	____	____	____	
Sex:	____	____	____	____	____	____	
Diagnosis or type of surgery:	____	____	____	____	____	____	
Yes No							

Figure 10.11. Sample of an instrument designed by nursing students in an observational study. (Courtesy of E. Dash, D. Willmann, R. Perpetua, D. O'Brien.)

endeavor. The nursing students who constructed the instrument similar to the one that is partially viewed in Figure 10.11 were interested in observing the crying behavior of children in the immediate postoperative period. They were going to be nonparticipant observers in a clinical situation in which it was possible to view 12 beds at the same time. To maximize their accuracy in making the observations, they set up the entire floor plan of the unit on their instrument so that each subject's crying incident could be easily recorded in the start and stop column on the tool.

Another group of students planned to gather data from kindergarten children regarding their recollections of a recent hospitalization for a tonsillectomy. They wanted to design a structured interview (a questionnaire was ruled out for obvious reasons), but also wanted some type of projective device to help put the children at ease and to help activate their memories of the event. They devised their own set of pictures that were shown to each subject at different stages of the interview with directions that encouraged them to "tell a story about what was happening in each picture" from the time the child was first sick until the postoperative departure from the hospital.

It is sometimes time-consuming to develop specialized instruments for a research project, but the return is usually worth the expenditure when the results are analyzed.

The researcher needs to be aware of the following guidelines in attempting to design instruments of this nature:

1. The instrument should be as simple and uncomplicated as possible.
2. The tool should present as unbiased a stimulus as possible.
3. Spend the time making the instrument appear to be a professional version. A sloppy tool may produce careless or unmotivated answers.
4. Seek a wide range of input and consultation about your device in the course of its development.
5. Pretest the tool extensively and revise it as needed.

If you are going to design your own questionnaire for gathering data, you should follow carefully the suggestions that have been discussed in this chapter.

Chapter 10 Problems for Solution (Answers are in Appendix J.)

1. What are the four general aspects of a questionnaire?
2. What do the terms mutually exclusive and collectively exhaustive mean in terms of a questionnaire design?
3. What are some of the tipoff words to ambiguous questions in a questionnaire?
4. Discuss the different ways of anticipating data-processing needs when constructing a questionnaire.
5. Name the four most common ways of gathering data.
6. What three factors must be considered in selecting a data-gathering method?

PART

IV

Interpreting Information

One of the first ways in which the nurse will be exposed to research in his or her field is likely to be through reading reports and articles in the professional nursing journals. Since many nurses may not get involved in research as practitioners, this may be the major way in which they keep up with developments in nursing.

is great enough to discourage the nurse from reading any further. Yet, a general understanding of statistical concepts is important if one is determined to intelligently read and evaluate a research report. To do this, it is not necessary to become proficient with mathematical calculations. However, confidence in dealing with numbers helps to make the comprehension of statistical procedures less awesome. A "Basic Math Review" has been included in appendix F for readers who need to brush up on these skills. Chapter 11 introduces the reader to the basic concepts of descriptive statistics. The following chapter explains the role of these procedures in making decisions about results of studies. Chapter 13 reviews the steps involved in presenting information by means of graphs and tables.

CHAPTER

An Introduction to
Descriptive Statistics

FREQUENCY DISTRIBUTION

Whenever you have collected a large amount of data, it is necessary to organize it in some meaningful way so that the data can be analyzed and discussed. One of the more useful methods of doing this is to construct FREQUENCY DISTRIBUTIONS of the data. In this context, the word frequency means how often some number occurs.

Table 11.1
Results of the State
Board Examination for a
Group of Student Nurses

MED NSG	PSY NSG	OBS NSG	SURG NSG	NSG CHL	MED NSG	PSY NSG	OBS NSG	SURG NSG	NSG CHL
440	563	516	371	493	531	479	489	471	583
607	600	609	592	683	558	479	563	521	583
510	489	278	457	455	343	396	220	258	192
684	600	590	599	688	531	600	526	450	493
517	544	618	535	553	600	655	526	627	561
280	331	322	343	463	406	489	304	428	508
572	535	572	570	613	524	433	405	400	410
440	581	452	450	388	350	415	341	414	403
621	535	609	599	576	718	674	711	620	696
656	590	646	663	696	489	359	553	464	583
593	276	479	599	568	517	396	498	506	463
579	479	516	450	561	558	572	572	583	583
607	563	683	620	651	517	498	442	371	448
593	553	452	563	523	454	581	572	620	553
419	553	452	528	523	482	479	433	471	312
579	563	479	464	455	628	655	683	585	576
531	507	563	528	500	503	526	507	656	598
628	609	609	640	628	628	609	600	556	638
468	535	535	585	493	413	396	581	300	380
399	637	470	421	425	496	479	553	535	598
392	470	424	393	410	621	609	674	613	636
552	470	526	542	538	614	553	664	599	636
621	646	553	592	643	315	415	415	236	335
246	387	304	201	290	642	664	618	620	636
433	461	544	485	508	517	544	461	535	530
510	572	516	592	523	364	489	359	314	380
384	387	387	329	418	565	572	526	387	523
357	452	479	471	583	482	452	452	450	463
461	470	507	549	448	371	331	378	371	373
510	461	581	542	418	558	572	535	506	470
621	609	637	563	621	531	452	489	329	433
635	692	701	606	568	531	489	461	585	530
489	498	526	521	418	419	618	479	464	455
426	470	479	371	485	489	470	683	585	636
496	479	479	442	485	322	350	313	407	395
371	304	350	471	455	670	590	526	592	643
496	609	609	570	530	628	563	479	585	561
426	396	489	343	320	572	646	563	542	561
600	581	609	500	606	399	304	350	350	388
593	489	609	514	561	419	452	433	336	342
385	498	507	506	508	635	683	618	606	651
440	424	359	464	463	558	507	516	478	621
468	498	433	435	448	593	692	526	542	546
482	461	442	450	388	440	498	563	521	470
545	637	646	634	623	600	553	461	563	470
517	378	535	471	373	552	581	609	514	553
371	405	359	414	500	600	731	637	620	643
468	507	452	478	493	447	489	489	414	530
718	600	701	691	711	357	424	452	364	418
392	452	322	203	410	322	507	479	400	485
586	600	572	563	591	642	600	553	634	651
406	359	516	542	500	496	452	507	386	470
552	544	609	528	523	343	378	387	421	455
					545	489	470	457	470
Number Taking Each Test & Exam					107	107	107	107	107

Table 11.1 contains the results of the state board examination for a group of student nurses. Their scores in each of five exams is given (medical nursing, psychiatric nursing, obstetrical nursing, surgical nursing, and pediatric nursing). The highest score one could obtain on a particular exam is 800. The passing grade is 350 for each exam.

We are sure that you can think of several questions about these results that you would be interested in having summarized. Some that immediately come to mind are:

1. How many students took the exams?
2. How many students passed each exam? How many failed?
3. What was the most frequent grade?
4. What was the range of grades?

There are, of course, many other questions that could be raised. We will address some of them in later sections.

As mentioned earlier, the first step to take when you are faced with organizing a large amount of information into a more meaningful format is to construct a frequency distribution. This could be done by first listing all of the scores that are possible for a particular test and then going through the data and counting how many times each score actually appeared. In cases where the possible choices are relatively small, this is exactly how you would proceed. However, with our state board examination results we could, theoretically, have results that go from 0 to 800. In fact, we are not really interested in every single possible score, but rather in ranges of scores. For example, we might like to know how many nursing students scored between 500 and 550. Let's begin with the scores for the medical nursing portion of the examination. In scanning the data we can see that the scores range from a low of 246 to a high of 718. To make our frequency table more compact and easier to use, we will divide the data into eleven "classes" of 50 points each, beginning with 200 and ending with 750. This will enable us to include all of our data. The class interval of 50 points is arbitrarily selected according to what groupings seem to make the data most useful.

To continue with our example, the data would be arranged in a format similar to that in Table 11.2. After making a column of the different class intervals, 200-249, 250-299, and so on you would go through the data sequentially and make a mark in the count column at the appropriate class interval. After completing this task, each set of count marks is added up and the number that results is placed in the frequency column. The next step is to add up the frequency column to determine how many pieces of data you had. Note that 107 students took the exam. Finally, you can express these frequencies as percentages simply by dividing each frequency by the total number of students who took the exam.

In summary then, the following steps are used in constructing a frequency distribution:

1. Find the lowest and highest numbers in the data for which you want to make a frequency distribution.
2. Decide what the class interval will be (it may be zero) and how many classes you will have. Arrange them in ascending order.
3. Prepare a table containing columns for a) each class b) a count c) a frequency, and d) a percentage.
4. Go through the data sequentially and make a mark in the count column at the appropriate class.
5. Add up the marks you entered for each class and put these totals in the frequency column.
6. Add up all these frequencies to get the total number of items in your data.
7. Complete the percentage column by dividing each frequency by the total number of data items.

The frequency distribution is very useful to the researcher in that it gives valuable summary data about the numbers in question (in this case exam scores). For example, you can see from the frequency distribution that most students scored between 600 and 649, although not by a significant margin. You also can see that seven students failed the exam (with scores below 350). The same table illustrates that 100 students passed the examination. The lowest score was below 250 and two students scored in the 700 range. Notice also, that 17 students scored between 500 and 550. As you see, we have answered the questions that were asked earlier in this section.

Table 11.2
Frequency Distribution of Medical Nursing
Scores on the State Board Examination

From–To	Count	Frequency	Percent
200–249	/	1	00.9
250–299	/	1	00.9
300–349	ⱵⱮ	5	04.7
350–399	ⱵⱮ ⱵⱮ ///	13	12.1
400–449	ⱵⱮ ⱵⱮ ////	14	13.1
450–499	ⱵⱮ ⱵⱮ ⱵⱮ	15	14.0
500–549	ⱵⱮ ⱵⱮ ⱵⱮ //	17	15.9
550–599	ⱵⱮ ⱵⱮ ⱵⱮ //	17	15.9
600–649	ⱵⱮ ⱵⱮ ⱵⱮ ////	19	17.8
650–699	///	3	02.8
700–749	//	2	01.9
		107	100.0

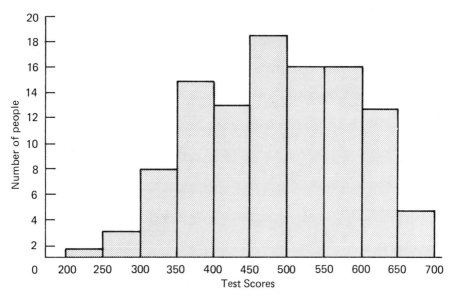

Figure 11.1. A histogram of the exam scores.

Often, it is helpful to display your results in a format different from that of a table. If you wish to present the same data in the form of a graph, the most appropriate graph is a histogram. To construct a histogram, first draw an axis similar to those you may have encountered in your first algebra course. The vertical line always contains, as labels, the frequencies. The horizontal line contains the class boundaries. Rectangles are then drawn over each class interval with a height equal to the frequency of that particular class. See Figure 11.1 for an illustration of the histogram for the same scores used in our previous example. Note that the histogram also provides the answers to the questions posed at the start of this section. In fact, many people feel that it is a more meaningful way to represent frequencies than the frequency table.

MEASURES OF CENTRAL TENDENCY

To proceed with a more precise analysis than that provided by summary techniques, you must familiarize yourself with the statistical concept of measures of central tendency. These measures are certain statistics (or numbers) that describe where a distribution of data tends to center itself.

Table 11.3
Psychiatric Nursing State Board
Examination Scores for Two Groups

	Group A Participated in State Board Review	Group B Did not participate in State Board Review
	563	470
	479	470
	489	572
	563	489
	563	470
	470	731
	563	498
	479	553
	572	553
TOTAL	4741	4806

As an example of what is meant by measures of central tendency and how these measures can be used, it is useful to compare two sets of data. For this purpose, let us assume that we have the psychiatric nursing test scores for two groups of nursing students. The first group participated in a state board review program prior to taking the test while the second group did not. The data for these two groups are summarized in Table 11.3.

It would seem, on the basis of the total scores, that Group B (the group that did not participate in the state board review), performed better. Their total score is 65 points above that of Group A. However, let us continue our analysis a little further. If you divide the total scores by the number of students, you will obtain the average score for each group. In our example, Group A has an average score of 526 and Group B has an average score of 534. Again, it would appear that Group B is the superior group.

This last measure, the average, is called the MEAN in statistical terminology. It is always obtained by adding a set of numbers and dividing that total by how many numbers there were in the set. In the example, the total of the scores for Group A was 4,741. When you divide this total by how many students there were (nine) the result is the average of 526.

Statistics, as a discipline, has its own set of symbols and formulas. Thus, the calculation of a mean for a set of data can be expressed as a formula. First, let us adopt the convention of algebra in which numbers are represented by a letter. We could then represent the data for Group A in the following form: (Note that the X represents a score and each is numbered by an arithmetic subscript.)

$$X_1 = 563$$
$$X_2 = 479$$
$$X_3 = 489$$
$$X_4 = 563$$
$$X_5 = 563$$
$$X_6 = 470$$
$$X_7 = 563$$
$$X_8 = 479$$
$$X_9 = 572$$

One way of indicating, symbolically, that we are adding up these numbers is to write

$$SUM = X_1 + X_2 + X_3 + X_4 + X_5 + X_6 + X_7 + X_8 + X_9$$

However, this is cumbersome and, if you had 1,000 numbers in a set of data, much too tedious. Therefore, a symbol is used to denote the summation process. This symbol is the Greek letter sigma (S for sum) and is written as Σ. To indicate that you were going to add up all of your X's you would simply write ΣX. (Meaning sum of all the scores.)

It is more appropriate to express such notation in a general form so that it is applicable for data sets with different amounts of data.

Thus, the proper way to express the summation of a set of data is

$$\sum_{i=1}^{n} X_i$$

where n is the number of numbers in your data set.

This is read as follows: sum up all the X's letting i go from 1 to n. Thus, in the example, you would write

$$\sum_{i=1}^{9} X_i$$

This would be equivalent to saying

$$X_1 + X_2 + X_3 + X_4 + X_5 + X_6 + X_7 + X_8 + X_9$$

(add up the scores for Group A.)

In order to symbolically express the mean of your set of data (which is what this explanation started out to do), you need to divide the sum obtained above by the number of numbers in your data set. Remembering that the symbol n represented how many numbers were in your data set, the formula for the mean would be written

$$Mean = \frac{\sum_{i=1}^{n} X_i}{n}$$

Finally, there is a symbol used in place of the word mean. This symbol is $\bar{X}$ (often called X-bar) or the Greek symbol μ. Thus, your statistical formula for the mean is:

$$\bar{X} = \frac{\sum_{i=1}^{n} X_i}{n}$$

But now let us get back to the problem of determining which group did better on the state board psychiatric examination. Thus far, as you may recall, Group B seems to be the superior of the two groups. You have looked at the total scores for each group, and the mean scores for each group.

On examining the data more closely, you will find that the most frequent result for Group A was 563 (it occurred four times) while for Group B the most frequent score was only 470. These results would seem to favor Group A. When you count which number occurs most often in a list (as we just did), you are finding the MODE of your set of numbers. If every number occurred only once, then there would be no mode. Also, it is possible for a set of numbers to have more than one mode. As you can see, the mode can provide some very useful information—which number occurs most frequently.

The final measure of central tendency that we will discuss at this time requires you to put the data into ascending order. Thus for Group A, you would rearrange the scores as follows:

470
479
479
489
563
563
563
563
572

Next, you locate the number in your list of data that has the same number of items above it as it has below it. That is, find the number in the middle of your list. When you have an odd number of items in your list, this is quite easy. However, when you have an even number of items, the number you are looking for is the average of the middle two items. For example, if we had a list containing the six scores below

500
550
570
590
620
630

Table 11.4
Summary Results of Applying Measures of Central
Tendency to State Board Psychiatric Examination Scores

	Group A Participated in a State Board Review Session	Group B Did not Participate in State Board Review Session
Total Score	4741	4806
Mean	526	534
Mode	563	470
Median	563	498

the number "in the middle" would be:

$$\frac{570 + 590}{2} = 580$$

This middle number is called the MEDIAN.

The median for our psychiatric examination example is 563 for Group A and 498 for Group B. The median score in this instance is very important in describing the level of success of Group A in comparison to Group B. The mean score for Group B has been affected by the very high score (73[1]) that one individual obtained.

These three measures, the mean, the median, and the mode are measures of central tendency. They indicate, each in its own way, where your set of data is tending to "center itself." If you apply these measures to the psychiatric state board examination example, the results would be as summarized in Table 11.4. On the basis of these results, Group A would appear to have performed both more consistently and at a higher level than Group B which did not participate in the state board exam review. This finding is different from our initial impression of the performance of both groups.

As you can see, making decisions based on one piece of summary information alone can sometimes be misleading. You must take great care in applying every statistical measure to be sure it is both appropriate to the situation and correct.

In the last example, the mean was actually misleading. This statistic indicated that Group B performed better on the examination (on the average, 12 points higher). In scanning the data, the reason for this becomes apparent. The sum of the scores was greatly affected by one of the entries— the score of 731. The most prevalent cause of this artificial inflation of the mean in this example is the small number of cases in the example. If the 731 had been one score in a group of 100, its influence on the average score would have greatly diminished. As you shall see in the next section, there are measures of variation in statistics that will be used to examine the specific characteristics of how a set of data varies.

In summary, we can comment on what each of these measures of central tendency can provide for the researcher.

The mean gives a (summary) composite picture of the data. It is designated by one figure that describes the average score in a distribution of numbers. The mean is probably the most utilized of the measures of central tendency since it is so easy to calculate.

The mode, since it is the most frequently occurring value, may be thought of as the single value that is most representative of all the values in a distribution.

The median is the item that is in the center of the distribution. It is therefore a more representative average than the mean when you have a distribution that contains some unusual data (for example, the score of 731 mentioned earlier).

MEASURES OF VARIATION

The measures of central tendency discussed in the previous section locate the center of a distribution. In many cases, this is not sufficient. The researcher needs to know more about how the data varied. For example, consider the two series of data below which represent the time spent each night for a week on homework for two different courses.

Time Spent on Homework (in Minutes)

	Community Health	Obstetrics
Monday	15	42
Tuesday	30	38
Wednesday	65	40
Thursday	45	37
Friday	40	38

The mean time spent on homework for each course is the same, 39 minutes. Yet, the data in each series are markedly different. The time spent each night on homework for the obstetrics course was always very close to the mean. The community health course, however, exhibited a large variation in the data. Some nights it took 15 minutes to complete the assignment and other nights it took 65 minutes. This section will discuss statistical measures that are available to analyze this variation.

The RANGE of a set of numbers is simply the difference between the smallest number in the distribution and the largest number in the distribution.

Let us return to the data on state board examination scores. The data for Group A (the group that completed a state board review course) is repeated below for convenience.

GROUP A
Scores on Psychiatric
Examination for Nursing Students who Completed a
State Board Review Course
563
479
489
563
563
470
563
479
572

The range for this set of numbers is 102. It was computed by subtracting the lowest score from the highest.

$$572 - 470 = 102$$

This number gives you some indication of the variation in performance by people in this group. Since only two numbers are used to get a very generalized idea of the spread of scores, the range is not a commonly employed measure. In addition, if there is only one large number in the distribution, the range will appear to be large when, in reality, it is not.

The VARIANCE of a set of numbers is the mean of the squared deviations of the individual items above their mean. That is, you subtract the mean from each number, square the result, and compute the average of these squares. This result is called the variance. If you take the square root of the variance, the result is called the standard deviation. Both the variance and the standard deviation will be of significant use when the topic of the normal distribution is discussed in a later chapter.

An example will help to clarify the calculation of these two measures of variation. Let us suppose that we want to calculate the variance and standard deviation for our sample of exam scores for Group A. The first requirement is to calculate the mean of the distribution. As you may recall from the section on measures of central tendency, the mean for these data was 526. Next, you must calculate the deviation by subtracting the mean from each item in the distribution. Then, you must square each of these answers. The process would unfold as shown in Table 11.5.

Table 11.5
Calculating the Standard Deviation

Scores	Subtract the Mean from Each Score	Square Previous Result
563	563 − 526 = 37	1369
479	479 − 526 = −47	2209
489	489 − 526 = −37	1369
563	563 − 526 = 37	1369
563	563 − 526 = 37	1369
470	470 − 526 = −56	3136
563	563 − 526 = 37	1369
479	479 − 526 = −47	2209
572	572 − 526 = 46	2116
4741 Sum		
526 Mean		

Once you have a list of the squared deviations, the next requirement is to get the average (or mean) of this list. Thus, we have:

$$\frac{1,369 + 2,209 + 1,369 + 1,369 + 1,369 + 3,136 + 1,369 + 2,209 + 2,116}{9}$$

$$\frac{16,515}{9} = 1,835$$

The variance is then equal to 1,835. Since the standard deviation is the square root of the variance, it is easily calculated. The standard deviation is equal to $\sqrt{1,835}$ or 42.84.

As with all measures in statistics, it is common to represent the formulas using symbols. For our example, the mean would be denoted by μ and the scores by the letter X (which is simply an alphabetic representation of our list of data). Thus, the column headings in the chart would be represented as:

X	$X - \mu$	$(X - \mu)^2$
563	563 − 526 = 37	1,369
479	479 − 526 = −47	2,209
.	.	.
.	.	.

If you recall the notation for summation that was discussed earlier in this chapter, you will notice that the variance can be represented by the following formula:

$$\text{Variance} = \frac{\Sigma(X - \mu)^2}{n}$$

where $\Sigma(X - \mu)^2$ indicates that you should add up all the squared deviations and n is the number of items you have.

The formula for the standard deviation is:

$$\text{Standard Deviation} = \sqrt{\frac{(X - \mu)^2}{n}}$$

since it is merely the square root of the variance.

It is important, at this point, to digress for a moment and review the concept of a population and a sample. A population (sometimes called a universe) is defined as each and every member of a particular group. Thus, all of the 107 nursing students who took the state board examination constitute a population. Once the population has been established, a sample can be described as some of the members of that population. Thus, a randomly selected group of ten students from that population would be considered a sample. Often, in a particular problem, you will not have the data for the population and will use information gathered from a sample to draw inferences or conclusions about a population.

Because of the fact that in one study the entire population might be utilized and in another study a sample might be utilized, it is important to convey to the reader which is the case. This is most easily done through the notation used in the statistical formulas. It is standard practice to use the following symbols:

| | Statistical Measure | |
	Mean	Standard Deviation
Population	μ	σ
Sample	$\bar{X}$	S

Thus, the formulas that have been presented in this chapter would correctly be written as follows:

Formula	If using population	If using sample
Mean	$\mu = \dfrac{\Sigma X}{n}$	$\bar{X} = \dfrac{\Sigma X}{n}$
Standard Deviation	$\sigma = \sqrt{\dfrac{\Sigma(X - \mu)^2}{n}}$	$S = \sqrt{\dfrac{\Sigma(X - \bar{X})^2}{n - 1}}$
Variance	$\sigma^2 = \dfrac{\Sigma(X - \mu)^2}{n}$	$S^2 = \dfrac{\Sigma(X - X)^2}{n - 1}$

Note that in the formulas for calculating the standard deviation and the variance for a sample, you divide by $n - 1$ (rather than n). An explanation of the reason for this will be left until later.

CHAPTER SUMMARY

The intent of this chapter was to introduce you to some descriptive measures in statistics. In particular, measures of central tendency and measures of variation were discussed. Some of the terms and concepts with which you should now be familiar are:

1. Frequency distributions
2. Class intervals
3. Percent calculations
4. Histograms
5. Measures of central tendency
6. Mean
7. Summation notation
8. Mode
9. Median
10. Measures of variation
11. Range
12. Variance
13. Standard deviation
14. Symbolic notation
15. Population
16. Sample

PROBLEMS FOR REVIEW (Answers are in Appendix J)

1. Two groups of patients were selected and given different treatments for pain. The time (in minutes) that elapsed until the remission of pain was as follows:

Group Receiving Treatment A	Group Receiving Treatment B
Patient 1: 53 minutes	Patient 10: 45 minutes
Patient 2: 47 minutes	Patient 11: 49 minutes
Patient 3: 51 minutes	Patient 12: 45 minutes
Patient 4: 40 minutes	Patient 13: 43 minutes
Patient 5: 40 minutes	Patient 14: 45 minutes
Patient 6: 68 minutes	Patient 15: 62 minutes
Patient 7: 61 minutes	Patient 16: 70 minutes
Patient 8: 52 minutes	Patient 17: 60 minutes
Patient 9: 55 minutes	Patient 18: 50 minutes

Using the measures of central tendency discussed in the chapter, which treatment would seem to be the most effective?

2. A doctor makes the following charges to medical patients for 15 hospital visits: $8, $7.50, $7, $12, $10, $9, $7, $8, $7.50, $9, $10, $8, $9, $7, $8

(a) Compute the mean, median, and mode for this distribution.
(b) What is the range?
(c) What is the standard deviation?

3. A student who is planning a nursing research study needs a preliminary estimate of the standard deviation for a particular population. A sample of ten observations was taken:

Observation	Value
1	21
2	16
3	17
4	23
5	13
6	17
7	20
8	18
9	20
10	19

(a) Find the sample mean.
(b) Find the sample standard deviation.

4. Discuss under what circumstances you would select the mean, the median, or the mode as the best measure of central tendency.

CHAPTER

12

Using Statistics to Make Decisions

THE NORMAL CURVE

If you were to take the data on test scores presented in Chapter 11 and plot them on a graph, when you connected the points and "smoothed" out the line you would have a figure remarkable like the one in Figure 12.1. This figure is called a normal curve (or a bell-shaped curve). When samples are taken from large populations, their histograms resemble a normal curve.

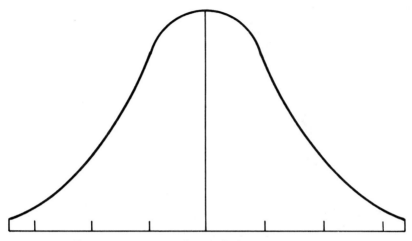

Figure 12.1. A normal (or bell-shaped) curve.

Heights of people, IQ scores, shoe sizes, length of stay in the hospital are all examples of data that have a normal distribution.

Some of the things that are known about the normal distribution are:

1. The mean is at the center of the distribution and divides the curve exactly in half (see Figure 12.2).
2. The mean and standard deviation of a set of data can completely describe a normal distribution.

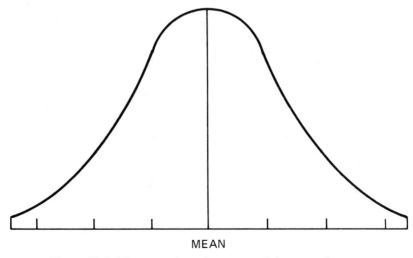

MEAN

Figure 12.2. The mean is at the center of the normal curve.

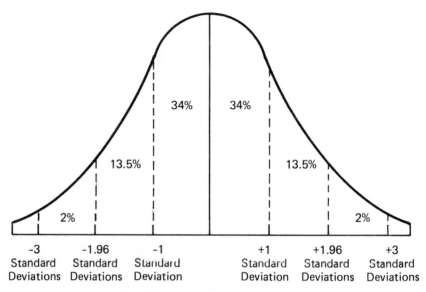

Figure 12.3. The areas under the normal curve.

There are, of course, distributions occurring in nature that do not constitute a normal distribution, but they are less frequent. Thus, if you calculate the arithmetic mean of a sample of items that is large enough to describe a normal distribution, you can infer that the arithmetic mean of the population could be approximated by the sample mean.

The usefulness of the normal curve can be seen in Figure 12.3. As this figure shows, 34 percent of the observations are found between the mean and +1 standard deviation. In addition, the following is true:

Percentage of Cases	Distance from the Mean
68	$\pm 1\sigma$
95	$\pm 1.96\sigma$
99	$\pm 3\sigma$

These percentages are the same for any normal curve. This last statement is of some significance. Because of this, the normal curve will be used to make estimates about the real world, since many events, if plotted on a graph, would resemble a normal curve.

For example, Figure 12.4 shows the distribution of scores for the psychiatric nursing state board examination. The mean (μ) is 500 and the standard deviation (σ) is 50. There are two scales shown on the graph, an X scale and a Z scale. The X scale represents actual scores, and the Z scale represents a standardized value that allows you to look up areas under any normal curve. The table of these areas is in Appendix B. The formula for the Z value is:

$$Z = \frac{X - \mu}{\sigma}$$

That is, the Z value is the distance from the true mean to the point X as measured in standard deviations. For example, you know by observation that the score of 600 is 2 standard deviations above the mean. (Each standard deviation is 50, so 600 is 2 standard deviations above the mean). The Z value also shows this:

$$Z = \frac{X - \mu}{\sigma} = \frac{600 - 500}{50} = 2$$

Let's try a few more. How far is the score of 500 from the mean? Since 500 *is* the mean, it should be zero standard deviations away from the mean. This is verified by the Z score.

$$Z = \frac{X - \mu}{\sigma} = \frac{500 - 500}{50} = 0$$

Since you also know that, by definition, 68 percent of all observations fall between ± 1 standard deviation of the mean, you can now say that it is likely that 68 percent of the students taking the exam scored between 450 and 550.

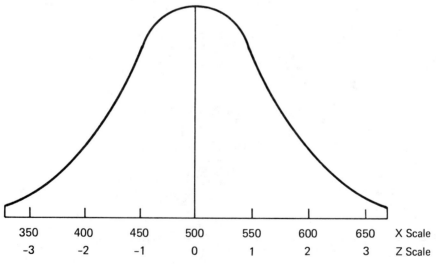

| 350 | 400 | 450 | 500 | 550 | 600 | 650 | X Scale |
| -3 | -2 | -1 | 0 | 1 | 2 | 3 | Z Scale |

Figure 12.4. Distribution of scores for the psychiatric nursing state board examination with a mean of 500 and a standard deviation of 50.

The areas corresponding to 1, 2, and 3 standard deviations are not the only ones that you can use. Appendix B contains areas for all Z scores from 0.00 to 4.00. This table of areas can be very useful in making estimates about a population.

The following examples will illustrate the kinds of questions that can be asked if you are dealing with a normal distribution and know its mean and standard deviation.

1. What is the probability that a student, selected randomly, has a score between 500 and 575?
    (a) First, identify the area under the curve in which you are interested (see Figure 12.5).
    (b) Second calculate the Z score (i.e., how far, in standard deviations, is 575 from the mean?)

    $$Z = \frac{X - \mu}{\sigma} = \frac{575 - 500}{50} = 1.5$$

    (c) Use Appendix B to find out the area under the curve that corresponds to a Z score of 1.5.
    The answer is .4332 or 43 percent.
2. What is the likelihood that a student selected at random will have a score greater than 625?
    (a) First identify the area that you are interested in (see Figure 12.6).

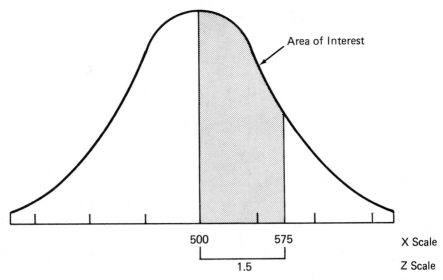

Area of Interest

500   575   X Scale

1.5   Z Scale

Figure 12.5. Calculating the Z score for a test score between 500 and 575.

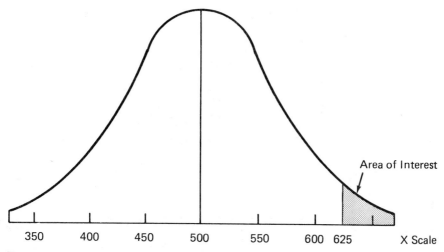

Figure 12.6. Finding the area of interest for the probability that a student will have a score that is greater than 625.

(b) Now calculate the appropriate Z score:

$$Z = \frac{X - \mu}{\sigma} = \frac{625 - 500}{50} = 2.50$$

(c) Look this value up in Appendix B and see that the area between the mean and a score 625 is .4938 or 49.38 percent.

(d) Because the normal curve is symmetrical, each half has an area of 50 percent. Since you are interested in the small area at the upper end of the curve (see Figure 12.7), you subtract the calculated area from 50 percent. Thus, only .62 percent of all scores will be greater than 625.

$$
\begin{array}{r}
.5000 \\
-.4938 = .62\,\text{percent} \\
\hline
.0062
\end{array}
$$

3. What percentage of the students are we likely to find scoring between 460 and 520 on the test?

Figure 12.8 illustrates the area of interest to us. You must be careful at this point since the area encompasses both sides of the distribution. Whenever you are looking up an area that fits this description, you need to calculate *two* Z scores. One is for the distance from the mean to the higher value and the other is for the distance from the mean to the lower value.

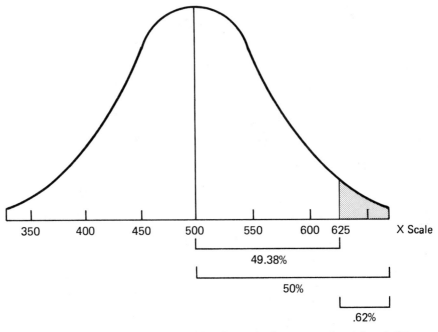

Figure 12.7. Finding the area under the normal curve to the right of 625.

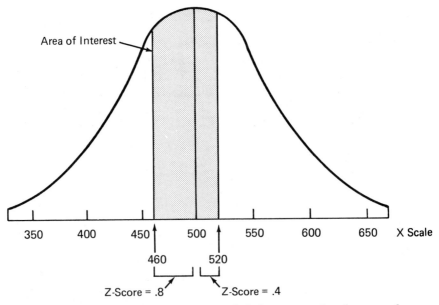

Figure 12.8. Calculating two Z scores to find the area under the normal curve between 460 and 520.

(a) $Z_1 = \dfrac{X - \mu}{\sigma} = \dfrac{520 - 500}{50} = .40$

$Z_2 = \dfrac{X - \mu}{\sigma} = \dfrac{460 - 500}{50} = -.80$

(b) The "upper" area (for Z_1) is .1554 or 15.5 percent.
The "lower" area (for Z_2) is .2881 or 28.8 percent.
(The minus sign is merely a reminder that this point is to the left of the mean.)

(c) Thus, the area between 460 and 520 is 15.5 percent plus 28.8 percent or 44.3 percent (see Figure 12.9).

4. If students who obtain a score greater than 645 or less than 360 are asked to take the test over, what percentage of the students would this involve?

(a) First identify the two areas of interest (see Figure 12.10).

(b) Once again, it is necessary to compute two Z scores:

$Z_1 = \dfrac{645 - 500}{50} = 2.90$

$Z_2 = \dfrac{360 - 500}{50} = -2.80$

(c) According to the tables, the area from the mean to Z_1 is .4981 or 49.8 percent. The area from the mean to Z_2 is .4974 or 49.7 percent.

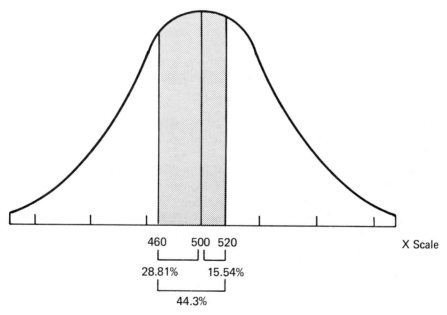

Figure 12.9. The area under the normal curve between 460 and 520 is 44.3%.

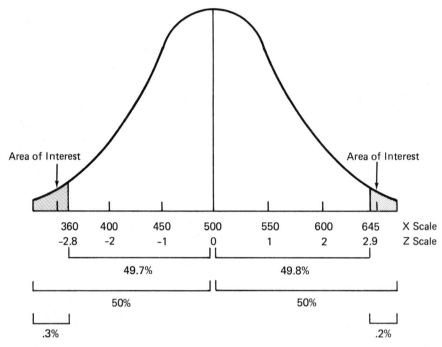

Figure 12.10. Finding the probability that a student selected at random scores either above 645 or below 360 on the test.

(d) What you are interested in, however, is the smaller areas at either end. Once again, knowing that each half of the distribution equals 50 percent, we have:
Right end 50 percent − 49.8 percent = .2 percent
Left end 50 percent − 49.7 percent = .3 percent
Thus only .5 percent of the students would be asked to take the test over again.

5. What percentage of the students will have scores between 525 and 600?
(a) Once again, draw a sketch of the area of interest (see Figure 12.11).
(b) Here also, two Z scores are needed. One is for the area from the mean to 600 and the other is for the area from the mean to 525. The *difference* between these two areas is the area wanted.

(c) $Z_1 = \dfrac{600 - 500}{50} = 2.0$

$Z_2 = \dfrac{525 - 500}{50} = -.50$

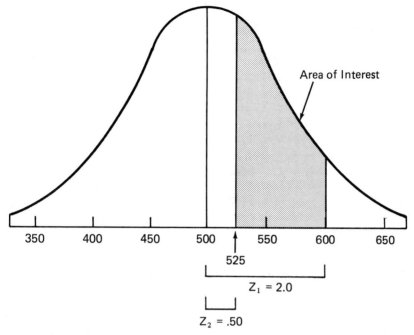

Figure 12.11. The area of interest for students with scores between 525 and 600.

(d) Appendix B indicates that the first area (from the mean to the point 600) is 47.7 percent. The second area (from the mean to 525) is 19.1 percent.

(e) Therefore, the area of interest is 47.7 percent − 19.1 percent = 28.6 percent (see Figure 12.12).

So, 28.6 percent of the students will have scores between 525 and 600.

6. If a state board review committee decides to change is passing grade, what score should be selected so that 70 percent of the students taking the test will pass?

In this case, you have been given an area, and are looking for a score. Figure 12.13 illustrates this example.

First you need to find out which Z score corresponds to an area of 20 percent (the left half of the distribution). Looking again at Appendix B, but this time in the body of the table, you search for the number (area) closest to .20. This corresponds to a Z score of 0.52. Thus, the point we are looking for is .52 standard deviations below the mean. Since a standard deviation is 50, .52 standard deviations is (.52) (50) or 26. Therefore, the score is 26 points below

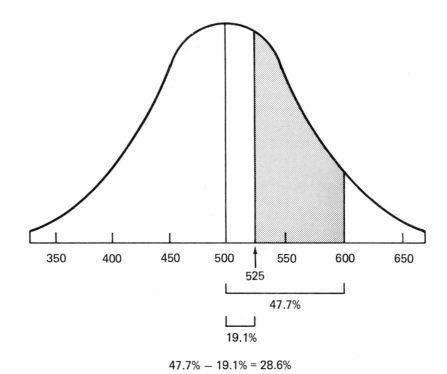

47.7% − 19.1% = 28.6%

Figure 12.12. Finding the area under the curve between 525 and 600.

the mean. The committee can be reasonably sure that 70 percent of the students will score above 474. The Z score formula could also have been used to obtain the same result. Thus, since you are looking for the value of X,

Formula: $$Z = \frac{X - \mu}{\sigma}$$

Substitute the known values: $$-.52 = \frac{X - 500}{50}$$

Multiply both sides by 50: $(-.52)\,(50) = X - 500$
Solve for X: $-26 + 500 = X$
$474 = X$

(Note that the Z value used was negative since it was to the left of the mean in Figure 12.13.)

As you can see, there are a variety of questions that can be answered about data that are normally distributed if we know the mean and standard deviation of the distribution.

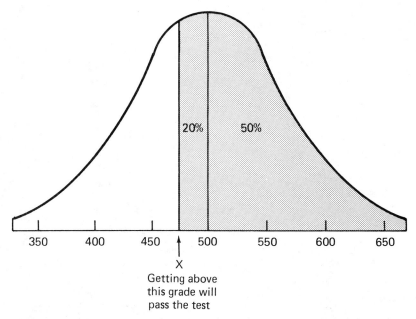

Figure 12.13. The area of interest is given as 70%.

In general, the steps that you followed were:

1. Draw the area of interest on a sketch of the normal distribution.

2. Calculate the appropriate Z score(s) using $Z = \dfrac{X - \mu}{\sigma}$

3. Use the appropriate tables to convert the Z score to an area under the normal curve.

4. Adapt the areas found in Step 3 to sketch drawn in Step 1.

The following exercises require the same techniques discussed in the examples in this section. You are encouraged to try them to demonstrate your understanding of the normal distribution.

1. Assume that the birth weights of infants are normally distributed with a mean weight of 7 pounds and a standard deviation of 1.5 pounds. Within which birth weights will 90 percent of all infants be found?

2. As a research project, a group of nursing students kept track of how long it took patients to complete their visit to an outpatient clinic. The data that they gathered are listed below.

Patient	Time for Visit (in Minutes)
1	65
2	85
2	70
4	25
5	78
6	92
7	115
8	120
9	120
10	98
11	118
12	117
13	122
14	115
15	112
16	95
17	60
18	15
19	98
20	101

   (a) Calculate the mean and standard deviation of these sample data.

   (b) What is the probability that a patient, selected at random, would have spent more than an hour and a half for his visit?

   (c) What percentage of the patients spent between 80 and 110 minutes?

   (d) What percentage of the patients spend less than an hour on their visit to the clinic?

3. Male students at a small eastern university have an average weight of 155 pounds, with a standard deviation of 10 pounds. What proportion of the male students weigh 145 to 155 pounds?

4. On a nursing research examination, Ms. Devereaux received a score of 85. The class mean was 74 and the class standard deviation was 9. What proportion of the students scored above her?

THE ACCURACY OF ESTIMATES

Since researchers rarely have the opportunity to examine the population for a particular study they are engaged in, it is necessary for them to take a sample from that population for analysis. The researchers must use the information gained from the sample to estimate the statistic of interest (e.g., the true population mean).

It has been demonstrated that the distribution of a statistic (*e.g.*, the mean) taken from a series of random samples will be a normal distribution. Thus, if you obtain one mean (via random sample) you can use its characteristics to infer something about the distribution of a large number of means drawn from the population and, hence, about the population mean itself. What is needed is a method for determining the accuracy of the estimated mean value.

In order to make this determination, it is necessary to examine what is called the STANDARD ERROR OF THE MEAN. This new measure is obtained by dividing the standard deviation by the square root of the sample size.

$$\text{Standard error of the mean} = \frac{\text{standard deviation}}{\sqrt{\text{sample size}}}$$

In symbolic notation, this formula would be written as:

$$SE = s_{\bar{x}} = \frac{\bar{s}}{\sqrt{\bar{n}}}$$

The letters $s_{\bar{x}}$ are used because the standard error (SE) is, by definition, the standard deviation of the sample means (hence s for the standard deviation of a sample, and $\bar{x}$ to remind us it is of the means).

This statistic will be used to tell you something about the accuracy o. your estimate of the mean. It is used very much like the standard deviation. The standard error of the mean indicates the dispersion of the sample means around the population mean.

For example, assume that a physician is interested in the coagulation time of the first drop of blood. He feels, based upon experience, that he knows what the time is for normal individuals. He records the coagulation time for 25 individuals in a random sample and gets a mean of 127.65 seconds and a standard deviation of 20.3 seconds. He asks you to analyze the results. As an estimate of the true standard error of the mean, you use

$$SE = s_{\bar{x}} = \frac{s}{\sqrt{n}}$$
$$SE = \frac{20.3}{\sqrt{25}} = \frac{20.3}{5} = 4.06 \text{ seconds}$$

To make your estimate, you take the sample mean and add one SE to it (*i.e.*, 127.65 + 4.06 = 131.7). Next, you take the sample mean and subtract one SE from it (*i.e.*, 127.65 − 4.06 = 123.59). Just as with the standard deviation, you can say that approximately 68 percent of the sample means would be between 123.59 and 131.71 (or, plus or minus one standard error of the mean). To continue,

Number of SE Around Mean	Range	Percentage of Distribution
±1	123.59 to 131.71	68%
±1.96	119.70 to 135.60	95%
±3	115.47 to 139.83	99%

Thus, you are able to say that you are 99 percent sure that the population mean is between 115.47 seconds and 139.83 seconds (for coagulation).

Now let us suppose that the physician had thought that the true mean coagulation time was 125 seconds. Was he correct? All you can really say is that there is a 68 percent chance that the true mean is between roughly 123 and 131, but not much else. The next section will discuss how to evaluate the physician's choice of 125 seconds.

In summary, this section has been discussing ways in which to make inferences about a population. The typical procedure it to take a sample randomly selected from the population and calculate the sample mean, the sample standard deviation, and the sample standard error. We can assume that the sample mean comes from a distribution of sample means that is a normal distribution.

Since these values are normally distributed, all we have to do to make an estimate of a mean that is 95 percent sure to include the true population mean is to add 1.96 standard errors to the sample mean (to get an upper bound) and subtract 1.96 standard errors from the sample mean (to get the lower boundary). Another way to think of the "95 percent sure" statement is that if 100 samples of the same sort were taken, the mean would be outside the above range only five times.

The process of finding an upper and lower bound on an estimate is usually referred to as "finding a confidence interval." The "percentage" of confidence is determined by the researcher. Most often, it is the 95 percent confidence interval that is found.

Suppose that a survey of 100 randomly selected patient records of patients with a certain disease indicates that the average length of stay in the hospital is 11 days. The standard deviation is calculated as 2.2 days. Find a 95 percent confidence interval for estimating the mean length of stay in the hospital. The first step is to find the standard error (SE).

$$SE = \frac{s}{\sqrt{n}} \qquad SE = \frac{2.2}{10} = 0.22$$

The confidence interval is obtained by the following formulas:

Lower Bound	Upper Bound
$\bar{X} - 1.96\ (SE)$	$\bar{X} + 1.96\ (SE)$

Thus, for the above example, the interval is:

Lower Bound	Upper Bound
11 − (1.96) (0.22)	11 + (1.96) (0.22)
11 − .4312	11 + .4312
10.56	11.43

Therefore, you can be 95 percent sure that the true population mean (of length of stay in the hospital for this particular disease) is between 10.56 days and 11.43 days.

The 1.96 figure represents how many standard errors from the mean are needed to encompass 47.5 percent of the area under the normal curve (see Section 12.1). When you add *and* subtract 1.96 standard errors, you encompass 47.5 percent plus 47.5 percent, or 95 percent of all observations.

Actually, any confidence interval can be calculated by referencing the normal distribution tables in Appendix B. The most common levels of confidence are:

> 99 percent ± 2.58 standard errors
> 95 percent ± 1.96 standard errors
> 90 percent ± 1.64 standard errors

For these different confidence intervals, you would simply substitute the appropriate constant for the 1.96 in the equations for the upper and lower bounds.

ESTIMATION USING SMALL SAMPLES

As discussed in the previous section, confidence intervals are used when the sample size is greater than 30. For many investigations, this is not the case. In a practical sense, there is often the opportunity to take only a sample of 15, 20, or 25 cases. For these situations, the normal distribution is not appropriate. Fortunately, we can base confidence intervals and estimations on a distribution that is very similar to the normal distribution. It is called the Student's t-distribution.

Using the t-distribution requires the use of a new table of values (Appendix C) and the use of a parameter called "degrees of freedom (df)." In our analyses, degrees of freedom will be equal to the sample size minus 1 (or, more commonly, $n − 1$). A discussion of the rationale behind the concept of degrees of freedom will be left to a more advanced text in statistical analysis.

Unlike the normal distribution, there is a different t-distribution for each sample size (see Figure 12.14). As the sample size (n) becomes larger, the t-distribution approaches the normal distribution in its appearance.

As an example of the use of the t-distribution, recall the example given

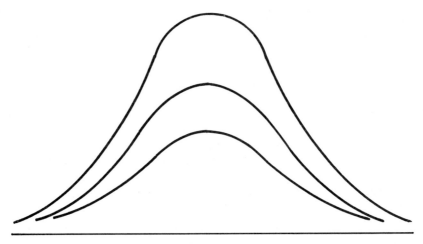

Figure 12.14. The t-distribution for different sample sizes.

in the last section on the doctor's estimate of the coagulation time of blood samples. Since the sample size is only 25, the t-distribution is appropriate when making estimates. Assume that you wish to place a 95 percent confidence interval around the true population mean. In this example, the mean was equal to 127.65 with a standard deviation of 20.3. As before, you first need to calculate the standard error of the mean.

$$SE = \frac{s}{\sqrt{n}} = \frac{20.3}{\sqrt{25}} = \frac{20.3}{5} = 4.06$$

Next, it is necessary to establish how many of these standard errors are needed around the sample mean to be 95 percent sure of the estimate of the true mean. Appendix C is used by first referencing the column corresponding to the desired level of confidence (95 percent). Then the row corresponding to the degrees of freedom for the particular problem is found. The sample size here is 25, so the degrees of freedom are 24. The t-value at the intersection of this row and column is 2.064. This represents how many standard errors need to be added *and* subtracted from the sample mean to obtain a range within which you are 95 percent sure to find the true mean.

Thus, for the current example:

Upper Bound	Lower Bound
$\bar{X} - (2.064)\ (SE)$	$\bar{X} + (2.064)\ (SE)$
$127.65 = (2.064)\ (4.06)$	$127.65 + (2.064)\ (4.06)$
$127.65 - 8.38$	$127.65 + 8.38$
119.27	136.03

The doctor can be 95 percent sure that the true mean coagulation time is between 119.27 seconds and 136.03 seconds.

ESTIMATES OF PROPORTIONS

In many studies or research projects, it is useful to estimate a proportion (or percentage) rather than a mean. For example, a person either suffers from motion sickness or he does not. Let us say that we have 100 people traveling on a train. The proportion of the passengers that became ill from motion sickness is 25/100 or 25 percent. What is the 95 percent confidence interval for the true population proportion?

Fortunately, much of what you have covered up to this point is still applicable. In order to construct a confidence interval you need to have:

1. A sample statistic (here you have the sample proportion p).
2. A degree of confidence (the example asks for a 95 percent confidence level).
3. A standard error of the estimate (for the proportion). The standard error for a proportion is given by the formula:

$$SE = \sqrt{\frac{p(1 - p)}{n}}$$

In this example,

$$SE = \sqrt{\frac{.25(.75)}{100}} = .043$$

The 95 percent confidence interval can now be constructed.

Lower Bound	Upper Bound
$P - (1.96)\ (SE)$	$P + (1.96)\ (SE)$
$.25 - (1.96)\ (.043)$	$.25 + (1.96)\ (.043)$
$.25 - .08$	$.25 + .08$
$.17$	$.33$

Thus, the researcher can be 95 percent sure that the true proportion of people getting motion sickness on the train ride is between 17 percent and 33 percent.

Some comments should be made at this point.

1. The 1.96 figure is, as before, the number of standard errors to be added *and* subtracted from the sample statistic to ensure that 95 percent of the observations will be included. It may be changed at the discretion of the researcher.

2. The 1.96 figure is for a normal distribution. It is known that the distribution of sample proportions (if this experiment were to be repeated over and over again) is approximately normal.
3. The distribution of sample proportions is approximately normal only when the smaller of np and $n(1 - p)$ is greater than 5. THIS TEST SHOULD ALWAYS BE MADE BEFORE USING THE NORMAL DISTRIBUTION TO ESTIMATE PROPORTIONS OR PROPORTION INTERVALS. (In our example, $np = 25$ and $n(1 - p)$ is 75. Since 25 is greater than 5, we may assume that the normal distribution can be used.
4. If the sample size is 30 or less, then the t-statistic should be used. The 1.96 would be replaced by the appropriate value from the t-tables (Appendix C).

As a final example, suppose that a nurse has developed a method for predicting the sex of an unborn baby six months before the baby is born. She tries out her technique on 26 women and correctly predicts the sex of 21 children. Construct a 99 percent confidence interval for this prediction technique.

First we calculate:

$$p = \frac{21}{26} = .807$$

$$\left.\begin{array}{l} 1 - p = .193 \\ np = 20.9 \\ n(1 - p) = 5.018 \end{array}\right\} \quad \text{normal approximation may be used}$$

$$SE = \sqrt{\frac{p(1 - p)}{n}} = \sqrt{\frac{(.807)(.193)}{26}} = .07$$

Degrees of freedom $= n - 1 = 25$
Confidence level $= 99$ percent

Lower Bound	Upper Bound
p − (2.78)(SE)	p + (2.78)(SE)

The 2.78 is obtained from the t-table in Appendix C for a confidence level of 99 percent and degrees of freedom equal to 25.

Lower Bound	Upper Bound
.807 − (2.78) (.07)	.807 + (2.78) (.07)
.807 − .29	.807 + .19
.617	.997

The nurse can be 99 percent sure that the proportion of correct predictions of a baby's sex will be between approximately 62 percent and 100 percent when she uses her technique.

COMPARING GROUPS (LARGE SAMPLES)

In many research projects, information is gathered from two independent samples, and the researcher wishes to compare these groups to see if they came from the same population. For example, is there any difference between the average score on state board examinations for students taking curriculum A and students taking curriculum B? Is there any difference between the mean respiration rate of patients taking a certain drug, and those who are not?

In order to answer these questions, and other questions involving the comparison of two groups, it is necessary to know something about statistical hypothesis testing. By a hypothesis, we mean an assumption about some population parameters (*e.g.*, the mean). This assumption will be accepted or rejected depending upon the information we gather from taking random samples.

Let us look more closely at the respiration rate example. Assume that 84 women were divided (in a random fashion) into two groups of 42 women each. One group was administered a drug that had a questionable effect on respiration rate. The other group served as a "control" group and did not receive the drug. An identical series of exercises was given to each group, and the respiration rate per minute recorded for each individual. The data are given below.

	Control Group	Group with Drug
Mean	16.2	14.1
Standard deviation	4.3	6.1

Step 1. State the hypothesis (in statistics, this is called the *null* hypothesis and is denoted by the symbol H_0).

In this example, the null hypothesis is that there is no difference between the two means (and thus, the drug has no effect on respiration rate). The hypothesis is stated symbolically as:

$$H_0 : \mu = \mu_2$$

where $\mu_1 = \mu_2$ represent the two means.

Step 2. State the alternate hypothesis. That is, the parameter has a value *other* than that described in the null hypothesis. There are three possibilities:
(1) $H_A : \mu_1 \neq \mu_2$
(2) $H_A : \mu_1 < \mu_2$
(3) $H_A : \mu_1 > \mu_2$

The alternate hypothesis selected is up to the researcher. In our respiration example, each alternate hypothesis would be described, in words, as follows:

The first alternate hypothesis ($H_A : \mu_1 \neq \mu_2$) states that if the mean respiration rate of the control group (μ_1) is not equal to the mean respiration rate of the drugged group (μ_2), it is *either* higher or lower than this rate.

The second alternate hypothesis ($H_A : \mu_1 < \mu_2$) states that if $\mu_1 \neq \mu_2$, the mean of the control group is less than the mean of the drugged group.

The third alternate hypothesis ($H_A : \mu_1 > \mu_2$) states that if the two means are not equal, the mean respiration rate of the control group is greater than that of the drugged group.

Each of these alternate hypotheses can be depicted on a graph of the normal distribution. Figure 12.15 illustrates the first alternate hypothesis. Note that the center of the distribution is labeled $\mu_1 - \mu_2 = 0$. This is just what you might expect since if the two sample means came from the same

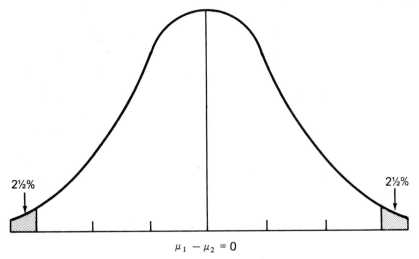

$\mu_1 - \mu_2 = 0$

Figure 12.15. Depicting the alternate hypothesis on a normal curve.

population, their difference should be zero. Now, it is possible that the second mean is too high (too far to the right on the curve) or that it is too low (too far to the left of the curve). If it is too far either way, we should reject the null hypotheses ($\mu_1 - \mu_2 = 0$). Well, how far is too far? This is yet another decision that must be made by the researcher. The decision involves selecting a parameter (usually devoted by the Greek letter α) called the level of significance. How much of a risk is the analyst willing to take of rejecting a true hypothesis? Generally, statisticians use a value of $\alpha = .05$. This is when the probability of rejecting a true hypothesis is less than 5 percent. In all of the discussions that follow, we shall assume a desired level of significance of .05. Now back to our example. Once again, reference Figure 12.15. Since we can be wrong in two directions (i.e., when $\mu_1 \neq \mu_2$) we need to "split up" that 5 percent margin of error. Thus the figure illustrates a shaded area at each end of the distribution that equals 2.5 percent.

Figure 12.16 illustrates the case in which the alternate hypothesis was $H_A: \mu_1 < \mu_2$ (i.e., if the two means are not equal, the control group mean respiration rate is less than the drugged group mean respiration rate). Note that since the rejection region is completely to the left of the distribution, we can use the entire 5 percent as the shaded portion of the curve.

The third possible alternate hypothesis $H_A: \mu_1 > \mu_2$ is illustrated graphically in Figure 12.17. Since the rejection region of concern is only whether the mean respiration rate of the control group is *greater than* the mean respiration rate of the drugged group, only one end of the distribution contains a rejection region.

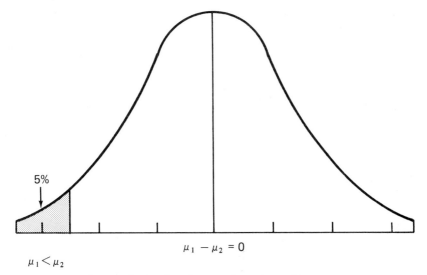

Figure 12.16. The alternate hypothesis $H_A: \mu_1 < \mu_2$.

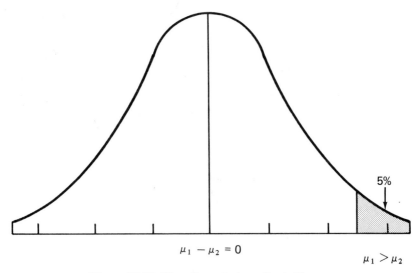

$$\mu_1 - \mu_2 = 0$$

$$\mu_1 > \mu_2$$

Figure 12.17. The alternate hypothesis H_A: $\mu_1 > \mu_2$.

The preceding discussion now allows us to state the next step in conducting a hypothesis test.

Step 3. Select a level of significance ($\alpha = .05$ is commonly used) and graphically construct the rejection region (i.e., depending on your selection of an alternate hypothesis).

You now must use the data gathered from the sample to see if the null hypothesis should be accepted or rejected. This is done by calculating a test statistic and seeing whether or not it falls in the rejection region for the particular problem being studied. You know how far (in standard errors) the rejection region is from the mean because of the area under the curve to that point.

Alternate Hypothesis	How Many Standard Errors
H_A:$\mu_1 \neq \mu_2$	-1.96 and $+1.96$
H_A:$\mu_1 < \mu_2$	-1.64
H_A:$\mu_1 > \mu_2$	$+1.64$

Thus, if the sample data reveal that the test statistic falls "beyond" these limits (or into the rejection region), you reject the null hypothesis. The test statistic is:

$$Z = \frac{\bar{X}_1 - \bar{X}_2}{\sqrt{\frac{s_1^2}{N_1} + \frac{s_1^2}{N_2}}}$$

Don't be discouraged by this seemingly complex equation; it is really the pinnacle of the mathematics you will see in this book and not all that difficult to use. Since you will have the values for the sample sizes (N_1 and N_2), the sample means ($\bar{X}$ and $\bar{X}_2$), and the sample standard deviations (s_1 and s_2), it is only a matter of substituting these values into the above equation.

Step 4. Calculate the test statistic.

The test statistic for the respiration example is calculated as follows:

$$Z = \frac{16.2 - 14.1}{\sqrt{\frac{(4.3)^2}{42} + \frac{(6.1)^2}{42}}}$$

$$Z = \frac{2.1}{\sqrt{\frac{18.49}{42} + \frac{37.2}{42}}} = \frac{2.1}{\sqrt{\frac{55.9}{42}}} = \frac{2.1}{\sqrt{1.32}}$$

$$Z = \frac{2.1}{1.15} = 1.82$$

The test statistic ($Z = 1.82$) falls into the rejection region on the right (see Figure 12.18). Therefore, you must reject the null hypothesis. That is, there is a significant difference between the two means.

Step 5. Accept or reject the null hypothesis.

In summary, the steps involved in performing a hypothesis test are:

1. State the null hypothesis.
2. State the alternate hypothesis.
3. Select a level of significance and sketch the acceptance and rejection regions.
4. Calculate the test statistic.
5. Accept or reject the null hypothesis.

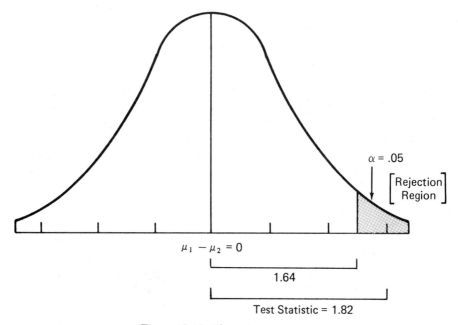

$\mu_1 - \mu_2 = 0$

1.64

Test Statistic = 1.82

Figure 12.18. The rejection region.

COMPARING GROUPS (SMALL SAMPLES)

When comparing groups that have a relatively small sample size (less than 30) a different test statistic is used. Section 12.3 introduced this statistic when discussing the t-distribution.

Initially, the same steps are followed in formulating the hypothesis as in the large sample comparisons.

1. State the null hypothesis (H_0).
2. State the alternate hypothesis (H_A).
3. Select a level of significance (α).
4. Calculate the test statistic (t).

The test statistic in this case will be

$$t = \frac{\tilde{X}_1 - \tilde{X}_2}{\sqrt{\dfrac{S_1^{\,2}}{N_1} + \dfrac{S_2^{\,2}}{N_2}}}$$

where,

$\bar{X}_1$ = the sample mean of Group 1.
$\bar{X}_2$ = the sample mean of Group 2.
S_1 = the sample standard deviation of Group 1.
S_2 = the sample standard deviation of Group 2.
N_1 = the sample size of Group 1.
N_2 = the sample size of Group 2.

Once the test statistic has been calculated, the t-tables in Appendix C are used to determine if the null hypothesis is to be accepted or rejected.

5.   Accept or reject the null hypothesis.

An example will help to illustrate the use of the t-statistic in comparing two groups (small samples).

Two hospital machines are being compared by the laboratory personnel. Machine 1 needs an average of 32 minutes to process 25 requests. The standard deviation is 6 minutes. Machine 2 needs an average of 36 minutes to process 30 requests. The standard deviation is 8 minutes. Is there a significant difference between the mean processing time of the two machines?

1.   State the null hypothesis (H_0).

This hypothesis is stated symbolically as

$$H_0{:}\mu_1 = \mu_2$$

That is, the mean processing time of Machine 1 is equal to the mean processing time of Machine 2.

2.   State the alternate hypothesis.

This is stated symbolically as

$$H_A{:}\mu_1 \neq \mu_2$$

That is, the mean processing time of Machine 1 is not equal to the mean processing time of Machine 2.

3.   Select a level of significance and construct the rejection region.

We shall use the commonly accepted level of $\alpha = .05$. The rejection region will be determined by referencing the t-tables.

4.   Calculate the test statistic.

In this problem, we have:

$$\bar{X}_1 = 32$$
$$\bar{X}_2 = 36$$
$$S_1 = 6$$
$$S_2 = 8$$
$$N_1 = 25$$
$$N_2 = 30$$

The formula for the t-statistic is:

$$t = \frac{\bar{X}_1 - \bar{X}_2}{\frac{S_1{}^2}{\mu_1} + \frac{S_1{}^2}{\mu_2}}$$

Substituting the given values:

$$t = \frac{32 - 36}{\frac{(6)^2}{25} + \frac{(8)^2}{30}}$$

$$t = \frac{-4}{\frac{36}{25} + \frac{64}{30}} = \frac{-4}{3.57}$$

$$t = \frac{-4}{1.89} = -2.11$$

5. Accept or reject the null hypothesis.

To determine whether or not we should accept or reject the null hypothesis, we must look at Appendix C. In this table of the t-distribution, the first step is to check the column in the table corresponding to the desired level of significance. Since $\alpha = .05$, we wish to be 95 percent confident. Since we have not indicated if we are interested in whether Machine 1 takes longer (or shorter) than Machine 2, a two-tailed test should be used. Figure 12.19 shows the rejection regions at this level of significance. Next, the number of degrees of freedom (the row value) must be found. When comparing two samples, the number of degrees of freedom is equal to the total sample size minus two (*i.e.*, $\mu_1 + \mu_2 - 2$). Thus, in this problem, the num-

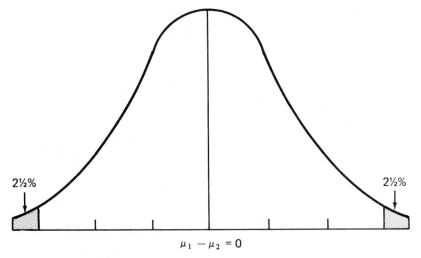

Figure 12.19. The rejection region at $\alpha = .05$.

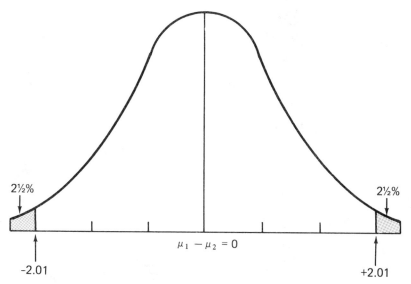

Figure 12.20. The rejection region when t = 2.01.

ber of degrees of freedom is $25 + 30 - 2 = 53$. The t-value at the intersection of the chosen row and column is approximately 2.01. This value defines the rejection region (see Figure 12.20).

Thus we would reject the null hypothesis if the t-statistic falls in the rejection region. Since our t-statistic of -2.11 falls in the rejection region to the left, we must reject the null hypothesis and conclude that there is a significant difference in the processing time of the two machines.

THE CHI-SQUARE STATISTIC

In the previous sections we have been discussing whether or not the observed difference between two sample means is significant. In this section, we shall discuss whether or not the differences between two sample proportions are significant.

As an example, let us suppose that a faculty member distributes an evaluation form to the 150 students in the basic nursing research class.

The form asks for the students' grade point average and whether or not they would take another course with this faculty member. The results of this experiment are as follows:

Nursing Research Class

Take Another Course with This Teacher	Grade Point Average		
	Below 2.0	2.0 to 2.99	3.0 to 4.0
Yes	12	30	31
No	8	45	24
Total	20	75	55

One question that might now be asked is whether or not students with a high cumulative average rate the faculty member differently than do students with a low cumulative average. The Chi-square statistic (pronounced "kye") will help to answer such questions.

Let us first set up a hypothesis test for this problem. Begin by letting,

P_1 = the true proportion of students with a grade point average of 3.0 to 4.0 who will take another course with this faculty member.

P_2 = the true proportion of students with a grade point average of 2.0 to 2.99 who will take another course with this faculty member.

P_3 = the true proportion of students with a grade point average of below 2.0 who will take another course with this faculty member.

The null hypothesis can be stated as follows: A student's grade point average does not have a bearing on whether or not the student will take another course with this faculty member.

This hypothesis can be stated symbolically as:

$$H_0 : P_1 = P_2 = P_3$$

The next step is to calculate which would be the expected number of students that would answer yes (and no) from these three grade point average groupings.

There were a total of 150 students and 73 of them answered "yes" to the question. Thus, we would expect $73/150$ or 48.6 percent of the students to take another course from this faculty member. How would this 48.6 percent be expected to be distributed over the three grade point average groupings? Since there are 55 students in the 3.0 to 4.0 category, we would expect that 55×48.6 percent would answer yes ($55 \times 48.6 = 26.73$ or 27 students). The remaining students ($55 - 27 = 28$) would be expected to answer no. If we apply this same logic to get the expected values for each entry in the table, we would now have the following (expected number of students is in parentheses):

Nursing Research Class

Take Another Course with This Teacher	Below 2.0	2.0 to 2.99	3.0 to 4.0
Yes	12 (10)	30 (36)	31 (27)
No	8 (10)	45 (39)	24 (28)
Total	20	75	55

The reader is encouraged to verify the figures in parentheses in the above table to ensure that she understands how these expected values are calculated.

If the original null hypothesis were true, we would expect there to be very little difference between the observed values and the expected values. The Chi-square statistic allows us to make this comparison. The symbol for the Chi-square statistic is x^2. It is defined arithmetically as follows:

$$x^2 = \frac{[\text{observed value}_1 - \text{expected value}_1]^2}{\text{expected value}_1} + \frac{[\text{observed value}_2 - \text{expected value}_2]^2}{\text{expected value}_2}$$
$$+ \frac{[\text{observed value}_3 - \text{expected value}_3]^2}{\text{expected value}_3}$$

Notice that this formula calculates the difference between the observed value and the expected value, squares this result and divides the new result by the expected value, for every cell of the original table.

An easier way to write this formula symbolically is:

$$\chi^2 = \Sigma \frac{(O - E)^2}{E}$$

where O represents an observed value, E represents an expected value, and Σ means do this calculation for all of the cells in your table and add them up.

For our particular problem the Chi-square statistic would be:

$$\chi^2 = \frac{(12 - 10)^2}{10} + \frac{(8 - 10)^2}{10} + \frac{(30 - 36)^2}{36} + \frac{(45 - 39)^2}{39} + \frac{(31 - 27)^2}{27} + \frac{(24 - 28)^2}{28}$$
$$\chi^2 = \frac{4}{10} + \frac{4}{10} + \frac{36}{36} + \frac{36}{39} + \frac{16}{27} + \frac{16}{28}$$
$$\chi^2 = .40 + .40 + 1.0 + .92 + .59 + .57 = 3.88$$

In general, if the Chi-square statistic is low, there is agreement between the observed values and the expected values. (If the statistic equals zero, the observed and expected values must be equal). On the other hand, if the value of this test statistic is large, there is a considerable difference between the observed values and the expected ones. The next question is "how large is large?" When is the value of the χ^2 statistically significant?

To determine the significance of a Chi-square statistic, reference the table of Chi-square values found in Appendix E. This table indicates the dividing line between accepting and rejecting a hypothesis. This dividing line (like the t-statistic) is based on two values.

1. The level of significance the researcher desires (*i.e.*, $\alpha = .05$, or $\alpha = .01$; review Section 13.5).
2. The degrees of freedom in the particular example (for our purposes, this will always be the number of proportions -1).

Let us say that we wish the probability of rejecting a true hypothesis to be less than 5 percent (i.e., $\alpha = .05$). We have three proportions in this problem so the degrees of freedom are $3 - 1 = 2$. We now look in Appendix E for that critical value (the dividing line) for the χ^2 statistic when $\alpha = .05$ and df = 2. This value is 5.991. If our test statistic is greater than this value, we reject the null hypothesis (there is, then, a significant difference). If the value of our χ^2 test statistic is less than this critical value, we *cannot* reject the null hypothesis.

In this particular problem, the calculated value of $\chi^2 = 3.88$ is less than the critical value of 5.991. Therefore the difference between the observed values and the expected values in our table was due purely to chance. There does not seem to be a relationship between a student's grade point average and his decision to take another course with this faculty member.

CONTINGENCY TABLES

One very useful application of the χ^2 is in connection with contingency tables. These tables are used when you are interested in whether two variables being analyzed are at all related. A contingency table is simply an arrangement of data into a table with two classifications. One of the classifications is identified by the column headings and one is identified by the row labels.

For example, if you were trying to determine if there was a relationship between a patient's sex and the dinner meal chosen while the patient was hospitalized, the data could be presented in a contingency table like the one below.

	Meal A	Meal B
Men	30	40
Women	20	60

This represents a tabular display of the meal choices for 70 men and 80 women.

When using contingency tables, the null hypothesis is always that there is no relationship. That is, the two ways of classifying the data are independent. To test this hypothesis, the χ^2 statistic is used. The one difference in calculating this statistic is that the expected frequencies are calculated somewhat differently.

The steps are as follows:

1. To find the expected frequency of a cell in a contingency table, multiply that cell's row total with that cell's column total. The product is then divided by the total sample size. Thus,
    (a) Calculate the row totals.
    (b) Calculate the column totals.
    (c) Calculate the total sample size.
    (d) For each cell, calculate

    $$\frac{(\text{row total}) \times (\text{column total})}{\text{total sample size}}$$

    (e) Place this value in parentheses in the appropriate cell.
2. Calculate the χ^2 statistic.
3. Calculate the number of degrees of freedom. This is equal to the product $(R - 1)(C - 1)$ where R is the number of rows and C is the number of columns.
4. Compare the calculated Chi-square statistic with the appropriate table value from Appendix E and accept or reject the null hypothesis at your chosen level of significance.

For the example presented at the beginning of this section, the calculations would be:

1. Place these calculations in parentheses in the appropriate cell (Step 1e).

	Meal A	Meal B
Men	30 (23.3)	40 (46.6)
Women	20 (26.6)	60 (53.3)

2. Calculate the Chi-square Statistic.
    The same procedures discussed in Section 12.7 are used to calculate the Chi-square statistic. The formula is:

    $$\chi^2 = \Sigma \, \frac{(O - E)^2}{E}$$

where O represents an observed value, E represents an expected value and Σ means do this calculation for all of the cells in your table and add them up.

For the current problem,

Calculate the row totals (Step 1a).

$$\text{Row 1 total} = 70$$
$$\text{Row 2 total} = 80$$

Calculate the column totals (Step 1b).

$$\text{Column 1 total} = 50$$
$$\text{Column 2 total} = 100$$

Calculate the total sample size (Step 1c).

$$\text{Total men} + \text{total women} = 150$$

Cell calculations (Step 1d).

First row, first column $\dfrac{70 \times 50}{150} = 23.3$

First row, second column $\dfrac{70 \times 100}{150} = 46.6$

Second row, first column $\dfrac{80 \times 50}{150} = 26.6$

Second row, second column $\dfrac{80 \times 100}{150} = 53.3$

$$\chi^2 = \frac{(30 - 23.3)^2}{23.3} + \frac{(40 - 46.6)^2}{46.6} + \frac{(20 - 26.6)^2}{26.6} + \frac{(60 - 53.3)^2}{53.3}$$
$$\chi^2 = 5.2$$

3. Calculate the number of degrees of freedom.

$$(\text{Rows} - 1)(\text{Columns} - 1)$$
$$(1)(1) = 1$$

4. Referencing the table for the Chi-square distribution in Appendix E for 1 degree of freedom and for a level of significance of .05, we find $\chi^2 = 3.841$.

Since our calculated χ^2 was equal to 5.2, we reject the null hypothesis and conclude that the sex of the patients and their choice of meals are *not* independent.

PROBLEMS FOR CHAPTER 12

1. Assume that a distribution of patient weights has a mean of 250 and a standard deviation of 20.0. If you were to select one patient at random from this distribution, what is the probability that the weight found will be:

(a) 250–270
(b) 230–270

(c) 270–280
(d) 100–400

(e)   0–280   (h)   250–100
(f)   270–600   (i)   245–265
(g)   0–250   (j)   250–290

2. Past experience with an examination in nursing fundamentals indicates
    that final scores are normally distributed with a mean of 130 and a
    standard deviation of 20. If a score of 100 is required to pass, what
    percentage can be expected to pass?

3. In a study in another country, a record was kept of the sex of children
    born to mothers who had been taking a birth control pill for at least two
    years before the child was born. There were 170 mothers of this type in
    the experiment. The number of boys born to this group was 58 (and the
    number of girls born was 112). Calculate a 90 percent confidence interval
    for the percentage of male babies expected from mothers of this type.

4. A research study performed by three psychiatric nurses at a large univer-
    sity obtained the following data on the attitudes of blue-collar workers
    who were employed in a large manufacturing plant:

	Active Patients	Former Patients	Classified Sick	Classified Well
Number Satisfied with Job	13	19	90	463
Sample Size	17	26	95	481
Percentage	76	73	95	96

    The two "patient" groups consisted of those who had been seen and
    diagnosed at the local hospital. The remaining workers were classified as
    sick or well on the basis of an index used to determine the mental health
    of workers through interviews.
    (a) Find a 95 percent confidence interval for the percentage of well
         workers who are satisfied with their job.
    (b) Find a 90 percent confidence interval for the percentage of sick
         workers who are satisfied with their job.

5. The following data give the gains in weight of 24 experimental animals
    that were split into two groups and fed two different drugs. Test the
    hypothesis that $\mu_1 = \mu_2$, assuming that $\sigma_1 = \sigma_2$.

x_1	66	64	52	48	42	44	54	58	62	74	58	54
x_2	82	50	74	58	52	60	68	50	58	72	58	66

6. A sample of 158 obese girls of average age 15 was analyzed with respect
    to various physical characteristics during early childhood. A control
    group of 94 nonobese girls of similar age and socioeconomic background
    was also analyzed. The following table gives the sample means and
    standard deviations for two characteristics of the two groups.

	Obese Group	Nonobese Group
Birth Weight	$\bar{x}_1 = 7.04, s_1 = 1.2$	$\bar{x}_2 = 7.19, s_2 = .9$
One-year Weight	$\bar{x}_1 = 23.3, s_1 = 2.8$	$\bar{x}_2 = 21.9, s_2 = 3.0$

(a) Use these data to test the hypothesis $H_0: \mu_1 = \mu_2$ for birth weight.

(b) Use these data to test the hypothesis $H_0: \mu_1 = \mu_2$ for one-year weight.

CHAPTER

13

Presenting Information in Graphs and Tables

One of the most effective ways to communicate the results of a study is to use graphs to describe the data being discussed and tables to summarize meaningful results. A great deal of information can be presented in this manner, and often the reader can better understand the author's intention in the study.

279

PREPARATION OF TABLES

There are two principle categories for classifying tables.

1. A table that is used for the analysis of data or presentation of findings is called an ANALYTICAL table.
2. A table that simply provides data for reference purposes is called a REFERENCE table.

Analytical tables usually appear in the body of the report while reference tables are often placed in the appendix. Table 11.2 (Frequency Distribution of Medical Nursing Scores on the State Board Examination) is an analytic table. The Table of Areas Under the Normal Curve found in Appendix B is more properly called a reference table.

The parts of a table can be clearly identified. Although every table need not contain all of the following elements, the list provides both a common standard for preparing tables and a useful reference.

The Table Number

The most common way to number tables is to use Arabic numerals. The first number usually represents the chapter in which the table can be found and the second number indicates which table in the chapter this particular one happens to be. Thus, Table 4.2 would be the second table in Chapter 4. In some cases, chapters within a manuscript are divided into "sections." A particular chapter may have Section 4.1, Section 4.2, Section 4.3, and so on. If tables are to appear in a manuscript organized in this fashion, a third number would be added to indicate which table in a particular section was being discussed. For example, Table 4.2.3 would be Table 3 in Section 4.2. The important point is to make each table number unambiguous so that every table can be easily found when discussed in a report or referenced elsewhere.

Since a research report is not often divided into chapters, tables are usually numbered consecutively. Thus, Table 4 is the fourth table in the report. Regardless of the numbering scheme used, all tables should be referenced in the text. If this is not done, the meaning and relevance of the table may be unclear to the reader. In addition, the publisher of a manuscript may not always be able to position the table in the precise location desired in the text, making reference in the text that much more essential.

The Table Title

The title of the table should convey to the reader what the table contains. It is necessary to be brief but, at the same time, to provide a complete description of what the table represents. After preparing titles for several tables, the "preparer" will become more adept at these descriptions. If you can answer the questions what, where, when, and how the data are classified, it is likely that the table title is complete.

For example, the following title is quite descriptive:

TABLE 6.3 SALARIES OF REGISTERED NURSES IN NEW ENGLAND, 1976–1978, BY STATE.

The Headnote

The headnote appears directly below the title and categorizes the data in the table. For example, the following are possible "headnotes":

(Thousands of Dollars)

(All Numbers Are Percentages)

The headnote, though not always required, should be enclosed in parentheses whenever used. It should be kept in mind that the headnote refers to the whole table.

Horizontal and Vertical Dividers

Usually, horizontal lines are placed above and below the column headings of a table but not used in the body of the table itself. Another horizontal line may be used to separate totals from the entries in the table. Vertical lines are not needed at the sides of a table but do appear as separators between columns.

While these rules may seem arbitrary, they are the most commonly used and, as such, should be followed whenever possible. Table 13.1 illustrates the format described thus far.

Table 13.1
Format of a Table

	COLUMN HEADINGS		Totals
LINE			
LABELS	BODY		
TOTALS			

Table XX.XX TABLE TITLE AND DESCRIPTION.

Column Headings and Divisions

The information in columns is identified by MASTER HEADINGS and COL-UMN HEADINGS as appropriate. The first column identifies the labels used for each row if they need to be labeled. The remaining column divisions are dictated by the nature of the data. Sometimes, the "total" column is placed at the left of the data for emphasis. Since a table is normally read from top to bottom and from left to right, it is useful to place information to be highlighted at the left side of the table. Table 13.2 illustrates the use of column headings and divisions.

The Body of the Table

The information or data contained in the table make up the "body" of the table. An individual entry in the table is identified by referencing a particular row and a particular column. Since horizontal lines are not used in the body of the table, many researchers insert a blank line after every five lines of data to improve their readability.

The Footnotes to the Table

Many times, an entry in a table needs amplification or explanation. In these cases, footnotes may be used and placed beneath the table. The footnotes can be numbered using numeric superscripts, letters, symbols, or even asterisks.

Table 13.2
Sample Set of Column Headings and Divisions

	MASTER HEADING		MASTER HEADING	
	COLUMN HEADING	COLUMN HEADING	COLUMN HEADING	COLUMN HEADING
LINE LABELS	BODY		BODY	
TOTALS				

The Source of the Data

Each table should contain a line at the bottom that indicates the source from which the data were taken. This not only gives credit to the "collector" of the data, but also provides direction to source material that may be more complete. In addition, the reader can evaluate the reliability of the source and any possible bias that might exist in the data.

Table 13.3 has been annotated to illustrate these eight principles of table preparation.

READING INFORMATION FROM A TABLE

Table 13.4 provides a good vehicle for examining ways in which the reader can obtain information from a table and also verify that the table was properly prepared.

This particular table contains both numbers and percentages. When percentages appear in a table, it is extremely important that they total 100 percent. Many tables fail to verify this and, as a result, confuse the reader. Sometimes, this happens as a result of having a computer prepare the calculations. Computers tend to "round" numbers during the calculation phase of the processing. Unless a computer programmer has "instructed the machine" (see Chapter 17) to ensure that all percentages total 100, totals can sometimes be 99.8 percent or 100.1 percent. This often leads to confusion on the reader's part. The point is that great care should be taken when preparing table entries, particularly if percentages are involved.

Let us look at Table 13.4. Suppose the reader was interested in knowing the answers to the following questions:

1. How many total graduates were there from baccalaureate programs in 1974 to 1975?

First, you must find the row entries that represent baccalaureate program data. (Note that the table has blank lines inserted to improve readability.) Next, find the column entry that indicates total graduations. (Note that this column is to the left of the table as suggested in the principles of table preparation.) This number is 20,241 students.

2. How many graduates were from accredited programs and how many were from nonaccredited programs?

Table 13.3

Salaries in Hospitals and Medical Schools in the United States, by Type of Institution and Position, July 1975

Type of institution and position	Starting monthly salary[1]				Maximum monthly salary[2]			
	Lowest	Highest	Midpoint	Average	Lowest	Highest	Midpoint	Average
Institutions combined								
Nurse anesthetist	$ 718	$1,530	$1,124	$1,176	$1,067	$1,917	$1,493	$1,480
Nurse practitioner	680	1,402	1,042	956	900	1,431	1,166	1,186
Head nurse	762	1,273	1,018	959	910	1,600	1,256	1,199
Staff nurse	638	1,100	870	806	795	1,350	1,073	1,024
Hospitals								
Nurse anesthetist	718	1,500	1,110	1,189	1,104	1,917	1,510	1,488
Nurse practitioner	910	1,402	1,156	1,035	999	1,431	1,215	1,233
Head nurse	762	1,144	954	958	910	1,471	1,190	1,177
Staff nurse	664	989	826	806	795	1,258	1,027	1,001
Medical schools								
Nurse anesthetist	1,105	1,325	1,215	1,183	1,370	1,835	1,602	1,566
Nurse practitioner	(3)	(3)	(3)	(3)	(3)	(3)	(3)	(3)
Head nurse	895	1,014	955	956	1,095	1,273	1,185	1,192
Staff nurse	690	859	774	792	884	1,260	1,072	1,014
Medical centers								
Nurse anesthetist	926	1,530	1,228	1,151	1,067	1,794	1,431	1,447
Nurse practitioner	680	981	830	859	900	1,281	1,090	1,121
Head nurse	790	1,273	1,032	961	961	1,600	1,281	1,236
Staff nurse	638	1,100	870	811	825	1,350	1,087	1,063

[1] Salaries normally paid in order to fill vacancies in a particular job class.
[2] Highest reported salaries actually paid to employees in a particular job class.
[3] Data excluded; insufficient number of schools reporting.
SOURCE: University of Texas Medical Branch at Galveston, 1975 National Survey of Hospital and Medical School Salaries.

Table 13.4

Graduations for Academic Years 1968–69 to 1974–75 from Initial Programs—R.N. in the United States and Outlying Areas,[1] by Accreditation Status on Succeeding January 1

Type of program and academic year	Total graduations	Accredited Programs[3]	Accredited Graduations	Accredited Percent of total	Nonaccredited[2] Programs[3]	Nonaccredited Graduations	Nonaccredited Percent of total
Total programs							
1974–75	74,536	932	58,478	78.5	480	16,058	21.5
1973–74	67,628	905	52,071	77.0	510	15,557	23.0
1972–73	59,427	898	45,268	76.2	530	14,159	23.8
1971–72	51,784	891	39,659	76.6	535	12,125	23.4
1970–71	47,001	878	36,269	77.1	541	10,732	22.8
1969–70	43,639	876	33,726	77.3	537	9,913	22.7
1968–69	42,196	843	33,072	78.4	535	9,124	21.6
Diploma							
1974–75	21,673	409	20,217	93.3	52	1,456	6.7
1973–74	21,280	430	19,631	92.3	65	1,649	7.7
1972–73	21,445	466	19,649	91.6	78	1,796	8.4
1971–72	21,592	497	19,575	90.7	91	2,017	9.3
1970–71	22,334	527	19,758	88.5	114	2,576	11.5
1969–70	22,856	560	19,937	87.2	137	2,919	12.8
1968–69	25,114	579	21,742	86.6	151	3,372	13.4
Associate degree							
1974–75	32,622	268	19,090	58.5	353	13,532	41.5
1973–74	29,299	236	16,484	56.3	368	12,815	43.7
1972–73	24,850	207	13,340	53.7	370	11,510	46.3
1971–72	19,165	181	9,619	50.2	361	9,546	49.8
1970–71	14,754	153	7,132	48.3	338	7,622	51.6
1969–70	11,678	129	5,184	44.4	317	6,494	55.6
1968–69	8,701	90	3,448	39.6	302	5,253	60.4
Baccalaureate							
1974–75	20,241	255	19,171	94.7	75	[4]1,070	5.3
1973–74	17,049	239	15,956	93.6	77	[4]1,093	6.4
1972–73	13,132	225	12,279	93.5	82	[4]853	6.5
1971–72	11,027	213	[4]10,465	94.9	83	562	5.1
1970–71	9,913	198	[4]9,379	94.6	89	534	5.4
1969–70	9,105	187	[4]8,605	94.5	83	500	5.5
1968–69	8,381	174	[4]7,882	94.0	82	499	6.0

[1] Includes Guam, Puerto Rico, and Virgin Islands.
[2] Included in this category are programs which applied but were never accredited and those which never applied for accreditation.
[3] Includes programs that closed during academic year: 1974–75, 37; 1973–74, 43; 1972–73, 55; 1971–72, 43; 1970–71, 56, 1969–70, 58, 1968–69, 39.
[4] Includes students graduated from one initial program leading to a master's degree.
SOURCE: National League for Nursing. *State-Approved Schools of Nursing—R.N., 1976* and previous years.

The proper row of the table has already been selected (*i.e.*, baccalaureate 1974 to 1975). You now look at the column labeled "Graduation" under the "Accredited" heading. This number is 19,171 students. Next, you look at the column labeled "Graduation" under the "Nonaccredited" heading. This number is 1,070 students. The sum of these two numbers should equal the total number of graduations in 1972 to 1973 baccalaureate programs. The sum of 19,171 and 1,070 is 20,241 students. This was the total found in answering Question 1.

3. What percentage of the baccalaureate graduates in 1974 to 1975 were from nonaccredited programs?

Using the same method as before, you reference the column labeled "Percentage of total" under the "Nonaccredited" master heading. The percentage is question is 5.3. The calculation of the 5.3 percent was made by dividing the total number of baccalaureate graduates for 1974 to 1975 (20,241) into the number of graduates from nonaccredited programs (1,070). Thus, 20,241 into 1,070 is equal to .053 or 5.3 percent. This should mean that the number of baccalaureate graduates in 1974 to 1975 from accredited programs was 94.7 percent. This was found by the following method: a graduate must be from an accredited or a nonaccredited program. This combined group represents 100 percent of the graduates. If 5.3 percent of them are from nonaccredited programs, then the balance (100 percent minus 5.3 percent) must be from accredited programs. This results in a figure of 94.7 percent. Note that this is precisely the figure found in the body of the table.

End of Section Practice Problems

Each of the following questions deals with Table 13.4.

1. What was the total number of graduations from diploma programs in 1972 to 1973?
2. What percentage of 1969 to 1970 graduates of associate degree programs were from accredited programs?
3. How many baccalaureate degree programs are there?
4. In the last year, which type of program (*i.e.*, diploma, baccalaureate, or associate) had the most closings? Which one had the most new programs?
5. Of all the nursing programs, what percentage are accredited?
6. How many nurses have graduated from baccalaureate programs since 1970?

GRAPHICAL PRESENTATION

Many times, a graph can convey information much more effectively than a table. The person reading the graph can often see trends or relationships that would not be as easy to detect with a tabular presentation of the data. However, most of us are somewhat reluctant to utilize graphs because of their perceived complexity. The intent of this section is to allay those fears.

Bar Graph

A bar graph consists of a number of rectangular bars where the height of each bar represents the frequency of a given category. Figure 13.1 presents four different examples of bar graphs. The bars in these graphs are usually the same width but may be either vertical (Figure 13.1 a) or horizontal

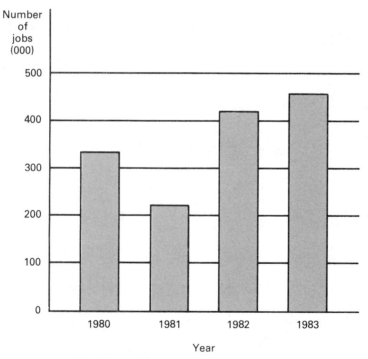

Figure 13.1a. Projected jobs available in nursing. (An example of a vertical bar graph.)

(Figure 13.1 b). By placing bars side by side as in Figure 13.1 c, two or more sets of data can be compared. Note that the different shading of each bar helps to distinguish one set of data from another. This is more critical in Figure 13.1 d. This figure includes a legend as an aid to the person reading the graph. Whenever you see a bar graph, look at it not just to verify a point made in the article that uses the graph, but rather to see what OTHER information is there. In this way, you will not only become more adept at interpreting bar graphs, but also you are likely to discover new facts and relationships.

The Histogram

The histogram is a form of the bar graph. It is used to present frequency data in graphic form. Figure 13.2 illustrates the use of a histogram to describe a frequency distribution. The interval (or item being measured) is marked off along the vertical axis. The height of a particular bar indicates the frequency of items found in that particular interval. Thus, 10 male patients weighted between 131 and 140 pounds. Note that in a histogram, the bars touch each other.

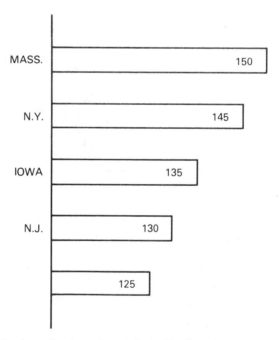

Figure 13.1b. Number of private hospitals in 5 selected states. (An example of a horizontal bar graph.)

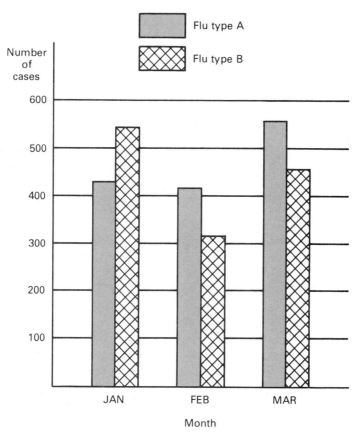

Figure 13.1c. Number of cases of two strains of influenza in the first three months of 1980 (City of Manchester).

Pie Diagrams

Figure 13.3 is a pie diagram. This technique divides up "a whole" into segments of a circle. It is a very effective way of comparing different components and their share of the whole.

Pictorial Charts

Pictorial charts use symbols to represent data. Figure 13.4 shows one such chart. Each symbol represents a certain amount of data and the number of these symbols represents the frequency. A wide variety of symbols (hearts, men, women, nurses, etc.) are available on transfer sheets at most stationery stores.

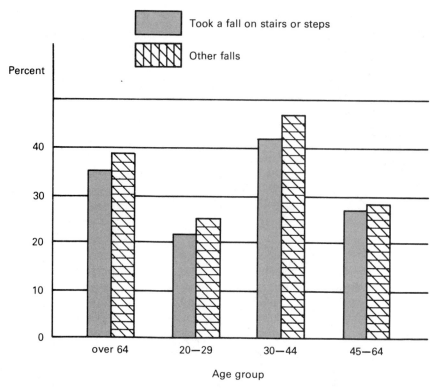

Figure 13.1d. Percent of different age groups injured and requiring hospitalization.

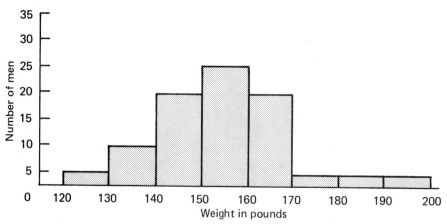

Figure 13.2. Frequency histogram of the weights of 100 male patients.

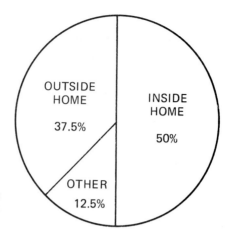

Figure 13.3. Pie diagram showing the percentage of injured children under 5 years of age by place of accident. Massachusetts 1970–1978 (fictitious data).

NUMBER OF EMPLOYEES

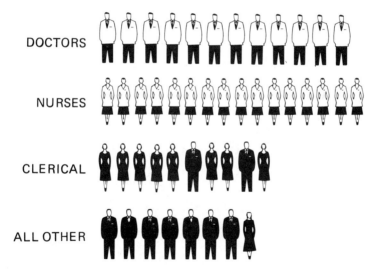

Each symbol represents 10 employees.

Typical distribution of employees in a large hospital.

Figure 13.4. Pictorial chart showing typical distribution of employees in a large hospital.

The Graph

Four different graphs are illustrated in Figure 13.5. Each graph contains an X axis (the horizontal line) and a Y axis (the vertical line). Note that each axis is clearly labeled as to what information is being measured and in what units the measurement is being done.

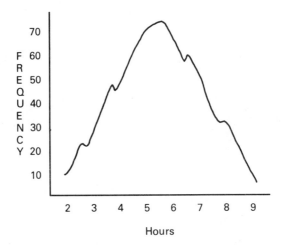

(a) Life of Medical Machine B (in hrs.)

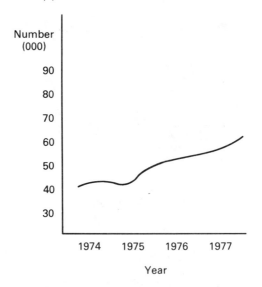

(b) Total hospital admissions in Texas.

Figure 13.5 cont.

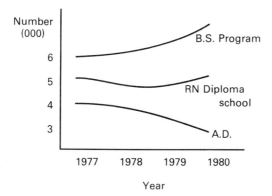

(c) Number of graduates from various Nursing programs.

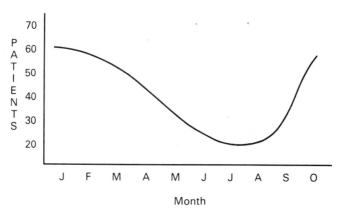

(d) Number of patients treated for flu in a small industrial firm.

Figure 13.5 Four examples of graphs (ficticious data).

A graph in this form requires (at least) two continuous variables. For example, let us suppose that the information in Table 13.5 is to be represented as a graph. The first step is to prepare each axis of the graph as in Figure 13.6 a. It is at this stage that the intervals along each axis are chosen (by referencing the range of values in the original table) and the labeling is done. Next, each pair of observations is used to find a point of the graph. That is, the X value is located on the X axis and the Y value is located on the Y axis. An imaginary vertical line is then extended upward from the point on the X axis and an imaginary horizontal line is extended out from the Y axis. Where these two imaginary lines meet, place a dot to represent the pair of observations you have just chosen. Figure 13.6 b illustrates this process.

Table 13.5
Approximate Weight for
Boys between the Ages of
Two and Ten Years.

Weight	Age
26	2
30	3
34	4
35	5
36	6
38	7
39	8
46	9
50	10

Finally, after having done this for all of the observations in your data set, you simply connect these dots to form a continuous line or curve (Figure 13.6 c). Now, you can read a variety of values from the graph that may be of interest to your study.

For example, if you are now given the age of a child you can quite easily find the corresponding weight figure. You first locate the age in question on the X axis, draw an imaginary vertical line until you intersect the line or curve on your graph. From this point, draw an imaginary line across until you hit the Y axis (weight). Read off the value that is represented by that

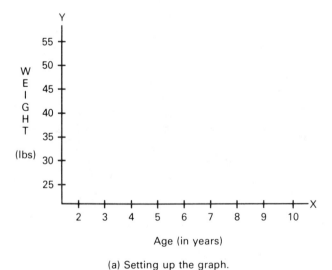

(a) Setting up the graph.

Figure 13.6 cont.

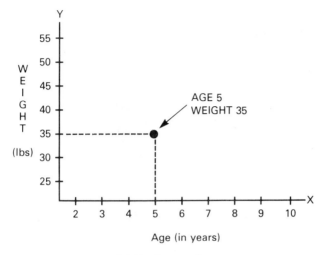

(b) Plotting a point.

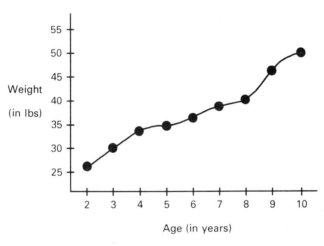

(c) The finished graph.

Figure 13.6 Preparing a graph.

point on the Y axis. This is the answer you were seeking. The procedure, of course, also works the other way around. That is, given a weight (Y axis value), you can determine the corresponding age (X axis value). Once again, practice brings expertise. Whenever you have an opportunity, thoroughly analyze a graph. Ask yourself questions about it. See how much information it contains.

Returning to Figure 13.5. Note that Figure 13.5 c has three different lines plotted on it. This is not unusual. However, care must be taken to clearly label each line so that the reader will know exactly what each line represents. As you can see, this technique is quite effective in comparing two or more variables.

There are, of course, a wide variety of other graphs and charts that can be used by researchers to present their findings. These have been a few of the more common ones. The choice of the form in which to present the information should depend, for the most part, on which method depicts the data and the desired relationships most clearly. Sometimes you may have to try several before choosing the one used in your final presentation.

Finally, we recommend that you take every opportunity to read tables, examine graphs, and construct charts. Ask yourself questions about the data that are presented. Find out what information they contain.

PART

V

Using the Computer

Computer applications in nursing and the health professions in general are so numerous that literature searches on this topic produce literally thousands of references. The next few chapters will concentrate on the use of the computer in a research environment. Chapter 14 will discuss some of the current uses of the computer in the health professions. Chapter 15 will introduce the reader to a typical computer facility, Chapter 16 will discuss using the computer, and Chapter 17 will suggest ways in which you may become more familiar with your own facility.

CHAPTER

14

Applications of Computers in the Health Professions

COMPUTERS IN HEALTH CARE

In the United States, health care is a $100 billion industry. Computers have been used in a variety of ways in a health care setting and many people feel that the computer will play an even more significant role in this industry in the attainment of quality health care at a reasonable cost. This role will include all types of functions from assisting with patient diagnosis to keeping track of information that is useful for hospital administration.

As you might expect, since hospitals are also businesses, their first use of computers was for keeping track of bills and preparing payrolls and financial reports. In more recent times, however, this use of the computer has begun to take a back seat to more sophisticated applications that are more directly related to patient care.

For example, automated patient monitoring is used in many coronary care units and pacemaker clinics to monitor electrocardiograms, analyze the information, and reduce the volume of data to manageable proportions. [1] It is speculated that, eventually, the memory of the computer would contain the names of patients with health problems who need specialized monitoring. Thus, if there were a period of heavy air pollution, the computer could print a list of people who were particularly susceptible to health problems in such a situation, and they could then be contacted and urged to have a checkup. Furthermore, the computer could maintain a list of patients who have had cardiac pacemakers implanted and produce a periodic list that would indicate when a particular pacemaker might be expected to run down. [2]

Commentary 14.1
Monitoring Patients

The primary features of a computer, speed, accuracy, and reliability, make it well suited for intensive care patient monitoring and routine diagnosis. It is only logical that once in the hospital, the computer be used for other applications for which it is well suited (*e.g.,* patient history). For example, Beehive Medical Electronic's system can perform intensive care monitoring, patient screening, electrocardiogram (EKG) interpretation, pulmonary analysis, patient history, and blood gas analysis functions. The intensive care monitoring system calculates various physiological parameters, allows keyboard entry of other parameters and of physicians and nurses comments, all of which are retained in the patients' computer files. All the data gathered on a patient can be recalled via computer terminals, so the physician can easily review the patient's progress over time and evaluate treatments. The EKG monitoring section examines every heartbeat for each patient around the clock. Special alarms are given for life-threatening arrhythmias, such as ventricular tachycardia. Respiratory parameters, such as respiration rate, airway resistance, tidal volume, pulmonary compliance, and respiratory quotient can be monitored. The keyboard entry parameters include the vital signs not monitored automatically and other items commonly found on nurses' reports. All data, whether automatically monitored or entered by doctors or nurses via the terminal keyboard, are retained in the patient's file. Data can be retrieved to display the latest measurement of each parameter, for trend displays, and for printed reports. The trend displays of a selected parameter are bar graphs for a seven-hour period. The most recent seven hours are displayed first, earlier data are trended with each button depression. Treatment indicators are displayed with the trends so the physician can easily observe the correlation between the treatments and change in the patient's condition. The area of EKG analysis by computer is receiving a lot of attention by computer scientists. The Beehive Medical system recognizes normal and 32 abnormal conditions. Distance need no longer be a factor in the diagnosis of electrocardiograms. If the local physician is not adequately trained in the interpretation of a specific EKG, he can dial a specialist, in a distant city if necessary, and transmit the electrocardiogram while it is being taken in the patient's home or the physician's office. The specialist's analysis can be augmented by computer analyzes. (Description of Beehive Medical computer system courtesy Beehive Medical Electronics, Inc.)

At the University of Florida's Teaching Hospital in Gainesville, an IBM computer system provides EKG readings via telephones to 13 remote Florida locations. The computer analyzes 30,000 EKGs a year. Computer-enhanced x-ray beams are used at Stanford University to help identify heart malfunctions, holes between chambers, and leaky valves. In fact, a new minicomputer-based diagnostic tool of this sort is making a significant impact in the health care industry. It is the computerized tomographic (CT) scanner. A CT scanner, using an x-ray beam, provides a cross-sectional view of a portion of the human anatomy. A scanner-produced image provides the type of view that would result if one could slice the body at the waist, for example, and look inside at the exposed organs. The photo produced by the CT scan is enhanced by the computer and displayed on a television screen (see Figure 15.1, page 340). This is done in much the same way as photographs taken in space are enhanced by computers at ground control centers. Not only does the scanner produce a significantly more valuable picture of the area of interest, but it promises to reduce drastically the painful procedures involved in injecting a radioisotope into a patient's bloodstream.[2]

The powerful and compact sensory, computational, and display capabilities of integrated electronics make possible exciting new avenues for prostheses to remedy blindness, deafness, paralysis, and loss of limb.[3] Some, especially sensory prosthesis, operate by copying the information normally gathered by the impaired sense onto an unimpaired sense. As a direct result of the computer, it is apparent that medical instrumentation is beginning a new era of revolutionary advances.

Commentary 14.2
Computerized Scanners

In a few hospitals, on-line terminals have become an accessible, if not totally accepted, medium for communications and data storage/retrieval among physicians, nurses, and technicians. But there's something catching on faster than the hospitalwide information system. A new minicomputer-based diagnostic tool that's the hottest thing in radiology is the computerized tomographic, or CT, scanner.

A CT scanner, using an x-ray beam, provides a cross-sectional view of a portion of the human anatomy. It overcomes the major shortcoming of a conventional x-ray image in which one organ is superimposed over another and where the density of a tumor, say, might vary only slightly from the density of the tissue surrounding it. Thus, it is often difficult to distinguish one from the other.

A scanner-produced image, instead, provides the type of view that would result if one could slice the body at the waist, for example, and look inside at the exposed organs. A scan of the chest area would show the ribs as white dots around the periphery of the oval-shaped image, within which are the various organs.

Using this technique, first developed in 1972 by EMI Ltd. of England, to scan the head, medical diagnosticians have at their disposal what is termed a noninvasive method of studying a patient's condition. It gets around the hospitalization of a patient, perhaps the injection into the bloodstream of some contrasting medium to highlight an area of interest, or even exploratory surgery. It promises to reduce drastically the use of such procedures as the injection of a radioisotope into a patient's bloodstream, an experience that can be traumatic.

In CT scanning, the x-ray source is made to rotate around the body of the patient. Opposite the source, on the other side of the patient, is an array of detectors that rotates along with the source. The detectors measure the intensity of the beam that has passed through the body, a value that varies with the density of the structures through which it has passed. The devices then increment by one degree and the procedure is repeated. At the end of 180 degrees of rotation in the case of some systems, or 360 degrees in others, the data for one slice have been accumulated.

Source: *DATAMATION*. September, 1976.

Commentary 14.3
The Neurosurgical Nurse and the Computer

In the Neurosurgical Intensive Care Unit at the University of Maryland Hospital, it has been found that the monitors and computer have been valuable assets to the nursing staff.[1] They have not replaced the nurses, but have made some of their tasks easier. By combining a good monitoring system with a computer, the nurses have more time for patient assessment as opposed to physical tasks, such as taking blood pressures, temperatures, and pulses.

Approximately four months after the introduction of a monitoring system, a Datapoint 2200 Minicomputer was installed. This system consists of a table console keyboard with a display screen, a printer/plotter, and a 23-inch television screen located above each monitored bed.

There are six physiological parameters monitored for each patient: arterial blood pressure (systolic, diastolic, and mean), intracranial pressures or central venous pressures (systolic, diastolic, and mean), heart rate, respiratory rate, PO_2 (partial pressure of oxygen), and PCO_2 (partial pressure of carbon dioxide).

Three forms of output are provided by this system: the television screen, the printer/plotter, and cassette tapes. Each bedside TV screen displays the monitored parameters in numerical form for that particular patient. Along with the parameters, the current time, the patient's name, the hospital number and the admission date are displayed. Of the ten parameters displayed, four are programmed to contain lower and upper alarm limits. The alarm limits on these four (systolic arterial pressure, systolic central venous or intracranial pressure, heart rate, and respiratory rate) are set and initiated by the nurse. If one of the parameter values goes outside of the limits set, an audible alarm is sounded. Although the alarm is the same for all of the parameters, an asterisk is displayed on the console display screen and the TV screen next to the limited value that has been crossed. Upon hearing the alarm, the nurse looks at the screen to identify the crossed parameter.

Graphs are plotted by the printer/plotter to give a visual trend graph of the measured parameters. These plots are averages of the parameters measured over a one- or five-minute interval. The nurse can select how often the parameters will be plotted.

Walleck, C. "The Neurosurgical Nurse and Computer Work Together." *Journal of Neurosurgical Nursing*, 7 (2): pp. 102–106, Dec. 1975.[9]

The data from the printer/plotter are also assembled and recorded onto cassette tapes. Each tape can record one 24-hour period. These data can be retrieved and replotted in the future.

The nursing staff does have to input some information into the computer. A patient needs to be logged into the system when admitted and logged out when discharged or moved to another bed. The nurse sets the alarm limits and enters certain lab test results. Each member of the nursing staff has been trained to input this information by using the typewriter keyboard on the desk console. These are relatively easy procedures and do not take much nursing time to accomplish.

There were many nurses who felt that all of these mechanical aids were taking time from the patient. It is true that until everyone became comfortable and confident working with the equipment, it did seem to take many nursing hours to set up and maintain it. But with experience, the nurses did find that they had more time to spend with the patient and his family.

Intensive care nursing is and has always been a complex challenge, especially with the added instrumentation. The nurses have adapted well to the challenge and are working toward becoming better neurosurgical nurses. Each ICU nurse is a "monitor" and the computer-monitored system has given the nurses the opportunity to improve themselves as monitors of neurological functions.

With the nurse and computer working together, patients are getting better neurosurgical intensive care.

COMPUTERS IN NURSING

Because of the computer's many advantages, its use in nursing will no doubt broaden and expand as nurses recognize the benefits that can be gained through their use. From the time computers were introduced in health care settings, nurses have been called upon to provide the information to be fed into the system for medical or administrative purposes. They need to become more cognizant of how computers can be utilized to help them provide up-to-date nursing care for patients. In an article in *Nursing Outlook*, Karolyn Hanna, R.N., M.S.N. urges nurses to become more aware of the impact of computers on their profession. "We must learn the functions and limitations of computers so that we can tell the programmer what we want the computer to do for nurses. It is important that nurses take an active part in the introduction of computers into the nursing world."[5]

It is no longer true that nursing-care-oriented computer-based information systems are situated primarily in large urban teaching hospitals. They are becoming quite common. The Nursing Coordinator of Data Processing at Charlotte Memorial Hospital in Charlotte, North Carolina stresses the importance of involving nurses in the design of nursing computer applications.

> Nurses, experienced in the actual care received by patients, were keenly aware that physician's orders (into the computer system) were complemented and supplemented by instructions for nursing care from registered nurses.[5]

The nurses developed a list of "initiators" for various types of patient care. When one of these initiators was keyed in at the computer terminal, a nursing care plan would be printed out by the computer. Other computer applications at Charlotte Memorial Hospital include handling room reservations, the admission of patients, preparation of medication plans, scheduling surgery, and providing lab summaries.

It is generally felt that computers bring added benefits to the nursing staff. Because computers tend to minimize clerical work and store large quantities of information, the nurse is relieved of these chores and, consequently, has more time for direct patient care, teaching, and planning. Another benefit of computers is the better control of the quality of patient care that often results from their use. Furthermore, since nursing notes can be fed directly into a computer via a terminal, the time spent by nurses during shift changes can be greatly reduced.

Perhaps the most important point that can be made is that there should be active nursing involvement as early as possible in the planning stages of developing an automated computer system for the hospital. In any case, it is clear that nurses can benefit substantially by becoming and remaining knowledgeable about this technology. The computer has enormous potential for assisting nurses in clarifying, teaching, implementing, and expanding the principles of high-quality patient care.

Commentary 14.4
Computerized Diet Planning

Central State Hospital, in Milledgeville, Georgia, is a city unto itself. Serving the population of some 8,300 are a fire department, security force, general hospital, chapels, and recreation facilities. Central State also has patient-operated stores, warehouses, a lumberyard, laundry, steam plant, and bus service.

A main kitchen, the size of two football fields, services (via truck)

68 dining rooms in 25 different buildings. The food service prepares and serves 31,000 meals a day (or in excess of 10 million a year). The annual food budget is approximately $3 million based upon $.25 a meal for raw food costs.

The key to food savings at Central State is computer-assisted menu planning (CAMP). Since CAMP was installed in 1969, menu items have been repeated less frequently and food costs have been cut by 5 percent.

Central State's CAMP system works with such constraints as nutrient value, separation ratio, dominant food attributes, and cost suboptimization. The hospital is capable of controlling eight nutrients. Once a food item has met the nutrient requirements, it is then checked to see when it was last served. For example, an item with a separation ratio of seven could be used once every seven days. Moreover, items that have met and passed the previous requirements are evaluated by cost. Prices are updated a minimum of every 30 days.

"It takes two dietitians, the food service director, and myself only one hour to review the print out and produce a satisfactory 90-day menu," reports the food service administrator. "In the past, it took ten people two hours every week to plan one week's menu."

When the 90-day menu is prepared, the data processing department prepares a food usage report itemizing day-by-day food requirements. Purchasing is now made easier. Items are bought out of need not out of habit.

The food item costs are based upon forecast information from publications such as the *Wall Street Journal* and trade magazines. Changes in the menu due to item availability, cost, food donations, and government surplus are fairly easy to make with the menu-planning system. Dietitians code the nutrient value and separation ratio of the new foods and can then substitute them in the menu without upsetting the preplanned balance. A nutritional analysis is run every 90 days to verify that each meal served met the nutrient specifications.

Abstracted from A few guests for dinner-like 8,000 plus. Data Processor XIII, 5 (December 1970/January 1971): 9.

It is not uncommon to find a computer terminal similar to the one in Figure 14-1 (a typewriterlike device that is directly connected to a central computer) at the nursing stations in a hospital.

The computer can handle many of the routine and repetitive tasks and free the nurse for other activities. A typical interaction at a nursing station might be as follows.[6]

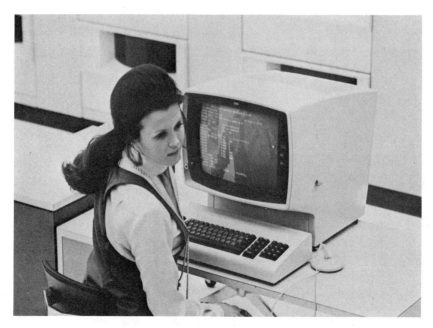

Figure 14.1. A computer terminal at the nursing station.

A medication order is written by a physician on a patient's chart. The nurse or ward clerk would want to transmit this information to the pharmacy. She would accomplish this by typing the instruction MEDICATION ORDER at the computer terminal. The computer would respond to this command by prompting the user for more specific information about the medication order. an example of this dialogue is shown in Figure 14.2.

Medication Order

TUESDAY APRIL 11, 1981
Please answer the following:

Nursing Station Location:	NORTH 1
Patient's Room Number:	135
Patient's Bed Location:	A
Drug Identification Number:	256
Dosage that was ordered:	0.25 mgm
Frequency of Dosage:	Q.D.
Duration of Medication:	CONTINUAL
Route of drug administration:	P.O.

Figure 14.2.
Medication order processing.

After this information is keyed in, the computer would display a message on the computer terminal at the nursing station asking for verification of the data just typed (see Figure 14.3). The nurse or ward clerk would carefully check this information against the patient's chart.

If the information is correct, the person at the computer terminal would type YES, and the medication order would be transmitted to the pharmacy and a copy of the order stored on computer tape. If there were any errors in

---

```
      COMPUTER  REQUESTS  VERIFICATION
         OF  THE  MEDICATION  ORDER

REQUESTED MEDICATION      (TUESDAY  APRIL  11,
ORDER                      1981)

NURSING  STATION          :  NORTH  1

PATIENT'S  ROOM  AND  BED
LOCATION                  :  135-A

PATIENT'S  NAME           :  JOHN  NEUHAUSER

PATIENT'S  HOSPITAL
ID  NUMBER                :  F406

DRUG  ORDERED             :  DIGOXIN

DOSAGE  ORDERED           :  0.25  MGM

FREQUENCY  OF  DRUG       :  Q.D.

DURATION  OF  MEDICATION  :  CONTINUAL

ROUTE  OF  DRUG
ADMINISTRATION            :  P.O.

IS  THIS  INFORMATION
ENTIRELY  CORRECT?
```

Figure 14.3.

the data, the nurse or ward clerk would type NO, and the computer would begin asking for the MEDICATION ORDER information all over again.

Note that this time the computer has displayed the patient's name (which was not typed in during the medication order request) and also the name of the drug. This can be done because the patient's name and room number were entered into the computer at the time of the patient's admission to the hospital. It is a simple matter for the computer to maintain "in its memory" a list of these name and room number assignments and look up the name of a patient when the room number is entered on a terminal at the nursing station. In a similar manner, the computer references a file of drug numbers that has an alphabetic description of the drug for each number. This list of drug-number codes was prepared just prior to the arrival of the computer system and entered into the machine during the first few days of its operation. The way in which the computer remembers data is not much different from the way a cassette tape or phonograph record works. This will be discussed in greater depth in Chapter 1.

At the same time that the drug-codes were developed, the physicians got together and assigned a "MAXIMUM DOSAGE ALLOWED" amount to each of the drugs. This limit was also stored in the computer along with the name of the drug. If a dosage order exceeds this amount, the computer will display the message illustrated in Figure 14.4 on the terminal at the nursing station.

Assuming that the MEDICATION ORDER was correct when the nurse or ward clerk typed YES to the computer's verification request, the order would be processed. This means that the order is automatically displayed on the terminal in the pharmacy. On the pharmacy order, the computer has printed an order number, the age and sex of the patient, the name of the patient's physician, and the dollar charge for the medication. Once again, this information is retrievable from the main files of the computer (created at admission time). Also, the computer prints a drug label that can be placed on the container itself (see Figure 14.5).

Another advantage of this kind of an integrated system is that the computer can keep track of all medications that have been ordered for a patient and alert the nurse if certain medications should not be given with certain other medications. While, once again, the data on what interactions are undesirable must be first entered into the computer; once done, the computer can keep referencing this list whenever necessary.

In addition to the kinds of interactions described above, the computer can also display schedules and care plans for use by the nursing staff.

For example, Figure 14.6 illustrates the use of the computer for preparing a daily care plan. This is done for every patient in the hospital, and when the nurse begins her shift at 7 A.M., she can have a daily care plan printed for all the patients at her nursing station.

```
                    DOSAGE LIMIT EXCEEDED

REQUESTED MEDICATION     (TUESDAY APRIL 11,
ORDER                    1981)

NURSING STATION          : NORTH 1

PATIENT'S ROOM AND
BED LOCATION             : 135-A

PATIENT'S NAME           : JOHN NEUHAUSER

PATIENT'S HOSPITAL
ID NUMBER                : F405

DRUG ORDERED             : DIGOXIN

DOSAGE ORDERED           : 025 MGM


     WARNING :   DOSAGE EXCEEDS MAXIMUM
                 ALLOWED AMOUNT.

     ORDER WILL NOT BE PROCESSED.

     OVERRIDE CODE NEEDED.

     RECHECK INFORMATION.
```

Figure 14.4.

In addition to the above applications, the computer terminal at the nurse's station could be used for the following:

1. Printing out a schedule of the lab work required each day and the instructions for each test.
2. Processing doctor's orders for lab tests (very much like the medication orders were processed).
3. Work sheets can be printed at the start of each shift indicating any special work or care that needs to be done.

MEDICATION ORDER REQUEST
DISPLAYED AT PHARMACY

ORDER NUMBER T18579   TUESDAY APRIL 11, 1981

NORTH 1 135-A   JOHN NEUHAUSER

HOSPITAL ID   F406

SEX   M

AGE   36

DRUG   DIGOXIN

DOSAGE   0.25 MGM

ROUTE   P.O.

FREQUENCY   Q.D.

DURATION   CONTINUAL

AMOUNT $7.50

PHYSICIAN   DR. DONALD MCHUGH

JOHN NEUHAUSER (F406)

135-A ORDER NUMBER T18579

DRUG NAME AND SUCH

DR. DONALD MCHUGH

Figure 14.5.

```
┌─────────────────────────────────────────────────────────────────┐
│                 COMPUTER GENERATED NURSING CARE PLAN              │
│                                                                   │
│                     FULTON MEDICAL CENTER                         │
│  ROOM 135-A       JOHN NEUHAUSER        TUESDAY APRIL 11, 1981    │
│  AGE 36           MALE                  HOSPITAL ID:   F405       │
│  PHYSICIAN:   DR. DONALD MCHUGH                                   │
│  DIAGNOSIS:   CONGESTIVE HEART FAILURE                            │
│  CARE PLAN                                                        │
│      (1)     BED REST. OOB FOR BATHROOM PRIVILEGES ONLY.          │
│      (2)     TAKE PULSE BEFORE ADMINISTERING MEDICATION.          │
│              WITHOLD IF PULSE BELOW 60. TEACH PATIENT TO TAKE     │
│              OWN PULSE.                                           │
│      (3)     LOW SODIUM DIET.  ENCOURAGE FLUIDS HIGH IN           │
│              POTASSIUM (ORANGE JUICE).                            │
│  OTHER ACTIVE ORDERS:                                            │
│              OBSERVE CLOSELY FOR SIGNS OF DRUG TOXICITY.          │
└─────────────────────────────────────────────────────────────────┘
```

Figure 14.6.

The applications are growing each day, as hospitals, physicians, and nurses discover the advantages of the computer. While most hospitals are currently using computers to process patient bills, maintain accounting data, and payrolls, more and more facilities are beginning to use the computer in other areas. Computers are now used for processing EEGs, EKGs, blood and urine analyses, and perhaps even for some diagnosis. When you consider that the introduction of minicomputers and microcomputers has significantly lowered the prices of these machines, the continued growth of these kinds of applications seems inevitable.

Commentary 14.5
A Computer Diagnosis

A medical diagnostic system designed at Leeds University has proved more accurate than doctors in assessing the most likely cause of acute abdominal pain among patients admitted to the university's department of surgery.

Between January and December of last year, 304 such patients were admitted to the unit, and the computer's diagnosis proved correct in 92 percent of cases, compared with 80 percent accuracy by the most senior doctor to see each case. The trial, organized by Dr. F. I. de Dombal, the university's leader in clinical information science, is described in the latest issue of the *British Medical Journal*.

The diagnostic system used in the English Electric KDF9 computer was designed on the assumption that busy doctors knew nothing about computers. After each patient had been seen by the doctor and examined, the findings were passed on to a technician, who translated them into language used by the computer.

Depending on the demands made on it by other university departments, the computer would list the likely diagnoses in order of probability within 30 seconds to 15 minutes. If the computer and the doctor in charge of the case disagreed, the computer would on request suggest further investigations that might be useful.

If none of the listed diagnoses was given high probability by the computer, it would again on request give a list of rarer conditions that might be considered by the doctor. In the year-long trial, the computer's diagnosis proved correct in 279 cases. In 15 it was wrong, in eight the patient's condition was not included in the diseases considered by the computer, and in two, no computer diagnosis was made because the doctors concerned with the case disagreed about the findings.

Whereas the computer advised an operation on six occasions when it would have proved unnecessary, in practice 30 such operations were carried out on the basis of the surgeon's own judgment. The computer system accurately classified 84 of the 85 patients with appendicitis, compared with 75 by the doctors, and its suggestion that no operation was necessary proved correct on 136 out of 137 occasions.

The computer team emphasizes in its report that the role of the doctor is undiminished by the use of the system, which is reliable only if accurate data are fed into it on the basis of the doctor's interrogation and examinations of the patient.

Use of the computer-aided diagnostic systems, the report says, has reemphasized the traditional values of accurate history taking and careful physical examination. It sees an increasing place for computer analysis as an adjunct to clinical assessment of difficult cases.

(Reproduced from *The Times*)

Commentary 14.6
Voice Response Systems

Terminal systems are being used by Bell Laboratories for control of inventory stock. Inventory records retrieved from a computer's memory via the terminal contain information, such as when and where inventory items were sent out, how long they will be gone, and if a particular item is available from the central stock.

A device that extends the applications of computers into new areas to which many people have easy access is the voice-response unit that uses the ordinary telephone for a terminal. These systems typically have such human voice characteristics as variable word and pause length and the ability to make new words form the existing vocabulary (*e.g.,* "pay," "install," and "—ment" words, such as "payment" and "installment," can be formed). To use the system, the caller dials it and a "ready" tone or spoken salutation is generated by the system. The user than keys in his inquiry using a Touch-Tone telephone and the voice response unit transmits the inquiry to a host computer that performs the actual search or computation. The voice-response unit then receives commands from the computer in the form of data track addresses that are used to locate specific words, phrases, or sentences on the vocabulary storage device in the response unit. The stored words are converted to audio and the caller hears the message. One can imagine a typical "conversation" between human caller and computer being as follows:

CALLER: Dials computer on a Touch-Tone telephone.

SYSTEM: "Key in access code."

CALLER: Keys in 60682531.

SYSTEM: "You entered 60682531." System performs authorization checks. "Access approved, enter request code."

CALLER: Keys 196, for driver's license check.

SYSTEM: "Driver's license check requested. Enter license number and state code."

CALLER: Keys AEK349 for license number and 42 for state code.

SYSTEM: Performs search of its files (*e.g.,* requires seven seconds). License holder is John M. Miles. Only want is seven-month old traffic violation—nonmoving. New York City P.D. Miles does have an emergency telephone call pending from area code 215 telephone number 564-5170. Press number 1 button for replay of telephone number. Press number 2 button for replay of want. Do you have any more requests? If so enter request code.

CALLER: Hangs up.

The application could be a surgeon calling his now-computerized answering service to request information on the blood count for a patient in a given room of a given hospital.

COMPUTERS IN RESEARCH AND EDUCATION

Many teaching hospitals, medical schools, and schools of nursing use computers both in their research and their teaching activities. By using a computer terminal in a classroom, students can become involved with a hypothetical patient, identify nursing problems, test solutions, and find out the results of their interventions without involving real patients.[7] Several computer manufacturers have developed computer programs that aid the instructional process (commonly called Computer Aided Instruction, CAI). The most sophisticated of these systems is called the PLATO system. With the aid of a very sophisticated computer terminal, the system can provide animated displays, and tie in to both audio cassettes and 35 mm. slide displays. The PLATO system has a variety of applications in the nursing area. These include programs that teach about drugs, instruct the student on the fundamentals of the fetal circulatory system, and test the student's knowledge of the working of the human heart. All of these programs are designed to proceed at the pace of the student. Thus, students proceed according to how they respond to questions posed during a particular lesson. If the computer detects the need for review of certain material, the computer program will automatically guide the student through an appropriate review.

In an article on research in *Science*, the journal of the American Association for the Advancement of Science, the authors comment on the computer in the research process:

> The revolution of the research process itself by computers is now well advanced. Computers have been adopted, adapted, and absorbed into every aspect of the research process, with aggregate consequences that are pervasive and profound.[8]

Commentary 14.7
Medical Education

The University of Southern California School of Medicine has developed a computer model of certain portions of the human body and uses the model and a human manikin to train clinical anesthesiologists. The manikin, called Sim One, is lifelike in appearance, having a plastic skin that resembles its human counterpart in color and texture. Sim One is in the position of a patient lying on an operating table with his left arm extended, ready for intravenous injection. The right arm is fitted with a blood pressure cuff, and a stethoscope is taped in place over the approximate location of the heart. Sim One breathes, has a heartbeat with temporal and carotid pulses, and a measurable blood pressure. He opens and closes his mouth, blinks his eyes, and "responds" to four intravenously administered drugs and two gases administered through mask or tube. Responses to the agents and method of treatment occur in real time, detected, controlled, and enacted under the control of the computer's program.

To illustrate this sequence of events, we may describe a typical case as follows. Oxygen is administered through a mask to Sim One for five minutes in order to raise the oxygen level in the tissues (to provide an extra margin of safety during the time in which a real patient might go without oxygen during the operation). Sodium pentothal is administered intravenously, which renders the Sim One "unconscious." Succinylcholine is injected which produces paralysis of skeletal muscles and indeed causes Sim One to stop breathing. The anesthesiologist then quickly slips off the mask and inserts the airway tube into the trachea, sealing it inside the walls of the trachea by inflating the balloonlike rubber cuff of the tube. Through this tube connected to the anesthesia machine, the anesthesiologist then administers oxygen and nitrous oxide by squeezing the inflated reservoir bag. During all this activity, Sim One's computer registers all of the anesthesiologist's action and the agents administered, and dictates the appropriate physiological responses to the manikin. At any time, the instructor has the option of "overriding" the physiological program in order to produce such problem situations as cardiac arrest, abnormally increased or decreased blood pressure, left or right block of the bronchus, increased or decreased breathing rate, cardiac arrhythmia, ventricular fibrillation, increased jaw tension, and even vomiting.

There are many ways in which computers are used to aid in the research process. In the neurological setting, surface electrodes attached to the head transmit EEG data directly into the computer for analysis. Several computer manufacturers have developed special computers to be used in the laboratory environment. These are usually connected directly with an experiment and provide instantaneous data for the researcher.

Commentary 14.8
Mind-Reading Computer

The experiment looks like some ingenious test of mental telepathy. Seated inside a small isolation booth with wires trailing from the helmet on her head, the subject seems deep in concentration. She does not speak or move. Near by, a white-coated scientist intently watches a TV screen. Suddenly, a little white dot hovering in the center of the screen comes to life. It sweeps to the top of the screen, then reverses itself and comes back down. After a pause, it veers to the right, stops, moves to the left, momentarily speeds up and finally halts—almost as if it were under the control of some external intelligence.

In fact, it is. The unusual experiment, conducted at the Stanford Research Institute in Menlo Park, California, is a graphic display of one of the newest and most dazzling breakthroughs in cybernetics. It shows that a computer can, in a very real sense, read human minds. Although the dot's gyrations were directed by a computer, the machine was only carrying out the orders of the test subject. She, in turn, did nothing more than think about what the dot's movements should be.

Brainchild of S.R.I. researcher Lawrence Pinneo, a 46-year old neurophysiologist and electronics engineer, the computer mind-reading technique is far more than a laboratory stunt. Though computers can solve extraordinarily complex problems with incredible speed, the information they digest is fed to them by such slow, cumbersome tools as typewriter keyboards or punched tapes. It is for this reason that scientists have long been tantalized by the possibility of opening up a more direct link between human and electronic brains.

Although Pinneo and others have experimented with computer systems that respond to voice commands, he decided that there might be a more direct method than speech. The key to his scheme was the electroencephalograph, a device used by medical researchers to pick up electrical currents from various parts of the brain. If he could learn to identify brain waves generated by specific thoughts or commands, Pinneo figured, he might be able to teach the same skill to a computer. The machine might even be able to react to those commands by, say, moving a dot across a TV screen.

Pinneo could readily pick out specific commands. But, like fingerprints, the patterns varied sufficiently from one human test subject to another to fool the computer. Pinneo found a way to deal with this problem by storing a large variety of patterns in the computer's memory. When the computer had to deal with a fresh pattern, it could search its memory for the brain waves most like it. So far the S.R.I. computer has been taught to recognize seven different commands—up, down, left, right, slow, fast, and stop. Working with a total of 25 different people, it makes the right move 60 percent of the time.

Pinneo is convinced that this barely passing grade can be vastly improved. He foresees the day when computers will be able to recognize the smallest units in the English language—the 40-odd basic sounds (or phonemes) out of which all words or verbalized thoughts can be constructed. Such skills could be put to many practical uses. The pilot of a high-speed plane or spacecraft, for instance, could simply order by thought alone some vital flight information for an all-purpose cockpit display. There would be no need to search for the right dials or switches on a crowded instrument panel.

Pinneo does not worry that mind-reading computers might be abused by "Big Brother" governments or overly zealous police trying to ferret out the innermost thoughts of citizens. Rather than a menace, he says, they could be a highly civilizing influence. In the future, Pinneo speculates, technology may well be sufficiently advanced to feed information from the computer directly back into the brain. People with problems, for example, might don mind-reading helmets ("thinking caps") that let the computer help them untangle everything from complex tax returns to matrimonial messes. Adds Pinneo: "When the person takes this thing off, he might feel pretty damn dumb."

Source: Time Magazine copyright, Time, Inc.[10]

Computer simulation is a technique whereby the computer is made to represent some corresponding set of events in the real world. By working with this computer model, the researcher can evaluate the impact of a variety of alternatives without affecting the actual experiment. For example, at the Stanford University Medical Center, researchers are using the computer to simulate a patient's need for heart surgery. By inputting a variety of data about the heart, the computer model can simulate (and graphically display) a working model of the heart and allow the physicians to see the effects of various treatments.

Most of us are aware of the numerical and computational power of computers. In this regard, the computer provides a tool for the researcher that can quickly perform a wide variety of statistical analyses in a very short time. If computers were not available, most research would take from ten to one hundred times longer to complete.

Effective research necessitates utilizing all of the resources available. Not only is the computer itself one of these resources, but it can make another one, the library, much easier for the researcher to use. The National Library of Medicine has the largest computerized index of biomedical research journals in the world. Over 500,000 articles have been entered into the data base of the computer. At remote locations across the United States, researchers with a computer terminal available can call the computer on the telephone, connect the telephone to their terminal, and then have access to the data base. Using a key word or two, they can then instruct the computer to print out a list of all references in the data base that contain these key terms. The system is also linked to Europe via satellite.

From all of the above, it should be clear that the computer has widespread application in the health care field. As nursing students, researchers or not, you would be ill-prepared should you be unaware of the ways in which the computer can be used to enhance the nursing process. Furthermore, you would be ill-equipped to cope with the technological revolution in health care without some knowledge and understanding of computers. The next few chapters will provide you with an introduction to computers and, it is hoped, prepare you to use them effectively in both research and nonresearch nursing settings.

Commentary 14.9
Predicting Suicide

People who have the potential for suicide can be helped—if they are identified in time. The Suicide Risk Prediction Program at the University of Wisconsin Hospitals in Madison now uses a computer to identify potentially suicidal people.

Questions appear on a screen and the patient types in answers. The interview takes from 45 minutes to three hours, and the computer makes a prediction on the likelihood of suicide in two and one half minutes.

A program developer, psychiatry professor John H. Greist, says that many people actually prefer discussing personal problems with the computer.

"If, for example, a person is talking about influenza symptoms, he usually prefers talking with a doctor. But when talking about problems that may be socially deviant, many prefer the computer. It's a nonjudgmental interviewer that doesn't raise its eyebrows at anything."

The computer makes fewer mistakes than a doctor since it records all comments. "In a study done to determine how accurate the computer is in determining potential suicides, we found that the computer was right 70 percent of the time, and the clinicians only 40 percent," Dr. Greist said.

Besides being available day or night, the computer is more economical than a clinician. Between 8 A.M. and 5 P.M. weekdays, a computer interview costs $3.00, and only $1.50 other times.

The patients who voluntarily agree to the computer interview are seen by the staff if the computer determines they are high suicide risks.

The Wisconsin Department of Health and Social Services reported 447 suicides in Wisconsin every year from 1966 to 1970.

"The actual rate is probably twice that. It's impossible to tell how many deaths attributed to other things are really suicides. There is a real need for suicide prediction," Greist said.

He developed the program in conjunction with the University of Wisconsin industrial engineering Prof. David H. Gustafson

Dennie Van Tassel. *The Compleat Computer.* University of California, 1976.

REFERENCES

1. On Time in the Hospital. Computing Report, January, 1968.

2. Bode R: Bigger Role for Computers in U.S. Health Care. *Think*, IBM: October, 1973, vol. 39, no. 8.

3. Control of Artificial Limbs. *MOSAIC*, July/August, 1978.

4. Hanna: Nursing Audit at a Community Hospital. Nursing Outlook, vol. 24, no. 1, 1976.

5. Zielstorff, R: The Planning and Evaluation of Automated Systems: A Nurse's Point of View. Journal of Nursing Administration, July/August, 1975.

6. See, for example, Smith E: The Computer and Nursing Practice. Supervisor Nurse. September, 1974.

7. DeTomay, R: Instructional Technology and Nursing Education. Journal of Nursing Education, Vol. 9, No. 2, April, 1970.

8. Baker W. O. et al. Computers and Research. *Science* 195: 18, 1977.

9. Walleck, C. "The Neurosurgical Nurse and Computer Work Together." *Journal of Neurosurgical Nursing*, 7 (2): pp. 102–106, Dec. 1975.

10. Source: Time Magazine copyright, Time, Inc.

CHAPTER

15

Taking a Tour of the Computer Center Facilities

Whether you visit a university computer center or one that is located in a hospital, the facility itself is likely to resemble the one in Figure 15.1.

While different facilities will have various combinations of equipment, all will include five fundamental parts: INPUT UNITS, OUTPUT UNITS, CENTRAL PROCESSING UNITS, MEMORY UNITS, and AUXILIARY STORAGE UNITS. All of these units are called HARDWARE since they are physical pieces of equipment one can touch. On the other hand, the term SOFTWARE refers to computer programs and instructions that inform the computer what needs to be done.

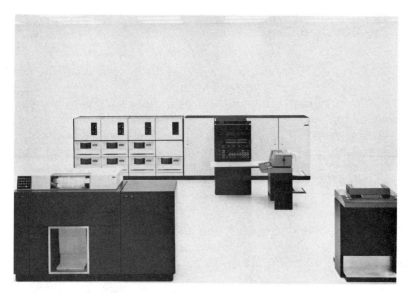

Figure 15.1. A typical computer facility.

INPUT UNITS

The primary input units are the CARD READER and the CONSOLE. These input units "put in" information for the computer to process. This is the first step of the computer processing cycle, and it is here that data, instructions, or computer programs are entered into the computer system.

The console shown in Figure 15.2 is very much like a typewriter and allows the operator of the computer to key in instructions directly to the computer. The operator may need to inform the computer which program is to be done next or which piece of equipment to start up or stop. The computer also "talks" or communicates with the operator by means of this console. Thus, if the computer detects an error in a user's request for computer processing, or senses a faulty piece of equipment, a message will be printed at this typewriter for the benefit of the operator. Since it would be impractical to have all users of the computer file into the computer room and use this "typewriter," most users prepare their instructions to the machine on punched cards. Figure 15.3 shows a punched card that has an instruction for the computer to process. This instruction tells the computer to add 20 to 35 and store the answer in the computer in a place called A. The interested reader may wish to look at COMMENTARY 15.1 for a further discussion of a "punched card."

Commentary 15.1
The Punched Card

The punched card may be found in virtually every type of commercial, scientific, or governmental agency.

The advantage of punched-card data processing over manual methods is that once the data have been punched onto cards, they may be used repeatedly to produce a variety of reports. Because each card represents a single unit or transaction, punched-card data processing is often called the unitrecord concept of processing data.

The two means of identifying punched cards are by color and by corner cut. Cards may be obtained in a variety of solid colors, or they may be obtained with a stripe of color. For example, a payroll card could be red, a billing card blue, and an inventory card white with a green stripe. The corner cut is another means of visually identifying a type of card. Although any of the four corners can be cut, cards often have an upper left or upper right corner cut. Another purpose of the corner cut is to ensure that all cards of the same type are facing the same direction or are right side up.

Punched-card data processing machines have the ability to read punches on cards; however, they cannot identify the type of card by color or corner cut.

The punched card is divided into 80 vertical columns called "card columns". Each card column may contain punching that represents a digit for 0 to 9, and alphabetic letter, or a special character (such as @&#%). The card columns are numbered 1 to 80 across the face of the card. Horizontally each card column is divided into 12 rows. These 12 rows are the designated areas in which a punch may be placed. Usually the rows 0 to 9 are visually identified by being printed on the card. The top two rows, the 11th and 12th rows, normally are not printed on the card as this area is sometimes used for the printing of headings or interpreted information.

The top edge of the card is referred to as the "12" edge, and the bottom edge is called the "9" edge. Cards are fed through the data-processing machines either 12 edge first or 9 edge first. Some machines require the cards to be face up, meaning that the printed side of the card is facing up. Other machines must have the cards placed face down, or the printed side of the card down. Proper reading of the cards will not occur unless they are placed within the machine correctly. Numeric information is recorded on a card by punching a single hole in a card column.

Alphabetic information requires two punches in a card column for each letter. A digit punch 1 through 9 is used with a zone punch 12, 11, or 0 to represent each of the 26 letters of the alphabet. The alphabet is coded as follows:

A 12 zone + 1
B 12 zone + 2
C 12 zone + 3
D 12 zone + 4
E 12 zone + 5
F 12 zone + 6
G 12 zone + 7
H 12 zone + 8
I 12 zone + 9
J 11 zone + 1
K 11 zone + 2
L 11 zone + 3
M 11 zone + 4

N 11 zone + 5
O 11 zone + 6
P 11 zone + 7
Q 11 zone + 8
R 11 zone + 9
S 0 zone + 2
T 0 zone + 3
U 0 zone + 4
V 0 zone + 5
W 0 zone + 6
X 0 zone + 7
Y 0 zone + 8
Z 0 zone + 9

Special characters are represented by one, two, or three punches in a card column.

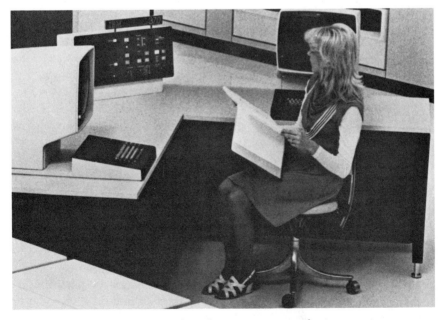

Figure 15.2. The computer console.

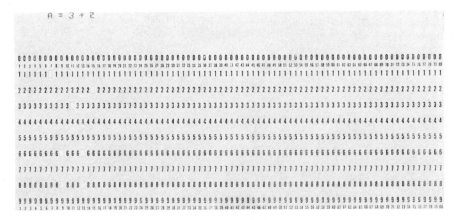

Figure 15.3. A punched card instruction.

A set of punched cards (containing instructions for the computer and/or data) is prepared by the person using the machine (yourself). This deck of cards is then placed in a CARD READER. One model of this machine is shown in Figure 15.4.

This device is connected by wires to the main computer. After the user places her deck of cards in the card reader and presses a start button, the machine automatically feeds the cards through the machine, sends the information contained on the cards to the main computer, and returns the cards to the owner at the opposite side of the card reader. All these steps are completed in rapid succession since card readers process from 600 to 2,000 cards per minute, depending on the particular model.

The card reader "sends" the information to the main computer by the process shown in Figure 15.5 Each card passes over a set of brushes. If there is a hole in the card, the brushes make contact with a metal plate and an electrical impulse is created. The computer has been programed to understand what letters are represented by certain impulses. In this way, the computer has "read" the information on the cards. At most computer centers, the user would return to the facility about an hour later to pick up her results (the OUTPUT). The time that elapses from the submission of the punched cards until the output is received is called TURNAROUND TIME. Turnaround time is a function of how many people are "ahead of you" in the computer's line of jobs to be done, the complexity of your program and several other factors.

Another device used for input at many computer facilities is the computer TERMINAL. These devices are quite similar to typewriters. Their biggest advantage is that the user can type in her instructions and data at the terminal, and answers will immediately be typed back at the terminal. Thus,

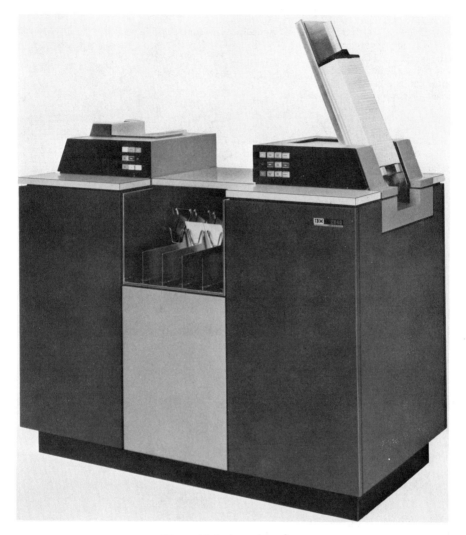

Figure 15.4. A card reader.

turnaround time can be reduced to a few seconds or minutes. In fact, many universities have several of these terminals located at various points throughout the campus. Because the larger, modern computers are so fast, several people could be at these terminals using the computer at virtually the same time. In addition, other people could be using punched cards for their programs (as discussed earlier). In fact, some large-scale computers can support

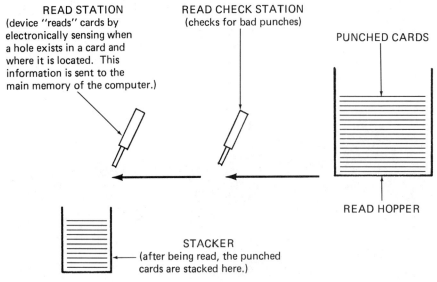

READ STATION
(device "reads" cards by
electronically sensing when
a hole exists in a card and
where it is located. This
information is sent to the
main memory of the computer.)

READ CHECK STATION
(checks for bad punches)

PUNCHED CARDS

READ HOPPER

STACKER
(after being read, the punched
cards are stacked here.)

Figure 15.5. The "reading" process.

up to 300 of these terminals and, again, with each user receiving her results almost instantaneously. This concept is called TIME SHARING. The users are "sharing the time" of the computer.

In addition to the console, the card reader, and terminals, there are a variety of specialized devices used for inputting information to the computer. These include punched paper tape readers, cassette tapes, optical readers (for reading lead pencil marks from a #2 pencil) and other sensing devices. Some of these machines are shown in Figure 15.10.

OUTPUT UNITS

After the computer has received the information from the input unit and has processed it, the next step is to print out the results. The primary output device is the LINE PRINTER. Figure 15.11 depicts a typical line printer. There are a variety of models available that differ with respect to the mechanism used to print a line of information. Printers can print up to 130 characters on a line at speeds ranging from 300 to 2,500 lines per minute. Research is currently underway to significantly increase these speeds.

As with input devices, there are a variety of other devices used for output. One, of course, is the computer terminal mentioned in the previous

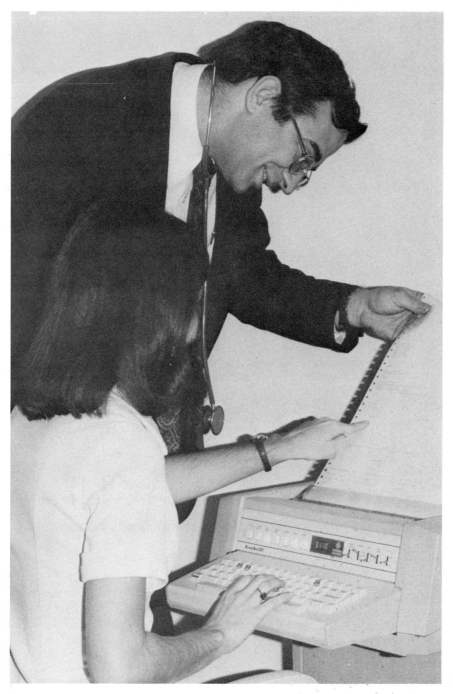

Figure 15.6. A teletype terminal.

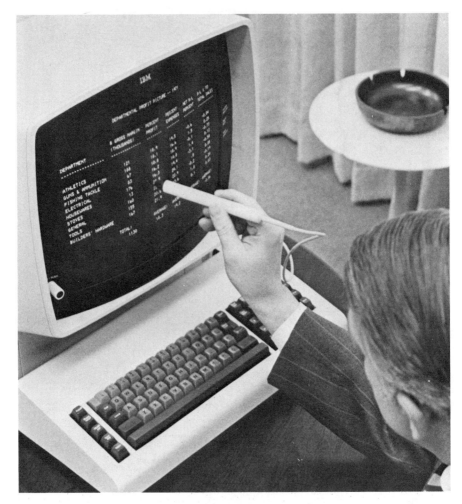

Figure 15.7. A CRT terminal.

section. Other devices include graph plotters, television screen displays (usually called a CRT-cathoderay-tube) voice response devices (often used by department stores for credit card approvals), display boards (such as those found in many modern sporting arenas), and also microfilm.

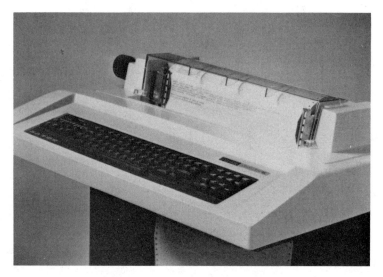

Figure 15.8. A DECWRITER terminal.

THE CENTRAL PROCESSING UNIT

The CENTRAL PROCESSING UNIT, usually called the CPU, is shown in Figure 15.12. This device is the "brain" of the computer. It has essentially three functions. An ARITHMETIC UNIT performs the additions, subtractions, multiplications, and divisions necessary to solve a particular problem. A CONTROL UNIT keeps track of which devices are being used (card readers, printers, terminals, etc.), whose program should be done next, and where to store information in the computer. The MEMORY UNIT has a limited number of places where information, instructions, or data may be "stored." All of these functions are handled by sophisticated circuitry inside the machine.

The computer can perform these operations incredibly fast. In fractions of a second it can complete tasks that would have taken humans several lifetimes to perform. Picture, if you will, someone knocking over your cup of morning coffee. Before the first drop hits the floor, a fairly large, modern computer could charge 2,000 checks to 300 different bank accounts *and* score 150 answers on 3,000 examinations *and* calculate the payroll for a hospital with 100 employees *and* examine the electrocardiograms of 100 patients *and* alert a physician if needed *and* have some time left over. All that before the first drop of coffee hits the floor! Because of this tremendous speed, new time units had to be developed. Operations like addition can be done in

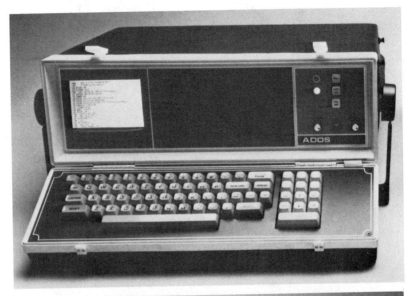

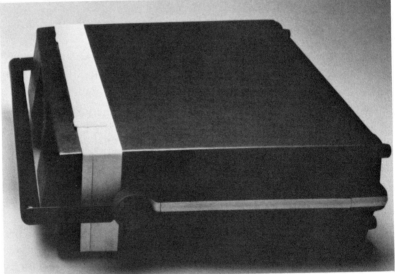

Figure 15.9. A portable terminal.

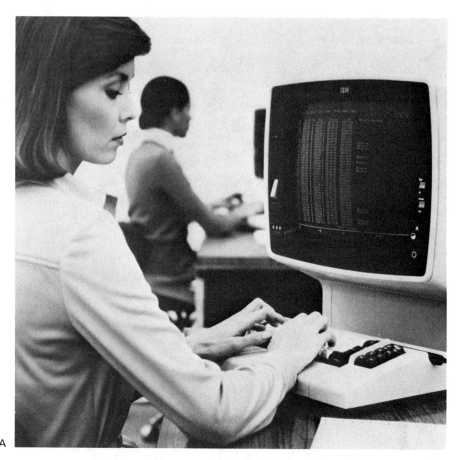

A

Figure 15.10. **A,** A cathode ray tube (CRT).

nanoseconds, or one thousandth of a millionth of a second. The newer computers operate in picoseconds (a trillionth of a second).

MEMORY UNITS

The memory unit is part of the CPU. Because of the limitations of space within the CPU, other memory devices called auxilary storage units have been developed. These will be discussed in the next section.

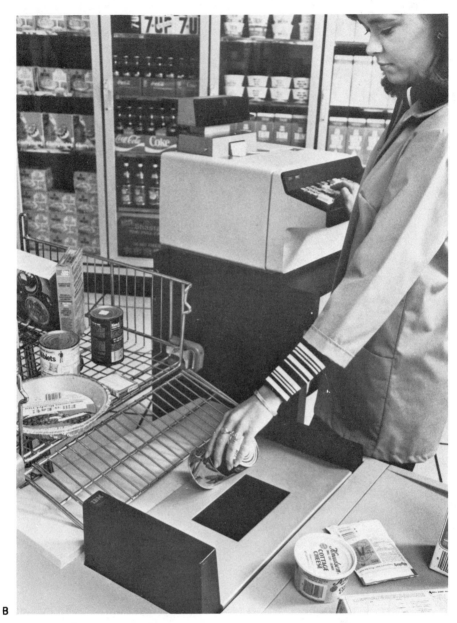

Figure 15.10. **B,** A computer used to scan a product code with the item's price.

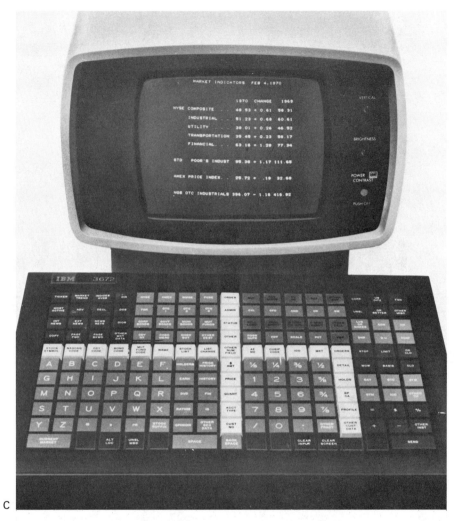

Figure 15.10. C, A custom-designed keyboard.

Memory is an appropriate term. The computer can "remember" things. This is not as surprising as you may first think since there are many common devices that remember things. The best example is your home tape recorder. It remembers what you have spoken. Phonograph records remember a song. A computer memory stores instructions and data. Just as it is not important to understand the technology of how a tape recorder "records," it is not necessary for us to examine the technological aspects of computer memory. This memory, called main memory, is small (in terms of how many data it

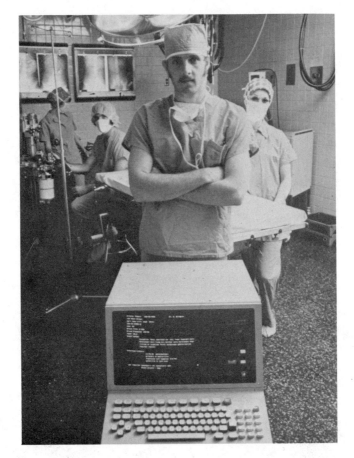

Figure 15.10. **D,** A patient-monitoring system.

can hold), but data can be retrieved from it quite fast. It is, however, very expensive. To compensate for these limitations, AUXILIARY STORAGE devices were developed that could be connected to the computer. These units are capable of storing very large quantities of information.

AUXILIARY STORAGE UNITS

The most common auxiliary storage unit is that for MAGNETIC TAPE. A magnetic tape unit is pictured in Figure 15.13. A reel of magnetic tape is put on this unit for the computer to process. Under the control of the

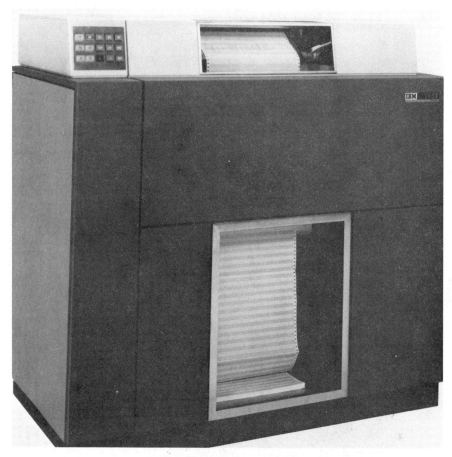

Figure 15.11. A line printer.

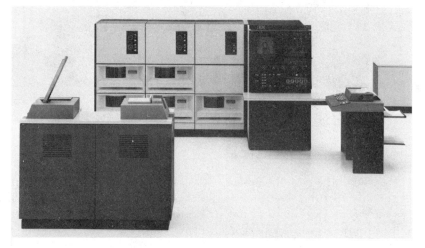

Figure 15.12. The central processing unit.

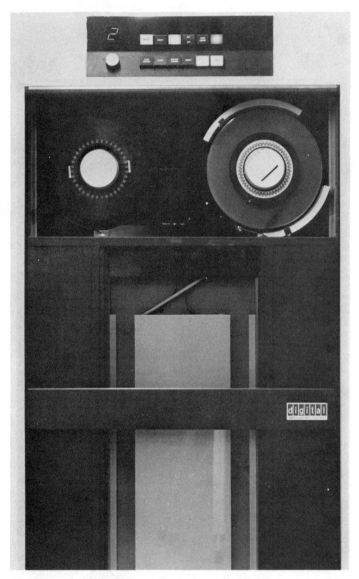

Figure 15.13. A magnetic tape unit.

CONTROL UNIT of the CPU, the tape drive will either record data onto the tape itself or read data from the tape into the computer's main memory. The tape itself (see Figure 15.14) is very much like the tape used in reel-to-reel tape recorders, only larger. A typical reel of magnetic tape holds 2,400 feet of ½-inch tape. These are manufactured with different capacities for storing

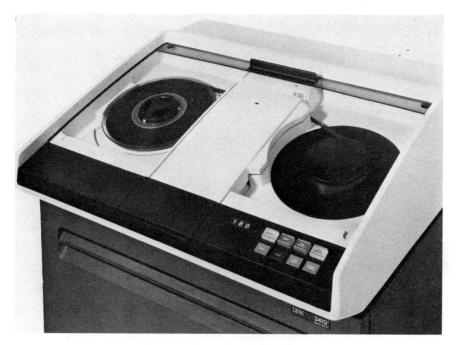

Figure 15.14. A reel of magnetic tape.

information. This "density" ranges from 556 characters per inch of tape up to 1,600 characters per inch of tape. As an example of how many data can be stored on a tape reel, suppose the tape could record 1,600 characters per inch of tape. Since a reel of tape has 28,800 inches (2,400' × 12") on it, the entire tape could hold 46,080,000 characters of data (1,600 characters per inch × 28,800 inches). While tapes can be processed very quickly, they have a limitation in that they must be processed sequentially. That is, if there were data on 100 patients on a tape and you wanted information of the 88th patient, you must first "pass by" the previous 87 patient records. This process takes considerably more time.

Another fairly common auxiliary storage device is the DISK UNIT. A disk unit is shown in Figure 15.15 and the disk itself is shown in Figure 15.16. The disk pack is very much like a stack of phonograph records sitting on a spindle. The stack is rotating very rapidly (about 40 revolutions each second). Because of this, a particular piece of information passes over the read-write mechanism 40 times *each* second. Thus, information can be retrieved much more quickly from a disk than from a tape. These devices also have very large capacities for storing data. These capacities range from a low of 250,000 characters (on a small "one-record" disk) to a high of 200,000,000 characters of data (on a modern disk pack).

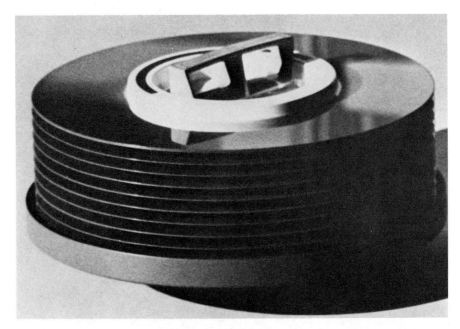

Figure 15.15. A disk pack.

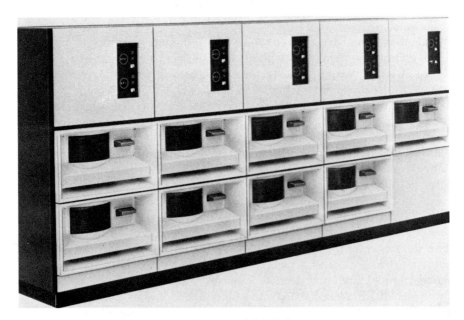

Figure 15.16. Several disk drives.

REVIEW OF COMPUTER SYSTEMS

These devices then, make up the equipment found at many computer facilities. Figure 15.11 showed how these pieces of equipment join together to form a computer system.

You are now in a better position to identify and understand the different components of the system. There are input units, output units, a central processing unit, and auxiliary storage units. The terms that you should be familiar with after reading this portion of the chapter include:

INPUT UNITS	HARDWARE
CONSOLE	SOFTWARE
CARD READER	CPU
PUNCHED CARDS	ARITHMETIC UNIT
COMPUTER TERMINAL	CONTROL UNIT
OUTPUT UNITS	MEMORY
TURNAROUND TIME	AUXILIARY STORAGE
TIME SHARING	TAPES
LINE PRINTER	DISKS

The next chapter will introduce you to ways in which you may use this valuable resource.

SOME ADDITIONAL COMPUTER TERMS

By this time, you have, no doubt, significantly expanded your computer vocabulary. Yet, there are still many other terms in the computer field that have not been explained. This section will present the most common of these terms, which you will certainly encounter in your travels around the computer center.

These final terms will be presented in alphabetical order in case they need to be referenced at a later date.

The computer can accept data that are either alphabetic, numeric, or a combination of these. Such a combination is called ALPHANUMERIC data. An example might be a patient's room number. Since a social security number contains hyphens, it would also be considered an alphanumeric piece of data.

One of the computer languages that we have not yet mentioned is ASSEMBLY language. It is a more cryptic version of some of the higher level languages. Thus, instead of the command PRINT, the command would be P. Every computer has some form of assembly language. It is usually longer and more difficult to learn than some of the other computer languages.

The term BINARY means "two states." All computers have their foundation rooted in the binary number system. A circuit may be open or closed; a switch may be on or off; a wire may be magnetized or not magnetized. It is by using codes based on the binary system that the computer is able to "remember" things.

The word BYTE is often heard in a computer facility. "That disk pack can store about 100 million bytes." "We have 256,000 bytes of main memory." A byte can be equivalent to a character of data. Thus, the disk pack mentioned above could store 100 million characters of data.

Some terminals that you will encounter at a computer center have no paper and display the results on a television screen. These terminals are called CRTs (Cathode Ray Tubes). They are exactly the same in every way to regular terminals except that there is no paper copy of what you do at the terminal. CRTs often print at faster speeds. The picture of the human brain in Figure 15.17 was made by taking a polaroid picture of the CRT during a computerized brain scan.

The computer program that resides in the memory of the computer and translates a particular Englishlike language into machine language is called a COMPILER.

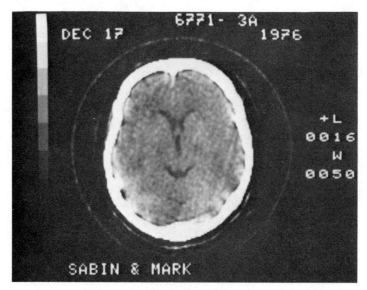

Figure 15.17. A computer-generated picture of the human brain.

There is a compiler for every language that is supported at a computer center. In addition to translating your computer program, the compiler checks your program for errors (in properly spelling or using commands) and prints out where they are in your program.

Sometimes you will hear the memory of the computer called CORE, or core memory. The term refers to the physical pieces that make up some memories. They are small iron cores (shaped like a wedding ring) that can be magnetized or unmagnetized to represent data in the computer. Figure 15.18 illustrates the concept of core memory. The newer computers make use of more modern technology for computer memory.

The words CRASH and DOWNTIME will be ones that you will no doubt become familiar with during your acquaintanceship with computers. Downtime is that period of time when the computer is not working. The machine can be "down" because of mechanical failure, for preventive maintenance, because of a power failure, or for a variety of other reasons. When the computer goes down unexpectedly, the result is usually called a crash. In either case, the computer is unavailable to the user.

A FILE is a collection of data that is usually made up of records and fields (e.g., if the hospital were collecting information on patients). A record would be all the information on a single patient and a field would be one piece of data within a record (e.g., the patient's name). Some people also call com-

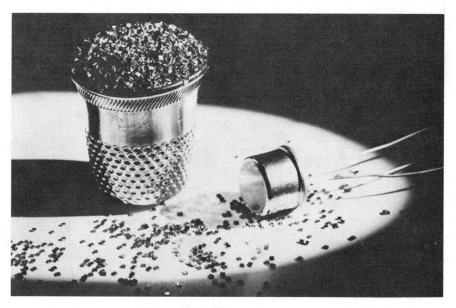

Figure 15.18. Computer memory.

puter programs "files" since they are a collection of commands. A file could be stored on paper in your filing cabinet or on punched cards, magnetic tapes, disks or any other suitable medium.

The letter K is a very common symbol in the computer field. It represents the number 1,000. Thus, the fact that a computer has "256K bytes of storage" simply means that the memory can store up to 256,000 characters.

The next few years in the computer industry will be characterized by an increasing role for MINICOMPUTERS and MICROPROCESSORS. Figure 15.19 depicts a microprocessor and Figure 15.20 illustrates a minicomputer.

Besides being a great deal smaller in size, these newer machines are significantly less expensive than their larger counterparts. The microprocessor, in particular, is likely to have a significant impact in the medical field (see Commentary 15.2).

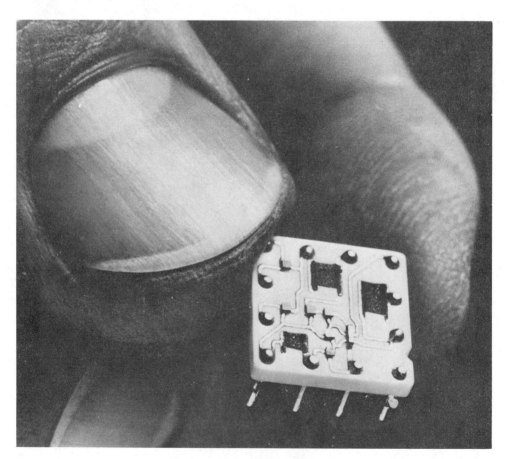

Figure 15.19. A microprocessor.

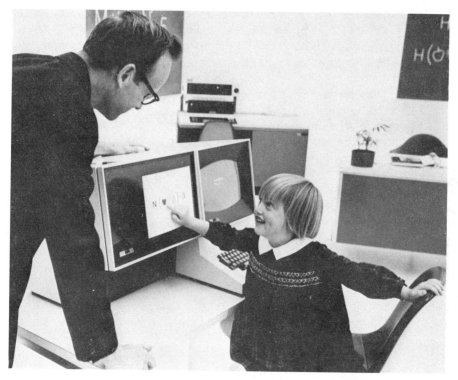

Figure 15.20. A minicomputer.

Commentary 15.2
Microprocessors

In most computers, the central processing unit is contained in a single cabinet. Modern electronics technology is continually advancing, resulting in ever smaller, faster, and more reliable central processing units. This has made possible the development of tiny processing units contained on a single semiconductor chip. These miniature CPUs are called microprocessing units, or microprocessors.

A comparison of the now-classic ENIAC computer with today's computer-on-a-chip reveals the remarkable advances that have been made in computer technology in just 30 years. The ENIAC filled an entire room. Its memory (some 18,000 vacuum tubes) was so large that a person could walk through it. Because of the vacuum tubes, the machine required an enormous amount of power and was not very reliable.

This unit contains a tiny central processing unit and memory, and (except for an input/output section) is truly a tinyl general purpose computer on a single chip. The chip is about the size of the first three letters of the word ENIAC. Yet this tiny computer can perform calculations many times faster than the ENIAC could.

Microprocessors can easily be mounted inside equipment, such as printers, terminals, and machine tools to control their operation. Their cost is falling dramatically—microprocessors are now available in quantity for less than $10 each (this does not include devices for data input or output).

Many experts predict that microprocessors will soon revolutionize our lives. The microprocessor industry is now a $50 million industry; by 1980 it is expected to jump to $450 million. Because of their small size and cost, these devices will be used to control the operation of almost all appliances and devices now controlled by electrical or mechanical means. Potential applications include the following:

Automobiles (carburetion, braking)
Home appliances (ranges, refrigerators)
Home heating systems (minimize energy consumption)
Traffic lights (optimum traffic flow)
Medical instruments (measuring blood pressure)
Toys (guiding electric trains)

One electronics company is already marketing a micro-computer-based control unit to be used in bars. The device precisely measures the ingredients for any type of drink. It also keeps close track of the inventory of ingredients on hand.

When you are seated at a terminal and using the computer, you are ON-LINE or connected directly to the computer. If you are working at a keypunch machine, however, you are OFFLINE.

In most college or university computer centers, one of the most frequently heard terms will be SPSS. The letters stand for the Statistical Package for the Social Sciences. It is a canned package of statistical programs that is quite popular with students. The programs are quite easy to use, very comprehensive, and in addition there is a very readable book on SPSS available.

While this chapter has not presented an exhaustive list of computer terms, it has covered those that are most frequently encountered by the new computer user. There are many sources available should you desire more information on the topics covered in the last few chapters. The university library and bookstore are, of course, two of the obvious choices. Some references that you might find particularly helpful are listed in Appendix G.

CHAPTER

16

Using the Computer as an Aid to Research

THE COMPUTER PROGRAM

Before discussing the ways in which you may use the computer for your own projects and analyses, it is important to discuss the concept of a COMPUTER PROGRAM. A program is a series of instructions that tells the computer to do something. Fortunately, these instructions can be in an Englishlike language. While the computer cannot understand English, there are other programs inside its memory units that translate the Englishlike language into "machine language" (i.e., turn on a switch, add something to a counter, etc.). Thus, if you wanted to have the computer add the numbers 25 and 35 and print out the result, the instructions might look like this:

1   A = 25 + 35
2   PRINT A
3   END

The instructions are numbered and are executed by the machine in ascending order. The first instruction commands the computer to add 35 to 25, put the answer in a memory location, and call that memory location A. The second instruction tells the computer to print out, on a piece of paper, whatever is in memory location A (this is, of course, the answer to the problem). Instruction 3 indicates to the computer that this particular program is finished.

The process of writing a series of instructions like the above is called PROGRAMMING, and the person performing that task is called the PROGRAMMER. Programming is taught at most colleges and universities and is certainly not at all beyond the capabilities of the readers of this text. The interested nursing student would be well advised to take an introductory computer programming course.

There are several Englishlike languages that the human can use to communicate with the computer. Each one has its own particular application and its own translator residing in the computer's memory. The most commonly found languages are FORTRAN, COBOL, PL/1, and BASIC.

FORTRAN is a shortened form of the words *formula tran*slation and is used most often in scientific applications where mathematical formulas are frequently encountered. COBOL stands for *Common Business Oriented Language* and is the computer language that is used in the business community. A COBOL program is structured in sentences and paragraphs and is very easy to follow. For instance, our previous addition example would in COBOL, read

ADD 35 TO 25 GIVING A.
WRITE A
STOP

Programming Language One (PL/1) was developed to include the best features of the COBOL language and the FORTRAN language, and a few new features of its own.

The final language in our list is BASIC and it is the simplest to learn. BASIC is most often used with terminals and in a time-sharing environment. Thus, the user would sit down at a terminal, type in a set of commands in BASIC and tell the computer to execute those commands. The machine would then perform the tasks requested and print the results of any computations back at the terminal.

WRITING YOUR OWN PROGRAM AT A TERMINAL

One way in which the nursing student may utilize the computer is to sit at a terminal and type in her own computer program. It would, of course, be necessary to have had a computer programming course or at least to have gone through a programmed instruction text on the subject.

To illustrate what would be involved in this process, we will introduce a relatively short and simple computer program. This program is to be used by the student to calculate the mean (or average) of 15 numbers.

The first step is to find an available computer terminal. Usually there are several located in the typical computer facility. The keyboard of a terminal very closely resembles that of a standard typewriter (see Figure 16.1).

While the specific steps outlined here will vary slightly from one computer facility to another, the general procedures will be the same.

After locating a terminal, the user merely turns the machine on, and the computer begins typing instructions to the user (sometimes the user must first type HELLO or a similar comment). The computer will usually ask for an ID number and a password (see Figure 16.2). The ID is a number assigned to the user by the computer center. It is used to keep track of who is using the computer (for accounting purposes only). An ID can be obtained from the computer center, a faculty member, or it may be assigned as part of an academic course. The password is a word that is made up by the user and appended to the ID number. The password would, presumably, be known only to that particular user and thus, unauthorized use of that person's ID number would be prevented. Some computer facilities charge the user for the amount of computer time they use while others provide the service free of charge (much like the library provides services). Readers will have to find out the particular policy in effect on their own computer facility.

When the ID number and password are typed in by the user, the computer checks them to see if they are valid. If they are not, the machine will simply retype the request for a valid ID number and password. If the information is valid, the computer usually types READY indicating that the facilities are ready to be used by this particular person.

In our example, the person would now type in her computer program. This is going to be a program in the BASIC language. When looking at figures

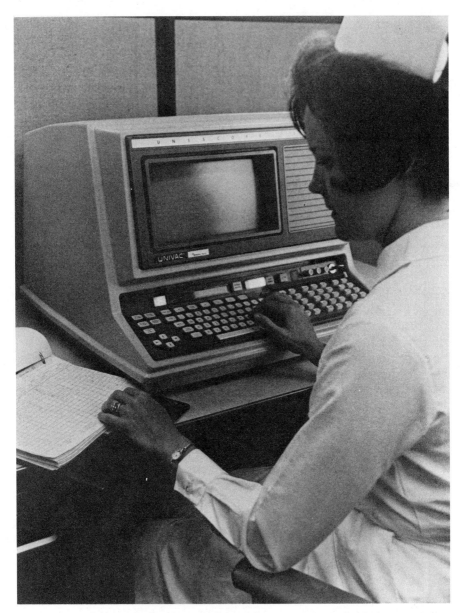

Figure 16.1. The keyboard of a computer terminal.

```
                    SIGNING ON TO THE COMPUTER

HELLO


TIME SHARING SYSTEM AT BOLTON UNIVERSITY    31 MAY 1980

PLEASE ENTER YOUR USER NUMBER AND PASSWORD:

USER NUMBER:   9652

PASSWORD:   HOSPITAL


WELCOME TO THE SYSTEM.


READY
```

Figure 16.2.

that contain actual computer listings, remember that anything in upper case was typed by the computer and anything in lower case was typed by the user.

Before illustrating the actual process of typing in the computer program, it will be listed below and explained in some detail. A program to calculate and print the mean of 15 numbers might look like this (the word might is used because different people would write this program in different ways, although each version would, of course, give the same answer).

```
1    REM A PROGRAM TO AVERAGE 15 NUMBERS
2    PRINT "PLEASE TYPE IN YOUR 15 NUMBERS"
3    PRINT "ONE AT A TIME. MAKE YOUR"
4    PRINT "LAST NUMBER -999 TO INDICATE"
5    PRINT "THAT YOU ARE THROUGH INPUTTING"
6    PRINT "NUMBERS"
7    INPUT N
8    IF N = -999 GO TO 11
9    S = S + N
10   GO TO 7
11   A = S/15
12   PRINT "THE AVERAGE=", A
13   END
```

A line-by-line explanation of this program follows:

Line 1   This instruction is a remark (as indicated by the word REM). The computer ignores this line. The programmer uses remarks to remind her what the program is about.

Line 2–6   The command PRINT tells the computer to print out on a sheet of paper whatever is between the quotes that follow the word PRINT. Thus, lines 2 through 6 print out some instructions for the user to follow.

Line 7   When the computer encounters the command INPUT, it will type a question mark (?) at the terminal and wait for the user to type in a number that the computer will then place in a memory location N.

Line 8   This instruction tells the computer that if the number typed in is a -999, it should go to line 11 for its next command. (If a -999 was typed in, the user is finished typing her 15 numbers and the average can be calculated.)

Line 9   This instruction is reached if line 8 is not true. The command is to add the number the user typed in (N) to a memory location called S. (S will eventually be the sum of all the numbers that we have.)

Line 10   The program then instructs the computer to return to line 7 for the next instruction (the process is repeated).

Line 11   This line can only be reached if all the numbers have been typed in (see explanation of line 8). Once this line is reached, the average (mean) can be calculated. The formula is rather simple: take the sum of all your numbers and divide it by how many numbers you had. In our example, the sum ended up in location S and there were 15 numbers. Thus the average is S divided by 15 (the 1 is the symbol for division in BASIC). The answer is stored in a memory location called A.

Line 12   Once again, the computer prints out whatever is contained in quotes (THE AVERAGE =) and also the contents of memory location A (which is the actual average).

Line 13   This command informs the computer that there are no more commands.

The reader should be fairly familiar now with what the instructions of this particular program will command the computer to do. The user types in these instructions, but the computer does not then execute them. It is only after *all* of the instructions have been typed in *and* the user has typed the command RUN that the computer actually begins to perform the task requested by each line. (In fact, before the computer executes the instruction, it checks that line for any mistakes. If the user has made a typing mistake—

for example, spelling the word PRINT as PRNT—the computer will type out a message informing the user of the mistake and requesting that it be corrected before processing continues!)

Let us now return to the nursing student sitting at a terminal. The ID and password have been typed in and accepted and the computer has typed READY. The user then types in the lines of the program that we have just reviewed. Figure 16.3 illustrates this process.

```
                  TYPING A PROGRAM IN BASIC

HELLO

TIME SHARING SYSTEM AT BOLTON UNIVERSITY   31 MAY 1980

PLEASE ENTER YOUR USER NUMBER AND PASSWORD:

USER NUMBER:   9652

PASSWORD:   HOSPITAL


WELCOME TO THE SYSTEM.


READY

NEW
NEW FILE NAME- AVER

READY

1     REM GIVING AVERAGE OF 15 NUMBERS
2     PRINT "PLEASE TYPE IN YOUR 15 NUMBERS."
3     PRINT "TYPE THEM ONE AT A TIME, MAKE YOUR"
4     PRINT "LAST NUMBER -999 TO INDICATE"
5     PRINT "THAT YOU ARE THROUGH INPUTTING"
6     PRINT "NUMBERS."
7     INPUT N
8     IF N = -999 GO TO 11
9     S = S + N
10    GO TO 7
11    A = S / 15
12    PRINT "THE AVERAGE IS", A
13    END
```

Figure 16.3.

```
                    RUNNING A PROGRAM

LIST
AVER            01:58 PM                31 MAY 80

1    REM GIVING AVERAGE OF 15 NUMBERS
2    PRINT "PLEASE TYPE IN YOUR 15 NUMBERS."
3    PRINT "TYPE THEM ONE AT A TIME. MAKE YOUR"
4    PRINT "LAST NUMBER -999 TO INDICATE"
5    PRINT "THAT YOU ARE THROUGH INPUTTING"
6    PRINT "NUMBERS."
7    INPUT N
8    IF N = -999 GO TO 11
9    S = S + N
10   GO TO 7
11   A = S / 15
12   PRINT "THE AVERAGE IS", A
13   END

READY

RUN
AVER            01:59 PM                31 MAY 80

PLEASE TYPE IN YOUR 15 NUMBERS.
TYPE THEM ONE AT A TIME. MAKE YOUR
LAST NUMBER -999 TO INDICATE
THAT YOU ARE THROUGH INPUTTING
NUMBERS
?  2
?  12
?  6
?  9
?  4
?  24
?  8
?  34
?  6
?  22
?  67
?  4
?  15
?  13
?  7
?  -999
THE AVERAGE IS 15.5333

READY
```

Figure 16.4.

After typing in the program, the user types the command RUN and the computer begins to execute the instructions (see Figure 16.4). First, the instructions are printed, and then the computer types a question mark (waiting for the user to type in the numbers). After the 15 numbers have been entered, the user types -999 (the signal that there are no more numbers). The computer then responds with the answer. The final line typed by the computer indicates how long it took the computer to solve that particular problem.

These concepts of a program are important to the nursing student for two reasons. First, they may help to dispel some of the mystique that surrounds computers and their use. Second, perhaps occasions may arise when the nurse researcher wishes to design programs to solve a particular assignment or problem. It is hoped that some of this material might motivate the student to pursue relevant computer courses.

USING OTHER PROGRAMS AT A TERMINAL

The nursing student does not have to take a computer course in order to be able to use the resources of the machine. Fortunately, there are a large number of computer programs that other people have written (and tested) that are "in the memory" of the computer. These programs are specially designed so that a person may use them without any knowledge of programming. When RUN, the programs ask questions of the user and, in response to these questions, perform the tasks necessary to fulfill the user's needs. These computer programs are usually called CANNED programs or LIBRARY PROGRAMS. Every computer facility has them. The extensiveness of a

Commentary 16.1
Just Relax on the Couch

The program that follows is a particular member of a family of programs that has come to be known as DOCTOR. The family name of these programs is ELIZA. This name was chosen because these programs, like the Eliza of Pygmalion fame, can be taught to speak increasingly well. DOCTOR causes ELIZA to respond roughly as would certain psychotherapists (Rogerians). ELIZA performs best when its human correspondent is initially instructed to "talk" to it, via the typewriter, of course, just as one would to a psychiatrist.

A typical conversation is the following:

Men are all alike.
IN WHAT WAY
They're always bugging us about something or other.
CAN YOU THINK OF A SPECIFIC EXAMPLE
Well, my boyfriend made me come here.
YOUR BOYFRIEND MADE YOU COME HERE
He says I'm depressed much of the time.
I AM SORRY TO HEAR YOU ARE DEPRESSED
It's true. I am unhappy.
DO YOU THINK COMING HERE WILL HELP YOU NOT TO BE UNHAPPY
I need some help, that much seems certain.
WHAT WOULD IT MEAN TO YOU IF YOU GOT SOME HELP
Perhaps I could learn to get along with my mother.
TELL ME MORE ABOUT YOUR FAMILY
My mother takes care of me.
WHO ELSE IN YOUR FAMILY TAKES CARE OF YOU
My father.
WHAT RESEMBLANCE DO YOU SEE BETWEEN YOU AND YOUR FATHER
You are not very aggressive but I think you don't want me to notice that.
WHAT MAKES YOU THINK I AM NOT VERY AGGRESSIVE
You don't argue with me.
WHY DO YOU THINK I DON'T ARGUE WITH YOU
You are afraid of me.
DOES IT PLEASE YOU TO BELIEVE I AM AFRAID OF YOU
My father is afraid of everybody.
WHAT ELSE COMES TO MIND WHEN YOU THINK OF YOUR FATHER
Bullies.
DOES THAT HAVE ANYTHING TO DO WITH THE FACT THAT YOUR BOYFRIEND MADE YOU COME HERE

(The above is not as difficult to program as it may seem, since it all revolves around two simple principles: repetition and key words. The repetition works as follows: If the user types something like
I hate my mother.
the computer can respond
WHY DO YOU HATE YOUR MOTHER
The computer has simply used the input sentence to phrase a similar sentence and carry on the conversation. This is what a "leader" on a talk show does or what a psychologist often does.

The second principle is scanning for key words. Each input sentence can be checked for common key words such as dislike, happy, depressed, and so forth. Then one of several "stock" responses can be generated. Even though the above computer conversation may look fairly intelligent on the machine's side, a closer examination will indicate that the computer program really contributes very little.

J. Weizenbaum: Eliza. From "Contextual Understanding by Computer". Communications of The ACM, Vol 10, no. 8, 1967

particular library will, of course, vary from facility to facility. For example, the following is a partial listing of programs at one computer center.

TALLY	Calculates the mean, range, highest value, lowest value and provides some summary statistics for a list of numbers entered by the user.
PLOT	Plots numbers on a graph.
TEACH	Teaches the user the fundamentals of computer programming.
INTEREST	Calculates the interest on a loan for a specified number of years.
CALENDAR	Provides the user with a calendar for any given year
TTT	Plays tic-tac-toe with the user.
HIST	Draws histograms of the user's data.
QUEST	Tallies the results of up to 100 questions on a questionnaire and presents the results in tabular form as percentages.
GRADER	Keeps track of student grades throughout a semester.
MEDIAN	Calculates the median for a list of numbers supplied by the user.
BANNER	Directs the computer to print a large sign of the user's choice
T-TEST	Performs the statistical t-test on the user's data
SUMUL	Solves a set of simultaneous linear equations

As you can see from this brief list, the applications include statistical analyses, mathematical applications, business programs, computer games, and some educational applications. The list is called brief because these particular programs were selected from a typical computer center library that contained over 700 programs in all.

What is more important is that these programs are quite simple to use. Once the user has signed onto the computer system (with the proper ID and password) and the computer has responded READY, one of these programs can be "called up." The user need only type the word RUN followed by the name of the library program she wishes to use. The computer then takes over and asks any appropriate questions about that particular application. Figure 16.5 displays an actual computer listing of a session in which the user wanted to use the canned program TALLY to obtain a mean for a set of numbers. After the user has typed RUN TALLY, the computer prints out the appropriate answers.

Note that the program "led" the user into supplying the appropriate information needed to solve the problem by asking questions. In many li-

```
                RUNNING A LIBRARY PROGRAM

RUN TALLY

THIS PROGRAM WILL COMPUTE THE MINIMUM,
MAXIMUM, RANGE AND MEAN OF A SET OF
NUMBERS THAT YOU TYPE IN AT THIS COM-
PUTER TERMINAL.

TYPE IN AS MANY NUMBERS AS YOU LIKE, ONE
AT A TIME.  WHEN YOU ARE THROUGH TYPING IN
NUMBERS, TYPE IN THE LAST NUMBER AS -999.

O.K. NOW TYPE IN THE NUMBERS.

?   5
?   10
?   15
?   20
?   50
?   100
?   75
?   25
?   25
?   25
?   -999

THERE ARE 10 NUMBERS IN THE SET
THE MAXIMUM IS 100
THE MINIMUM IS 5
THE RANGE IS 95
THE MEAN IS 35

READY
```

Figure 16.5.

brary programs, if a question is unclear to users, they may type HELP (or some other code) in response to the question. Naturally, all of these capabilities have to be built into the computer program by the programmer.

Let's carry through one final example from start to finish. Suppose that the nursing student has sent out the questionnaire illustrated in Figure 16.6.

A NURSING RESEARCH QUESTIONNAIRE

PLEASE CIRCLE THE ANSWER THAT BEST DESCRIBES YOUR
RESPONSE TO EACH OF THE FOLLOWING QUESTIONS. A '1'
MEANS STRONGLY DISAGREE, A '2' MEANS DISAGREE, A '3'
MEANS AGREE, AND A '4' MEANS STRONGLY AGREE.

1. I do not expect to ever use my nursing research skills.
    1   2   3   4

2. I expect that computers will have a significant impact on my profession.
    1   2   3   4

3. I consider myself to be strong in mathematics.
    1   2   3   4

4. I enjoy doing statistics.
    1   2   3   4

5. I enjoy reading mystery stories.
    1   2   3   4

6. I chose nursing because of the job opportunities in the field.
    1   2   3   4

7. I plan to continue in nursing even if I raise a family.
    1   2   3   4

8. I am satisfied with the nursing education that I received.
    1   2   3   4

9. I would enjoy being a nursing supervisor.
    1   2   3   4

10. I think that graduate school is necessary in order to move up in the
    nursing profession.
    1   2   3   4

Figure 16.6.

In this example, there are ten questions. Each question has five possible
answers. In order to present the results of the study, the student wishes to
know how many people answered 1 to question 1, how many people answered 2, to question 1, and so on for all the questions. In fact, it would be
preferable if all of the results were tabulated as percentages. For example, for
question 1 the results might be:

QUESTION	1	2	3	4	5
1	25	15	40	20	0

Thus 25 percent of the people circled 1 as their answer to the first question.
Fortunately, there is a library program available to perform this analysis for
the student.

Let's assume that the nursing student has 12 questionnaires returned. (While this number of questionnaires could just as easily have been tabulated by hand, it is selected here solely because of limitations of space. This example would work in the same way if 1,000 questionnaires had been returned.)

For convenience, the nursing student has the stack of questionnaires at the terminal. After signing on the system with the ID and password, the student types the command RUN QUEST. The computer retrieves the program QUEST from its program library (in memory) and executes it for the student. Figure 16.7 illustrates the execution of this program.

The data that are typed in by the student are copied directly from each of the questionnaires in the pile beside her. Thus, the first line of information

```
                RUNNING THE QUESTIONNAIRE ANALYSIS PROGRAM

RUN QUEST

QUEST    11:30 AM                                    11 JUNE 80

DO YOU NEED INSTRUCTIONS ABOUT HOW TO USE THIS PROGRAM ? YES

THIS PROGRAM WILL PERFORM AN ELEMENTARY ANALYSIS OF A SIMPLE
QUESTIONNAIRE.  THE PROGRAM ACCEPTS YOUR DATA AND PREPARES
A FREQUENCY DISTRIBUTION FOR EACH QUESTION.  EACH QUESTION
MUST HAVE NUMERIC ANSWERS AND THESE ANSWERS MUST BE BETWEEN
0 AND 9.  YOU MAY HAVE UP TO 100 QUESTIONS ON YOUR QUESTION-
NAIRE AND AS MANY QUESTIONNAIRES AS YOU WISH.

TO USE THE PROGRAM, YOU SHOULD TYPE IN (WHEN ASKED) ALL OF
THE ANSWERS TO ONE QUESTIONNAIRE.  THIS PROCESS IS REPEATED
UNTIL ALL OF THE DATA ON ALL OF YOUR QUESTIONNAIRES HAS BEEN
ENTERED.  THE PROGRAM WILL THEN PRINT THE FREQUENCY DISTRIBU-
TION FOR EACH QUESTION.

IT OFTEN HELPS TO DO ALL QUESTIONNAIRE CODING BEFORE ENTERING
YOUR DATA INTO THE COMPUTER.

YOU MUST KEEP TRACK OF WHAT A PARTICULAR RESPONSE TO A QUESTION
REPRESENTS SO THAT YOU CAN INTERPRET THE OUTPUT.  THAT IS,
YOU WILL HAVE TO REMEMBER THAT AN ANSWER OF '4' TO QUESTION 3
MEANT 'STRONGLY AGREE".  THE COMPUTER WILL ONLY BE TELLING YOU
WHAT PERCENTAGE OF ALL YOUR RESPONDENTS ANSWERED '3' (NOT
WHAT IT MEANS).

TO BEGIN THIS PROGRAM, TYPE RUN QUEST AND DO NOT ASK FOR THE
INSTRUCTIONS TO THE PROGRAM.


READY
```

Figure 16.7.

```
        ENTERING DATA TO THE QUESTIONNAIRE ANALYSIS PROGRAM

RUN QUEST

QUEST        02:30 PM                          11 JUNE 80

DO YOU NEED INSTRUCTIONS ABOUT HOW TO USE THIS PROGRAM
? NO

HOW MANY QUESTIONNAIRES DO YOU HAVE
? 12

HOW MANY QUESTIONS ON EACH QUESTIONNAIRE
? 10

PLEASE TYPE IN THE ANSWERS TO EACH QUESTIONNAIRE.  THAT IS,
EACH TIME A ? APPEARS YOU SHOULD ENTER THE 10 ANSWERS TO THE
NEXT QUESTIONNAIRE.  SEPARATE ALL NUMBERS BY A COMMA.

PLEASE BEGIN ENTERING YOUR DATA

?   1,3,2,4,2,2,1,2,3,3
?   2,2,1,2,3,4,3,2,3,2
?   2,2,2,2,3,3,1,2,1,1
?   3,3,2,2,3,4,4,4,2,1
?   1,1,1,1,1,2,3,2,1,3
?   1,4,4,4,4,2,3,2,3,4
?   1,2,2,2,2,4,3,4,4,1
?   3,2,3,2,3,3,3,3,1,2
?   4,4,4,4,1,1,1,2,1,3
?   4,3,3,3,2,1,4,3,2,1
?   3,2,1,4,1,1,4,2,3,2
?   3,2,1,1,1,3,2,4,4,1
```

	% OF PEOPLE RESPONDING			
QUESTION	1	2	3	4
1	33	16	33	16
2	8	50	25	17
3	33	33	16	18
4	16	41	8	35
5	33	25	33	9
6	25	25	25	25
7	25	8	41	16
8	0	58	16	26
9	33	16	25	26
10	41	25	25	9

Figure 16.8.

typed in corresponds to the questionnaire shown in Figure 16.8 (the first one in the pile).

After the student has typed in the data for all 12 questionnaires, the computer types out the table of percentages that were desired. Again, all of this was possible without any knowledge of programming. The only requirement was for the nursing student to know how to sign on to the computer system and which library program to use. Since there are a large number of library programs available, there is a strong likelihood of there being several applications that are useful to the student.

These, then, are the two major ways in which nursing students can utilize terminals that are connected to their computer. They may write their own programs or take advantage of library programs already stored in the computer. A similar situation would exist in the hospital environment where there are "canned" programs for clinical care. The nurse would type in certain information on a particular patient, and the computer would type out an appropriate nursing plan. Chapter 17 will discuss ways in which you can find out more about what computer resources and programs are available to you.

Commentary 16.2
A Medical Information System

Success is the word used most often to describe El Camino Hospital's computerized medical information system. Operational since 1972, the system has gained total support from virtually all hospital personnel. Physicians, nurses, and administrative people use the system routinely as part of their day-to-day activities. Studies sponsored by HEW have heralded the system for its impact on improving patient care and containing costs. There is vast information available to hospital professionals through simple light pen selections on a CRT screen. The system handles most manual activities, reduces errors, and replaces the nurses' Kardex files. Automated systems technology is vital to the future of health care, and it is a valuable tool for enhancing the quality of patient care and improving the use of labor resources.

The bulk of professional use of the system is the nursing service. Not only do nurses have access to all physician functions (to act as their agents), but many other categories as well. These include all scheduling and preparation functions, nurse charting, central supply ordering, and, most important, a whole new concept of nursing care.

This concept revolves around the building of nurse care plans from expected outcomes contained within the computer system. The care plan helps the nurse to be aware of the expected status of her patients for each day of hospitalization and makes it easier to detect deviations from normal. These same data are then used to carry out nursing audits for quality assurance. The data in the nursing care plan, along with an appropriate list of physicians' orders, are printed at the beginning of each shift for each patient and the care plan is the working document for the oncoming shift. While this is an expensive document in terms of computer time, its use is unquestioned.

Secondary gains for the nurse from this system are overwhelming and easily explain the complete nursing acceptance. New nurses coming on the staff are given a total of eight hours training on the system using didactic and "hands-on" methods. It is considered that this time is roughly equivalent to that required to teach the previous manual system.

Evaluation of a Medical Information System in a Community Hospital. U.S. Department of Health, Education and Welfare, 1976.

USING PUNCHED CARDS FOR YOUR COMPUTER WORK

If your computer facility does not have terminals available, or if you prefer not to use them, the procedures that you follow will vary somewhat from those described above. The same analyses can usually be performed, the only difference is that the turnaround time is usually somewhat longer.

Before discussing in detail the steps you would follow in using punched cards with the computer, it would be useful to discuss how those cards are prepared. Figure 16.9 shows a keypunch machine. The keypunch is not connected to the computer. It is merely a machine (not unlike a typewriter) that punches holes in cards that correspond to the keys that are pressed by the typist. All commands, instructions, and data must be punched on these cards and then read into the computer's memory through the card reader. The reader may wish to refer back to Commentary 15.1 for a review of the punched card.

It does not take long to get used to using a keypunch. Figure 16.10 is a schematic of the keypunch machine. Blank cards are placed in the card-feed hopper. As the keypuncher types information, a card passes through the punching station and ends up in the card stacker. When the keypuncher has completed all the necessary typing, the card stacker will contain the punched deck. A close up view of the keyboard of this machine is shown in Figure 16.11 Notice how similar the keyboard is to that of a typewriter.

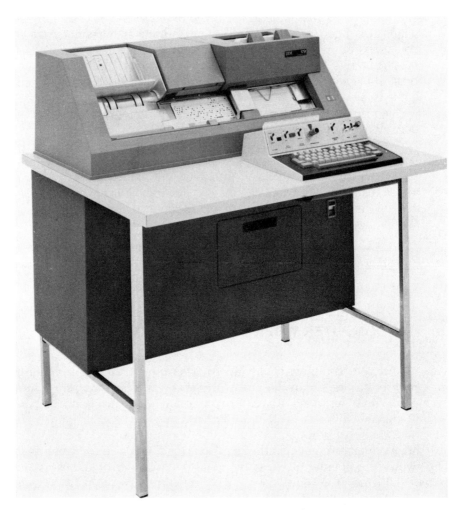

Figure 16.9. A keypunch machine.

The detailed steps that one would follow in preparing cards for keypunching would be:

1. Turn on the machine (the switch is underneath the desklike top, on the right-hand side).
2. Turn on the PRINT and AUTO FEED switches located above the keyboard. The PRINT switch ensures that what you type is also printed on the card. The AUTO FEED switch ensures that blank cards are continually fed into the punching station.

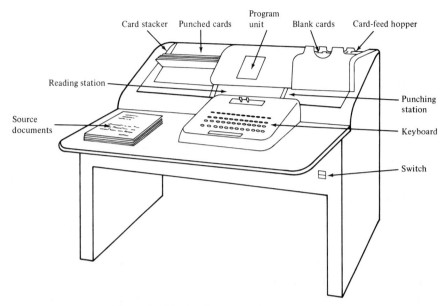

Figure 16.10. A schematic of the keypunch.

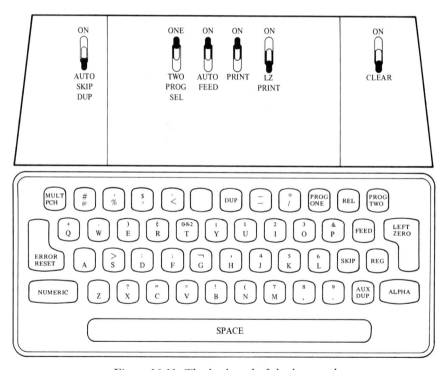

Figure 16.11. The keyboard of the keypunch.

3. Make sure the cards in the card-feed hopper have not previously been punched.
4. If the card-feed hopper is empty or you desire different cards, place your cards in the hopper facing forward with the 9 edge down.
5. Press the FEED button twice. This will prepare your first card for keypunching.
6. Keypunch your information. Press the NUMERIC key for all upper case symbols and numbers.
7. Press the REL (release) key to position the next card for keypunching.
8. Continue this procedure until all the necessary cards have been prepared.

After a few sessions of actual keypunching, you will be expert at preparing these data. One word of caution. When punched cards are used, the computer is very particular about where on the card the information may be punched. When working at the keypunch, it is often useful to know which of the 80 columns you are about to use. This can be determined by looking at a pointer located in a glassed area in the center of the machine. The arrow will be pointing at the number of the column to be punched next. Since corrections cannot be made on a punched card, if you make a mistake while typing, press the REL key to skip to the next card and begin typing that card over again. (Be sure to remove the error card from your final punched deck).

If large amounts of data need to be prepared, many people find it more convenient to have their data punched by a professional keypunching service. Sometimes this group is part of the computer center itself, and other times one must refer to the Yellow Pages for a nearby office. Although there is a charge for this service, it is often quite reasonable and the time saved coupled with virtual error-free preparation often compensates for the charges.

Suppose the nursing student wishes to prepare the program for calculating the mean (discussed earlier) on punched cards. First, it is necessary to comment that the BASIC language is not available using punched cards, so some other computer language will have to be used. We will use FORTRAN. You will see that, for such a simple program, there are very few differences.

The same program listed at the beginning of this chapter is shown as a deck of punched cards in Figure 16.12. The numbers that appear in columns 73 to 80 are sequence numbers that indicate the order of the cards. The c punched on card 1 indicates that this card contains a COMMENT and should be ignored by the computer. Card 2 commands the computer to read a number, place it in a memory location, and call that memory location NUMBER. The number can be found on a punched card following the END command.

Card 3 instructs the computer that if the number 999 is found on a data

```
            A  FORTRAN  PROGRAM  TO  AVERAGE
                     FIFTEEN  NUMBERS

C          AVERAGE  OF  FIFTEEN  NUMBERS      001

     7   READ,  NUMBER                        002

         IF  (NUMBER  .EQ.  -999)  GO         003
         TO  11

         SUM  =  SUM  +  NUMBER               004

         GO  TO  7                            005

    11   AVG  =  SUM  /  15                    006

         PRINT,  AVG                          007

         END
```

Figure 16.12

card, the computer should go to the command labeled 11 for the next command. (This command is to begin calculating the average.)

If the number is not equal to -999, the next card is processed. The command here is to add the contents of the memory location NUMBER (our number) to another memory location called SUM. Thus, the numbers are being added up.

Card 5 commands the computer to go to the card labeled 7 for the next command (i.e., read the next number from the next data card).

Card 6 is reached only when all of the numbers that were to be added up have been processed by the computer. This card then calculates the average.

Card 7 instructs the computer to print the answer and card 8 signifies that there are no more instructions for the computer to follow.

Once again, while the nursing student should be able to follow what is taking place in the above sample program, a thorough understanding of a computer programming language necessitates taking an introductory programming course.

Let's assume now that our nursing student has the deck of punched cards illustrated in Figure 16.13. Every computer facility requires that at least two cards be added to the beginning of the user's deck. The first gives the user's name and account number and the second gives the name of the computer language being used (in this case FORTRAN). The account number is necessary so that computer usage can be accounted for. The language name is required so that the computer can know which language translator will be needed for which program. Armed with this deck of cards, the student is now prepared to use the computer. The procedure would be something like the following.

The user would bring the deck of cards to the card reader. (At some facilities, this machine is operated by the computer center staff, while at other facilities it is operated by the users themselves). After the cards have been processed through the card reader, the user retrieves the deck (the computer has copied what was on the cards into its memory) and returns later to pick up the results. Once again, the time between the submission of the deck of cards and the retrieval of one's output (TURNAROUND time) varies from computer center to computer center. You will become aware of the best times to submit your programs as you become more familiar with your facility.

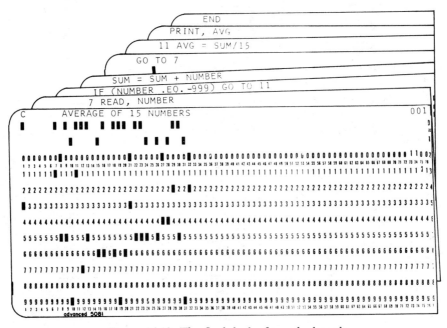

Figure 16.13. The final deck of punched cards.

BOSTON   COLLEGE   COMPUTING   CENTER   3:30 PM   9/30/80

```
C     AVERAGE OF FIFTEEN NUMBERS
    7 READ, NUMBER
      IF (NUMBER .EQ. -999) GO TO 11
      SUM = SUM + NUMBER
      GO TO 7
   11 AVG = SUM / 15
      PRINT, AVG
      END
```

35.0

Figure 16.14. The output from the card oriented program.

In our current example, the output that would result from the program is pictured in Figure 16.14. Just as with programs typed at a terminal, the computer will identify any typing errors you might have made and on which card they occurred. If errors were made, new cards will have to be keypunched to replace those with errors, and the entire deck resubmitted.

Commentary 16.3
Drug Monitoring

Rockland State Hospital in New York is a mental institution with a 6,500-bed capacity and a staff of about 2,000 employees. As a mental hospital, much of its treatment is drug therapy. Thus keeping track of the use of drugs is important to the hospital both to analyze the effects of its treatments, and as a matter of operational control. It is part of a multistate, multifacility network of mental hospitals and community health centers that uses a computer communications network to share data and data-processing facilities.

The Rockland State drug-monitoring system provides a complete record of the patient's pharmacological treatment. Record is kept of the ward location, treating physician, legal status, diagnosis, and drug therapy. The basic input documents are patient status and location change forms and the drug order form.

Let us follow a typical patient into the system. When he arrives at the reception center, the evaluation of his illness and therapy begins. He may stay at the reception center anywhere from a week to several months, and that is where the record begins. That patient's history and results of the mental exam are recorded. His need for medication is determined by a doctor and recorded by the computer, and the computer also completes a number of legally required forms. When the patient's stay at the reception center ends, he may be transferred to one of the treatment centers, discharged from the hospital, or moved to another dormitory. All of these changes are recorded in the computer, which fills out the appropriate forms. When a patient is transferred from one building to another, his drug orders are cancelled and new ones must be created by a doctor, thus preventing inappropriate treatment. Any change in the patient's drug regimen is instituted by a doctor giving an order to the computer. If the patient is given leave to visit home, the number of days of absence granted is noted in the computer. If he doesn't return on the scheduled date, his drug orders are cancelled.

In many people-processing systems the basic transaction involves a legal document. The drug order form is a legal document that must be part of the patient's medication orders. The administration of the hospital takes great care to check these orders by hand and uses many administrative review steps to be certain that errors of type and dosage are not made. For example, each week, lists of every patient's drug regimen are produced for each physician and supervisor, by building and ward. The nursery staff also uses this same list for individual patient treatment.

Again, the operational data provide the administrative data. An inventory of drugs is kept at the pharmacy and in each building. Each patient's drug dosage is subtracted from this record. Monthly physical inventory and records of drug use are checked to determine reorder levels and budgets required to buy drugs. This kind of tight control also helps prevent theft.

After many years of use, the hospital has established the advantages of its drug control system: relief from routine, time-consuming paperwork, accurate reports on the drug regimen and history of each patient, close administrative control of the stocking and use of drugs, and statistical analysis of the results of treatment.

Source: Charles Mosmann and Stanley Rothman. Computers and Society. California, SRA, 1976.

USING OTHER COMPUTER LIBRARY PROGRAMS

One package of programs that is quite widely used is the Statistical Package for the Social Sciences (commonly called SPSS). This set of computer programs is very popular because

1. It is very easy to use.
2. It is widely available.

3. It can perform a detailed analysis of data.
4. It can prepare extremely good tables and charts.
5. It is excellent for summarizing the results of a questionnaire.

While space is too limited for a thorough presentation of the uses of SPSS, we shall cover one application in detail.

First, any serious user of SPSS must obtain a copy of the major reference guide: *Statistical Package for the Social Sciences* by Nie, et al (McGraw-Hill 1975).

Let us assume that a researcher has received the results from the questionnaire pictured in Figure 16.15 and wishes to summarize the findings. The following steps indicate what may take place in order to get from the "completed questionnaire" to the "computer output."

STEP 1: Code the Questionnaire

The questionnaire may have to be coded. That is, numeric values may have to be assigned to the answers on the questionnaire. Open-ended questions may have to be categorized and so forth. The data must ultimately be in a "machine readable" form and this form is most often "numbers." Figure 16.16 illustrates how this particular questionnaire might be coded. Note that coding is different from scoring (adding up the results of several questions). Scoring can be done more easily by the computer. In fact, if there are any

---

Sample SPSS Questionnaire

Please answer the following questions:

1. In the presidential election of 1976 did you favor Mr. Ford, Mr. Carter or neither candidate?
(Circle one)
    (F) Mr. Ford
    (C) Mr. Carter
    (N) Neither candidate
2. What is your sex? (Circle one)
    (F) Female
    (M) Male
3. What was your approximate letter grade in your political science course? (Circle one)
    A   B   C   D   F
4. What was your income in 1979?

Figure 16.15

Coding a Questionnaire			
Questionnaire	Presidential Favorite	Sex	Grade	Income (000)
1	F	M	B	23
2	C	M	B	18
3	C	M	B	15
4	F	F	A	15
5	F	M	A	28
6	C	M	B	15
7	C	F	B	20
8	C	M	B	20
9	F	M	A	16
10	F	M	A	34
11	N	F	A	15
12	C	F	A	30
13	N	M	B	26
14	C	F	A	18
15	C	M	B	20

Figure 16.16

"calculations" that must be performed on the data, the researcher should leave them for the machine.

In any case, the data can be coded on the user's own coding form or directly on the questionnaire itself. The objective is to make the data easy to read for the person who is preparing the data for input to the computer program. Chapter 10 discussed some of the techniques that could be used to ease the entire coding process.

Let us assume that these particular data are to be keypunched onto cards for input to an SPSS program. The key point to remember here is that the data must be punched consistently—that is, each questionnaire should have its information punched in the same locations on each punched card. For example, if the answer to question 5 was being punched in column 9 of a punched card, every question should have question 5 punched in column 9 of its corresponding punched card.

STEP 2: Select the Software Package To Be Used

SPSS is not the only set of computer programs available for processing and analyzing data. Other common packages are BMD (Biomedical) and DATATEXT. Researchers should use the package that is available to them in their particular setting.

STEP 3: Which programs from the package seem appropriate?

The answer to this question depends entirely on the objectives of the study. There may be a need to summarize the data in tables, prepare histograms, or perhaps perform some statistical tests to verify a hypothesis of the researcher.

Some of the programs available with spss are:

DESCRIPTIVE STATISTICS	PARTIAL CORRELATION
FREQUENCY DISTRIBUTIONS	MULTIPLE REGRESSION ANALYSIS
CROSSTABULATIONS	ANALYSIS OF VARIANCE
T-TEST	DISCRIMINANT ANALYSIS
CORRELATION ANALYSIS	FACTOR ANALYSIS
SCATTER DIAGRAM PLOTS	

For this particular presentation we will be using the FREQUENCIES program and the CROSSTABULATION program. It should be noted that the spss manual mentioned earlier provides a thorough explanation, with examples, of all of the programs in the package.

```
                        SPSS PROGRAM LISTING

(A)   RUN NAME           QACS SURVEY
(B)   VARIABLE LIST      PRES,SEX,GRADE,INC79
(C)   INPUT FORMAT       FIXED (A1,1X,A1,1X,A1,1X,F2.0)
(D)   N OF CASES         15
(E)   INPUT MEDIUM       CARD
(F)   VALUE LABELS       PRESS ('F') FORD ('C') CARTER ('N')
                         NEITHER/SEX ('F') FEMALE ('M') MALE
(G)   FREQUENCIES        GENERAL = PRES GRADE
(H)   OPTIONS            8.9
(I)   STATISTICS         ALL
(J)   READ INPUT DATA
(K)   F M B 23
      C M B 18
      C M B 15
      F F A 15
      F M A 28
      C M B 15
      C F B 20
      C M B 20
      F M A 16
      F M A 34
(L)   FINISH
```

Figure 16.17.

STEP 4: Writing the spss Program

Writing a "program" for spss is not at all like writing a computer program in a computer language (BASIC, FORTRAN, COBOL). Actually, most of the spss program consists of describing your data. What do they look like? What should things be called? Perhaps the best way to illustrate this concept is by looking at an actual spss program. Figure 16.17 shows an spss program that will process the data from the questionnaire. The numbers at the extreme left in brackets are *not* part of the program itself, but are only provided as a reference for the discussion that follows. Note that each line is divided into two "fields." The information in the first field begins in column 1 of the card and the information in the second field begins in column 16.

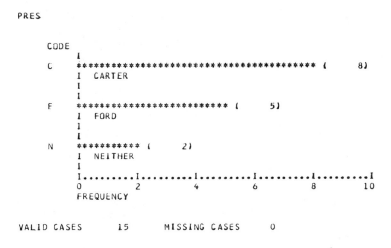

Figure 16.18. SPSS program output.

GRADE

CATEGORY LABEL	CODE	ABSOLUTE FREQ	RELATIVE FREQ (PCT)	ADJUSTED FREQ (PCT)	CUM FREC (PCT)
A	6	40.0	40.0	40.0
B	9	60.0	60.0	100.0
	TOTAL	15	100.0	100.0

GRADE

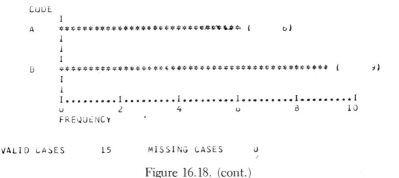

VALID CASES   15   MISSING CASES   0

Figure 16.18. (cont.)

Item	Description

(a)   The RUN NAME is a name you give this particular project. This name will be printed on the top of every page of your computer generated output.

(b)   The VARIABLE LIST card is where you identify the names of the variables used in your study. These are name that you make up. They must, however, be listed in the same order in which they were punched onto the punched cards (refer back to Figure 16.16).

(c)   The INPUT FORMAT card informs the computer of exactly where on the punched card the above variables were punched. There are three symbols that may appear in this statement

A represents a column of alphanumeric data
X represents skipping a column
F represents numeric data

There are two digits after the F; the first indicates how many total digits there are in the variables; the second indicates how many of these are decimals. Thus, a variable with a value of 16.35 would have F4.2 as its input format. Note how the description in parentheses corresponds to the way in which all the data were punched.

(d)   N OF CASES informs the computer how many sets of the data were to be analyzed. Thus, for our example there were 25 questionnaires.

(e)   The INPUT MEDIUM card lets the computer know whether the data can be found on magnetic tape or on punched cards.

(f)   VALUE LABELS are optional but can greatly enchance the computer output by having your choice of labels printed with each table. Note that the value labels inform the computer what each of the coded values represent. Thus, for the variable AGE, a 1 means "under 25," a 2 means 25 to 34, and so on. As a result, wherever a 2 might appear as a label for one of your tables, the words 25 to 34 will also appear.

(g)   The FREQUENCIES card is, actually, the request for the program called FREQUENCIES. This program prints out the frequency of each response to any of the variables in your study. For example, you might wish to have the percentage of male and female respondents, or perhaps the percentages of responses to each possible answer to question 1. The FREQUENCIES program will do this for the researcher. If the user puts the word ALL after the GENERAL = statement, frequencies will be provided for all the variables in the study. If only certain frequencies are needed, these would be listed instead of the word ALL.

(h)   The OPTIONS card allows the user to select from a variety of options available with the program. Each program has its own set of options. The options available with the FREQUENCIES program are:
          Option 1: Ignore missing values.
          Option 2: Do not print labels.
          Option 3: Print in 8½ by 11 inch space.
          Option 4: Save answers on a tape or disk.
          Option 5: Type everything in condensed format.
          Option 6: The two page tables are printed. (used with option 5).
          Option 7: No tables printed (just statistics).
          Option 8: Print a histogram.
          Option 9: Print a reference dictionary.
          Foir this particular request, only options 8 and 9 were discussed.

(i)   STATISTICS may also be requested with each run and they, too, vary from program to program. The statistics available with the FREQUENCIES program are:

MEAN	KURTOSIS
STANDARD ERROR	SKEWNESS
MEDIAN	RANGE
MODE	MINIMUM
STANDARD DEVIATION	MAXIMUM
VARIANCE	

(j)   The READ INPUT DATA card must be placed immediately before the data.

(k)   These are the data from the 25 questionnaires.

(l)   The last card is the FINISH card. This signifies the end of your program.

The output for this program is shown in Figure 16.18.

Usually, one or two additional cards are required by the computer center processing your work. These cards provide miscellaneous billing information to the computer center. You are encouraged to find out what these "Job Control Cards" are and to actually prepare and run the sample program presented in this chapter.

CHAPTER

17

Finding Out What Computer Resources Are Available to You

This chapter is less of a chapter and more of a series of questions the nursing student should ask as she continues to become more familiar with the computer facility available to her. Space has been left for recording the answers to these questions directly in the text. In this way, the material will be immediately available to the nursing student when needed. These questions can be addressed to the computer center staff, faculty, or students in the computer science department, your course instructor, or your friends.

376

WHAT KIND OF COMPUTER IS IT?

Is it an IBM machine? A Honeywell system? Are there tape units? Disks? What are the model numbers? All of this information can be helpful to the user.

Description of computer system:

WHERE IS THE COMPUTER LOCATED?

Sometimes the computer is located in a place other than where the students use it. It is useful to find out where it is and to visit this facility and arrange for a tour.

BUILDING	ROOM NUMBER

DURING WHAT HOURS IS THE COMPUTER AVAILABLE?

At many facilities, time-sharing services are available 24 hours a day, whereas card-processing facilities are more restricted. Weekend hours often differ. When are the buildings locked? What types of services are available during which hours?

DAY	HOURS	SERVICES
MONDAY		
TUESDAY		
SUNDAY		

WHO ARE THE STAFF MEMBERS OF THE COMPUTER CENTER?

Knowing who to go to when you have a question or a problem can be invaluable.

NAME	RESPONSIBILITY	OFFICE	PHONE

WHAT ARE THE HOURS OF THE USER ASSISTANTS?

Most computer centers have user assistants (sometimes staff members, sometimes students) who have regularly scheduled hours posted for assisting users with any problems (large or small) that may occur. These are good people to get to know. They can often save you much time and wasted effort.

USER ASSISTANT	HOURS	DAY

WHAT ARE THE KEY COMPUTER CENTER PHONE NUMBERS?

At times, the machine may be shut down for maintenance or have a particular problem that needs attention. Calling ahead of time can often save a wasted trip to the center from off campus.

PLACE	PHONE NUMBER
MACHINE ROOM	
USER ASSISTANT'S DESK	
SECRETARY	

ARE THERE ANY INTRODUCTORY COMPUTER COURSES AVAILABLE?

You should talk to as many people as possible to find out what courses are available, who are the best teachers, and when the courses are given.

COURSE NAME	PERSON TO CONTACT

WHAT COMPUTER LANGUAGES ARE SUPPORTED BY THIS COMPUTER FACILITY?

If you know what languages are available, you will be in a better position to choose courses. This will also tell you how broad the applications are likely to be.

LANGUAGE	YES	NO
BASIC		
FORTRAN		
COBOL		
PL/1		

IF THE COMPUTER SYSTEM SUPPORTS TIME-SHARING AND HAS TERMINALS, WHERE ARE THEY LOCATED?

Since it is likely that your heaviest use of the computer will be with terminals, it is important to find out all you can about them.

BUILDING LOCATION	HOW MANY TERMINALS	TIME WHEN BUILDING IS AVAILABLE

IF THERE IS A COMPUTER CENTER USER'S MANUAL, WHERE CAN IT BE LOCATED?

Most computer centers make up their own user's manual describing the services provided to customers. This can be an invaluable source of information, particularly to the new user and should be utilized in a similar fashion to a hospital procedure manual.

ROOM NUMBER	PRICE

WHAT STEPS ARE NECESSARY TO GET A USER'S ID NUMBER?

You can't use the computer without an ID number so this may in fact be the most important step.

PERSON TO CONTACT	NAME: OFFICE:
FEE CHARGED FOR ID	
TIME-SHARING ID, NUMBER ASSIGNED	
PERIOD FOR WHICH NUMBER IS VALID	ID NUMBER EXPIRES MONTH DAY YEAR

CARD-PROCESSING ID NUMBER ASSIGNED	
PERIOD FOR WHICH NUMBER IS VALID	ID NUMBER EXPIRES MONTH DAY YEAR

WHAT PROCEDURES ARE NECESSARY TO OBTAIN A LIST OF THE PROGRAMS AVAILABLE IN THE TIME-SHARING USER'S LIBRARY?

Make sure you get a list of all the canned programs in the computer system. Some students who fail to do this waste a lot of time writing their own program or doing a job manually when programs already existed and were "in the library." Know your resources!

PROCEDURE FOR GETTING A DESCRIPTION OF LIBRARY PROGRAMS AVAILABLE VIA
COMPUTER TERMINALS:

WHAT PACKAGES AND PROGRAMS ARE AVAILABLE FOR CARD-PROCESSING USERS AND WHAT ARE THE PROCEDURES FOR USING THEM?

There are many services and programs available to you as a card user. Find out what they are. What are the statistical packages called? What math routines are available? Are there manuals that describe how they work?

PACKAGE OR PROGRAM	REFERENCE

PROCEDURE FOR GETTING A DESCRIPTION OF ALL THE CARD-ORIENTED LIBRARY
PROGRAMS:

WHAT JOB CONTROL CARDS ARE NEEDED AT THE BEGINNING OF EVERY DECK OF CARDS THE USER PROCESSES THROUGH THE COMPUTER?

Every card-oriented job needs at least two computer center job control cards at the beginning of every deck. The first contains the user's ID number and the second tells the computer which language or package is going to be used. Make sure you find out exactly how the information on these cards should be punched (i.e., which columns). Typing any of this information in the wrong columns will cause your program to be ignored.

FIRST JOB CONTROL CARD

INFORMATION	COLUMNS ON CARD

SECOND JOB CONTROL CARD

INFORMATION	COLUMNS ON CARD

OTHER CARDS NEEDED:

WHERE ARE THE KEYPUNCH MACHINES LOCATED?

If you are ever going to do any card-oriented jobs or prepare data on cards, you will need to know where the keypunch machines are located.

BUILDING	ROOM	NUMBER OF MACHINE

FIND OUT IF THE COMPUTER CENTER PRODUCES A MONTHLY NEWSLETTER. IF SO, GET YOUR NAME ON THE MAILING LIST.

Many times, new programs, equipment or services are announced in the computer center's newsletter. If no newsletter is available, find out where the announcements are posted.

NEWSLETTER EDITOR	OFFICE LOCATION

WHERE DOES A USER PICK UP HER OUTPUT FROM A CARD-PROCESSING JOB?

Since the user must wait for some time before results from a card-processing job are ready (turnaround time), it is necessary to know where to go to pick up those results when they are ready.

LOCATION(S)

If you have carefully obtained the answers to all of the preceding questions, you are well on your way to becoming a regular computer user. Keep the notes you made handy, and refer to them as often as necessary until the information becomes second nature to you. Be on the look out for changes that may be made in any of the above material and update your lists accordingly.

PART

VI

Communicating Research Results

    This final section covers the last, and one of the most overlooked, parts of the research process. The results of research studies will only be utilized by nurses when they are presented in an organized and clearly stated fashion. Chapter 18 explains the process of organizing results and drawing appropriate conclusions from the findings. Chapter 19 provides an example of the steps which are commonly taken to turn questionnaire responses into succinct statements that describe a whole sample group. This process is illustrated by using a questionnaire that was administered to a group of undergraduate nursing students. The chapter also contains an analysis of the results that was prepared by two students in the class. Chapter 20 gives guidelines for refining research skills and gives suggestions for ways of staying actively involved with research.

CHAPTER

18

Analyzing and Interpreting Research Results

ORGANIZATION OF COLLECTED DATA

The first step in handling data for a study should include measures to ensure the most efficient use of your research time. Some of the preliminary steps have been covered in Chapter 10 in relation to instruments that have been independently designed by the researchers. The next steps may be important safeguards for novice researchers to follow after the subjects have provided the data:

1. Put all the instruments together in one place. Make sure it is a safe place to which you can gain easy access. Some nurses prefer a locked file and some have been known to use the trunks of their cars, but the key aspect is to keep them all together to prevent any data from being lost.
2. Write down an identification number on each instrument, classify it according to the group in which it belongs. Also, record the total number of questionnaires in each subgroup you may have. This little "key" can save immeasurable hours of confusion when you are analyzing large groups of questionnaires. A group of nursing students who were studying the attitudes of students toward the elderly began their analysis or results with the key in Figure 18.1.
3. Take a blank instrument and prepare an answer key. Be sure to write down the meaning of a high or low score in terms of the overall results. (For instance, place at the top of the questionnaire: high score = positive attitude, if that is the direction of your scoring key.)
4. Prepare "dummy" tables of the results you are anticipating. The example in Figure 18.2 was set up while the questionnaires were being processed. It not only facilitates the actual processing of data, but makes the researchers focus on the kind of information they are seeking.
5. If you are transferring scores from various parts of the instrument, be prepared to put them all (with proper labels) on the page that you will be using the most. In many instruments, this means putting the total scores of the questionnaire on the page containing the demographic data. The less the amount of shuffling through the pages of each individual questionnaire, the better.

Sample Key of Questionnaire

Identification Numbers and Group Representation

Group	I.D. Number	Actual Number in Group (Completed and Returned Questionnaires)
Freshman Nurses	001–050	47
Freshman Non-nurses	051–100	46
Senior Nurses	101–150	44
Senior Non-nurses	151–200	42
TOTAL	200	179

Figure 18.1.

Sample Dummy Table of Expected Results

Class and Major	Attitude Toward Elderly			
	Positive Attitude		Negative Attitude	
	n	x	n	x
Freshman Nurses				
Freshman Non-nurses				
Senior Nurses				
Senior Non-nurses				

Figure 18.2.

SCORING YOUR INSTRUMENT

This process will vary according to the type and style of instrument, but does have several common themes. The major concern here is for accuracy. If the tests are machine scored, make sure the answer key you have constructed is correct. Process the hand-scored questionnaires in an environment that is conducive to concentration. The one overall score you derive for each instrument is the quantification of that instrument. It is a shorthand method for handling a large mass of data (a number of items for each individual) and condensing it into a form that can describe the position of each subject with regard to the factor you are measuring. The process of "scoring" information from interviews or open-ended written questions is somewhat different.

In order to process open-ended material, the researcher should set up categories by sorting the answers according to the major themes present in the responses. This process is best carried out by several individuals so that a group consensus can be established for each heading. The steps involved in this process are as follows:

1. Read over *all* the responses to a particular question to get an idea of the scope of items mentioned. Look for broad trends.
2. Set up categories that are exhaustive (there should be a category available for each and every response—this is generally handled by including

the category *other* or facsimile) and mutually exclusive (each response should clearly fit into only *one* possible category if you have them set up correctly).

3. Place the subject's responses into the categories while keeping track of the number of responses in each one. When you finish, these subtotals should sum to the total number of responses made.

4. Inspect the categories to see if they are truly mutually exclusive (perhaps you can combine two that proved to be very similar).

5. List the categories in order from the most predominant responses to the least popular so you will be able to put the proper emphasis on the categories when you combine them with the other information you have processed.

List of responses by Public Health Nurses to "What is the thing you dislike most about your present nursing position?"

Boring, unchallenging work.
Too many patients to provide quality care.
Paper work
Working environment (i.e., insufficiently equipped clinic).
Lack of recognition of my abilities.
No pats-on-the-back from supervisor.
Forms, forms and more forms.
Forms too lengthy.
Low pay.
No staff education programs.
Too much paper work.
Lousy hours.
Not enough pay.
Length of referral forms.
Travel time to see patients.
Daily log to be filled in by each nurse.
The way my supervisor assigns me my patients.
Always assigned the most difficult cases or the patients who are not wanted by any other nurses.

Not enough time for wholistic approach to patient care.
Huge, unwieldy caseload.
Repetitive data forms to be filled out for each patient contact.
Papers to fill out.
Performing non-nursing clerical duties.
Making out accident reports.
Large number of people to work with in varied clinics.
Lack of intellectual stimulation.
Lack of time for total patient care.
Wasted time on non-essential nursing chores.
Many partial nursing functions which could be completed by an aide.
Lack of a good role model in my supervisor.
Desk type duties.
No intellectual stimulation.

Figure 18.3

The responses listed in Figure 18.3 are actually answers given by 32 public health nurses on one item contained in a questionnaire measuring work satisfaction. The question and each response are listed exactly as they were written.

The researchers who were analyzing the data constructed eight categories and counted the number of responses for each one. The categories were then listed in decreasing order of frequency as follows:

Category	Number of Responses in Category
Paperwork—desk-related duties	10
Lack of time for total patient care	5
Dissatisfaction with supervising personnel	5
Decreased intellectual stimulation	4
Time spent on non-nursing functions	3
Characteristics of the work environment	2
Dissatisfaction with pay	2
Hours	1
Total Responses:	32

Some studies rely on raters, judges, or coders to make judgments about the research data and classify some of the results. The judges should be making accurate appraisals if the results are to be counted upon. The researcher should examine the following areas if proceeding with this type of study.

1. Document the following points:
   · The selection process in securing the judges.
   · The competency they may or may not have in the area.
   · The training they have undergone in specific aspects of this research project.
   · Whether they worked on the project individually or in groups.
2. Check factors affecting the accuracy of the data prior to the judging process:
   · Check the clarity of the rating instructions.
   · Examine the difficulty in executing the task.
   · Are the category labels clear?
   · Consider the amount of agreement between the judges (inter-rater reliability).
   · Is one judge consistently making decisions that are out of line with the rest of the group?
   · Check the setting in which the judgments are being made.

STEPS IN ANALYZING DATA

After ensuring that the responses from each subject have been properly scored or categorized, the researcher should proceed to the next level. This level entails examination of the composite of responses from the entire group of subjects. There are a few steps in the process of analyzing data that can greatly simplify the process if enacted:

1. Look over the information and see what kinds of responses you got from the subjects. This is a quick, overall impression.
2. Review the objective and the scoring of the instrument so you are thoroughly familiar with both.
3. Determine the overall score or rating for the entire group of subjects. In determining the attitude of students toward the elderly, you need to assess whether the overall attitude of the entire subject pool is positive or negative. The first step in analyzing the questionnaires used for the study mentioned in Figure 18.2 is to determine a mean score for all subjects. Then separate the data according to groups if appropriate so that you can get a distinct feeling for the way each one fell. For instance, in examining the data related to Figure 18.2, you might want to look at the attitudes of the sophomore and senior non-nursing students toward the elderly separately in order to get an idea about each group. You would then look at both groups (combined) as "non-nursing students" (both sophomores and seniors) to see how they fared as a total group.
4. Jot down notes to remind you of key points as you proceed.
5. If it is a multipart instrument, break it down into sections that you can comfortably handle and proceed one step at a time with each section.
6. Examine the responses in-depth.
   · Examine each section in detail according to the type of data you have and make comments on what you find.
   · Keep rough notes on each part of your analysis.
   · Fill in dummy tables you prepared before the actual analysis.
   · Recheck to see that you have scored the instrument in such a way to make the most effective use of the responses.
   · After you have reviewed the results of each section, make logical comparisons between the different sections as appropriate.
7. Note any unusual responses.
   If for some reason you notice that a subject gives an unusual response, make note of it. If subjects are giving clues, such as writing in unsolicited responses to a coded question or leaving one particular question blank, jot this down because it may have an influence on your results and can

be noted in the discussion section of the study report. Unusual responses to open-ended questions may add an element of "color" to your discussion section. You may want to "flag" several for later quoting. Normally, the results section deals with the responses of the entire group. Individuals are cited only in special circumstances.

8. Write down your results in as objective a fashion as possible. Remember to describe the entire group and then appropriate subgroups as you see fit. You need to combine questions on the instrument for this process rather than look at the results in terms of each individual item.

9. It may be helpful to put all results on one instrument or in one table (if space permits), so they may all be visualized at once.

10. Construct any figures or tables that would graphically represent a point about your results. Use these devices for something you particularly want to emphasize.

The more organized you can be in inspecting and tabulating the results, the easier the job will be. An example of utilizing some of these steps may help to clarify some of the major points. The authors of this book had always assumed that students were apprehensive about research and some of the allied facets of the research process (statistics and computers). This was based mainly on their personal student experiences, the reports of friends, and the apparent nonverbal messages transmitted by students at the beginning of each semester. But was this really true? Do students have a "negative" attitude toward the research process and is this attitude any different after exposure to a course that attempts to present research in a positive fashion? An attitudinal questionnaire was constructed to find out more objective information on the attitudes of the students. The instrument can be seen in Figure 18.4.

A scoring key was then devised by the authors to ensure accuracy in processing the responses. Note that the Likert scale answering system is utilized and that the key was set up to produce a high score for a positive attitude. This means that some items (1,2,3,5,7,8,10,12,13,15) are scored in a "reverse" fashion to yield a high score for a positive attitude. A copy of the scoring key can be found in Figure 18.5.

The attitude survey was administered to a group of students prior to enrolling in the junior level research course to determine their initial attitude. The questionnaire was given to the same students the semester after the completion of the research coursework (which included experience with statistics and computers) to see if any changes had occurred by the end of their senior year.

The tabulation of results for the student groups according to the time intervals (sophomore - senior) on each item of the questionnaire is presented in Table 18.1. There are separate headings according to the sophomore and senior time interval. All responses are in percentages.

Table 18.1

For each of the following questions, please circle the response that you feel most closely represents how you feel.
(SA = strongly agree, A = agree, U = uncertain, D = disagree, SD = strongly disagree.)

Question	SA		A		U		D		SD	
	sen.	soph.	sen.	soph.	sen.	soph.	sen.	soph.	sen.	soph.
1. The idea of learning about computers makes me uneasy.	0	2.4	32	8.4	8	10.8	44	61.4	16	16.9
2. Computers are of no interest to me.	0	7.2	4	2.4	16	16.9	68	53.0	12	20.5
3. I am not the type who can easily learn how to use computers.	0	1.2	16	7.2	28	20.5	44	54.2	12	16.9
4. A one semester course on computers should be required for all nursing students.	8	4.8	20	25.3	44	42.2	20	21.7	8	6.0
5. Computers will have little influence on my day to day nursing activities over the next few years.	4	1.2	16	6.0	28	44.6	32	32.5	20	15.7
6. I am confident that I can carry out a small research study.	12	1.2	72	1.2	16	13.3	0	68.7	0	15.7
7. Research is of no interest to me.	0	2.4	12	8.4	20	8.4	56	62.7	12	18.1

#	Statement	SA		A		U		D		SD	
8.	I get apprehensive when I think about reading a research report.	0	3.6	12	16.9	8	21.7	72	51.8	8	6.0
9.	Every nursing student should take a required one semester course in research.	8	1.2	68	12.0	8	32.5	12	39.8	4	14.5
10.	You have to go into a specialized field of nursing to do research.	4	4.8	8	15.7	0	32.5	64	37.3	24	9.6
11.	A statistics course should be required for all nursing students.	4	3.6	52	21.7	12	53.0	24	20.5	8	1.2
12.	I feel uncomfortable with numbers and symbols.	16	6.0	28	20.5	4	8.4	36	48.2	12	16.9
13.	A nurse could perform her professional duties just as well without any knowledge of statistics.	4	4.8	20	12.0	48	51.8	24	28.9	4	2.4
14.	I feel comfortable with extracting information from graphs and tables	0	3.6	40	27.7	20	14.5	40	49.4	0	4.8
15.	I skip over the sections on statistical analysis when I read research reports in journals.	4	7.2	52	28.9	12	19.3	32	38.6	0	6.0

Questions # 1, 2, 3, 5, 7, 8, 10, 12, 13, 15 are scored SA(1) A(2) U(3) D(4) SD(5)
Questions # 4, 6, 9, 11, 14, are scored SA(5) A(4) U(3) D(2) SD(1)
Number of students responding: sophomores = 100
seniors = 100

Research Attitude Survey

For each of the following questions, please circle the response that you feel most closely represents how you feel. (SA = strongly agree, A = agree, U = uncertain, D = disagree, SD = strongly disagree.)

1.	The idea of learning about computers makes me uneasy.	SA	A	U	D	SD
2.	Computers are of no interest to me.	SA	A	U	D	SD
3.	I am not the type who can easily learn how to use computers.	SA	A	U	D	SD
4.	A one semester course on computers should be required for all nursing students.	SA	A	U	D	SD
5.	Computers will have little influence on my day to day nursing activities over the next few years.	SA	A	U	D	SD
6.	I am confident that I can carry out a small research study.	SA	A	U	D	SD
7.	Research is of no interest to me.	SA	A	U	D	SD
8.	I get apprehensive when I think about reading a research report.	SA	A	U	D	SD
9.	Every nursing student should take a required one semester course in research.	SA	A	U	D	SD
10.	You have to go into a specialized field of nursing to do research.	SA	A	U	D	SD
11.	A statistics course should be required for all nursing students.	SA	A	U	D	SD
12.	I feel uncomfortable with numbers and symbols.	SA	A	U	D	SD
13.	A nurse could perform her professional duties just as well without any knowledge of statistics.	SA	A	U	D	SD
14.	I feel comfortable with extracting information from graphs and tables.	SA	A	U	D	SD
15.	I skip over the sections on statistical analysis when I read research reports in journals.	SA	A	U	D	SD

Figure 18.4

Overall - More positive attitude about computers, research and statistics after academic coursework and related learning experienced.

Computing:
+favorable attitude overall.

More seniors uneasy in learning about computers after learning exercises with them. (More realistic about it than when sophomores?)

Majority are undecided about having a required Course. (fairly even distribution of those for and against).

Research:
Confidence in ability to carry out a study greatly increased between sophomore and senior years.

A required research Course was favored by more students as seniors (74%) than as sophomores (13.2%)

Experience produced more comfort in reading research (80% as seniors vs 57.8% as sophomores).

Statistics Course:
A required statistics course favored by more than half after actual course work (56% as seniors vs. 25.3% as sophomores).

Not much change in discomfort with numbers and symbols.

More students skip over statistical sections on research reports as seniors (56%) than as sophomores (36.1%). What caused this? Do more students read reports now?

Figure 18.6

High Score = Positive Attitude				
1.	1	2	3	4	5
2.	1	2	3	4	5
3.	1	2	3	4	5
4.	5	4	3	2	1
5.	1	2	3	4	5
6.	5	4	3	2	1
7.	1	2	3	4	5
8.	1	2	3	4	5
9.	5	4	3	2	1
10.	1	2	3	4	5
11.	5	4	3	2	1
12.	1	2	3	4	5
13.	1	2	3	4	5
14.	5	4	3	2	1
15.	1	2	3	4	5

Figure 18.5. Scoring Key for the Research Attitude Survey

The responses can be examined in this table and comparisons made on individual items, subsections (the five questions in the research, computer, and statistical sections are separated by a line), and finally in light of overall attitude change. The notes in Figure 18.6 were made by the authors while they were analyzing the data presented in Table 18.1.

INTERPRETING AND EVALUATING RESEARCH FINDINGS

The interpretations of the data consist of explanations of or probable meanings given to the results by the researchers. Investigators should utilize both their critical-thinking abilities and their creative talents for viewing results in a variety of ways. There are a number of aspects of the overall study that should be reviewed and considered when constructing this section of a report.

· Do the results coincide with your expectations?
· How do the results relate to the broad problem and the specific purpose of the study?
· Do they make sense in light of reality? Common sense? (If not, the first action should be to recheck the scoring and the analysis of results.)
· Was there some outstanding feature of the data that you noted in the process of analyzing the raw data?
· How do the results of subsections relate to the overall findings of the study?
· What is the real meaning of what you've found?
· Are there alternate explanations that could have contributed to the results?
· Were there any unexpected outcomes of the study?
· What is the relationship of your results to the literature in the field?
· How would you comment on the results if you were willing to adopt an adventurous ("far out") position?
· What possible relationships are there between the results and real-life nursing practice?
· Are there any practical applications of the results?

This final step in dealing with study results must include more than running through a checklist that reviews the more technical aspects of research methodology. The researchers should make every attempt to view and comment on the findings so that the applicability to actual nursing practice will be clear to all readers. One model for establishing evaluative criteria, such as feasibility, fit, and congruence with the theoretical basis for practice, is clearly presented in *Nursing Outlook* in an article by Cheryl Stetler and Gwen Marram.[1] Investigators should attempt to go beyond the mere reporting of numbers and place some perspective on the meaning of the data. An example of the presentation of large amounts of numerical tabulations without the loss of meaning or reader interest can be found in two issues of *Nursing 76* and *77*. The two-part presentation of results stems from a questionnaire on the Quality of Health Care in the United States that was answered by over 10,000 nurse readers.[2,3]

The investigator should wrap up a research report with suggestions for conducting future research studies. By the time this step has been reached, the researcher has usually said, "I wish I had done it a different way," numerous times. The researcher is familiar with the various issues involved in the study of this particular problem, and can usually make several useful suggestions that other nurses may heed in designing studies of a similar nature.

REFERENCES

1. C. Stetler and G. Marram: Evaluating research findings for applicability in practice, *Nursing Outlook* 24,9 (1976): 559–563.

2. G. Funkhouser and Nursing 76: Quality of care. Part one, *Nursing 76* 6, 12 (December 1976): 22–31.

3. G. Funkhouser and Nursing 77: Quality of care. Part two, *Nursing 77* 7, 1 (January 1977): 26–33.

CHAPTER

19

A Descriptive Study of and by Undergraduate Nursing Students

One of the best ways to gain an understanding of the research process is to follow an example from beginning to end. This chapter will present part of an actual project that was given to nursing students. The section presented here has been reproduced to demonstrate many of the techniques that may be used to process, analyze, and present results on a particular topic. The introductory material (such as the development of the problem and review of the literature) has been omitted in this write-up and the project will be picked up at midpoint. The example will also show the close integration within the research process of research principles, utilization of statistics, and computer science concepts.

THE PURPOSE OF THE STUDY

The purpose of the study was to describe a group of nursing students on the basis of selected personal and professional characteristics. In addition, the nursing student would get experience in looking at different types of data and gain some facility with analyzing those data and presenting them in a meaningful way.

GATHERING THE DATA

To gather the data necessary to evaluate certain personal and professional characteristics of nursing students, a special questionnaire was designed. This questionnaire included:

1. Biographical questions (some of which were closed-ended or precoded and some of which were open-ended).
2. Questions describing the respondent's ego strength.
3. Questions describing the value profile of the respondent in relation to the particular value of individualistic tendencies.

Several sources were used to create the instrument that is illustrated in Figure 19.1. Part I contains the open-ended and closed-ended biographical questions and describes some of the respondent's personal characteristics. The answers for Part I were recorded directly on the questionnaire. Part II was adapted from the Thomas-Zander Ego Strength Scales.[1] They describe ego strength as being conceptualized in two parts. First is a person's ability to be self-directing and to translate intentions consistently into behavior. Second is the ability to control and discharge tension without disrupting other psychological processes. The form has 27 items answered true or false.

Note that the instructions for Part II indicate that a standard answer sheet will be used to record the answers. A sample standard answer sheet is illustrated in Figure 19.2. This is particularly useful with true-false or multiple choice type questions. Eventually, the answers to Part II will have to be scored to obtain a respondent's score on the ego strength scale. The use of a

Personal and Professional Nursing Characteristics Questionnaire

PRIOR TO FILLING IN THE QUESTIONNAIRE:

Place your ID number in two separate places. First write it on the line provided in the upper right hand corner of this questionnaire. Second, place it in the space labeled identification number in the lower right hand corner of the IBM answer sheet. Do not place your name on any of the papers. Use the NO. 2 Pencil to fill in all the answers.

PART I

Directions: Place your responses directly on this questionnaire. Please answer all questions. Circle only one answer for each question.

1. Nursing Education:
   a. Basic student
   b. RN student
2. When did you decide to become a nurse?
   a. When I was a child (under 12 years old).
   b. In my early teens (13–15 years old).
   c. In the last years of high school (16–18 years old).
   d. After completing high school (19 years old and over).
3. How important is nursing to you?
   a. I regard nursing as my primary, lifelong professional career.
   b. Nursing is interesting, and I will continue in it as long as it fits into other aspects of my life.
   c. Nursing is only a way of earning a living.
   d. I would leave nursing if given an opportunity to do so.
4. What do you think might interfere with or disrupt your nursing plans?
   a. dissatisfaction with nursing.
   b. marriage and/or children.
   c. another career option.
   d. nothing that I can foresee.

Directions: Place your responses in the space provided. Please print or write clearly.

5. What was your primary motivation for choosing nursing as a profession? _____ .
6. What was your reason for selecting a baccalaureate program?____
   _____
7. What appeals least to you about nursing?_____ .
8. What appeals most to you about nursing? _____ .
9. Describe the type of position you plan to work in immediately after graduation from the baccalaureate program: _____
   _____ .

(Continued)

Figure 19.1

10. What professional goal (or goals) do you plan to fulfill within 5 years after graduation from the baccalaureate program? _____
_____ .

11. What is your degree of confidence that you have made the right decision in selecting nursing as a career?
    a. 0–20%.
    b. 40–60%.
    c. 60–80%.
    d. 80–90%.
    e. 90–100%.

PART II
Directions: Fill in all answers for this section on the IBM answer sheet provided. Please make no further marks on this questionnaire.
    Read each of the following statements and decide whether it is *ture* or *false* as applied to you. Mark the answer in the appropriate col-on the IBM answer sheet.

1. I am a very ambitious person.
    a. True
    b. False

2. I am very stubborn and set in my ways.
    a. True
    b. False

3. No one can change my beliefs in which I have strong faith.
    a. True
    b. False

4. I frequently find myself worrying about the future.
    a. True
    b. False

5. I frequently worry about things that never happen.
    a. True
    b. False

6. I give everything I have to what I undertake to do.
    a. True
    b. False

7. I am a calm person in almost any emergency.
    a. True
    b. False

8. Often I feel tense without any good reason.
    a. True
    b. False

9. I am restless or irritable when people make me wait for them.
    a. True
    b. False

(Continued)

Figure 19.1 (cont.)

10. I am always self-reliant and independent in doing my work.
    a. True
    b. False
11. I am one who likes actively to keep busy.
    a. True
    b. False
12. I have an inferiority complex about my abilities to do things.
    a. True
    b. False
13. I have strong beliefs which I will always stand by.
    a. True
    b. False
14. One of my greatest troubles is that I cannot get down to work when I should.
    a. True
    b. False
15. I can work in the midst of a number of distractions.
    a. True
    b. False
16. Whenever I am upset I always get over it right away.
    a. True
    b. False
17. Often I feel that my time is spent aimlessly.
    a. True
    b. False
18. When I decide to do something, I go right to work on it.
    a. True
    b. False
19. I don't like to have to work hard to get things done.
    a. True
    b. False
20. I never persist at things very long without giving up.
    a. True
    b. False
21. I have very definite, established goals in life which I intend to pursue at all costs.
    a. True
    b. False
22. Often I find myself doing and saying things that turn out to be things that shouldn't have been done or said.
    a. True
    b. False
23. Sometimes I don't care whether I get anywhere in life or not.
    a. True
    b. False

(Continued)

Figure 19.1 (cont.)

24. There are odd moments now and then when I suspect I might go to pieces.
    a. True
    b. False
25. Every now and then I lose my temper when things go wrong.
    a. True
    b. False
26. Every now and then I can't seem to make up my mind about things.
    a. True
    b. False
27. I am one who *never* gets excited when things go wrong.
    a. True
    b. False

PART III
Directions:
  These questions have been designed to measure the extent to which you hold each of several general attitudes or values common in our society. Please read each of the statements and select the response which best represents your immediate reaction to the opinion expressed. Select the response which most clearly approximates your *general* feeling.
  Note that this set of questions starts at question 30 on the IBM answer sheet. Follow set up of question 30 for all answers. (a) Strongly agree, (b) Agree, (c) Neither Agree or Disagree, (d) Disagree, (e) Strongly Disagree.
30. To be superior a man must stand alone.
    a. Strongly Agree
    b. Agree
    c. Neither Agree or Disagree
    d. Disagree
    e. Strongly Disagree
31. In life an individual should for the most part "go it alone," assuring himself of privacy, having much time to himself, attempting to control his own life.
    a, b, c, d, or e.
32. It is the man who stands alone who excites our admiration.
    a, b, c, d, or e.
33. The rich internal world of ideals, of sensitive feelings, of reverie, of self knowledge, is man's true home.
    a, b, c, d, or e.
34. One must avoid dependence upon persons or things, the center of life should be found within oneself.
    a, b, c, d, or e.
35. The most rewarding object of study any man can find is his own inner life.
    a, b, c, d, or e.

(Continued)

Figure 19.1 (cont.)

36. Whoever would be a man, must be a non-conformist.
   a, b, c, d, or e.
37. Contemplation is the highest form of human activity.
   a, b, c, d, or e.
38. The individualist is the man who is most likely to discover the best
   road to a new future.   ·
   a, b, c, d, or e.
39. A man can learn better by striking out boldly on his own than he
   can by following the advice of others.
   a, b, c, d, or e.

Copyrighted portions of Part II and Part III reprinted with permission.

Figure 19.1 (cont.)

separate answer sheet will allow for ease in hand scoring since all the answers
appear on a single page. It also paves the way for machine scoring if desired.

Part III of the questionnaire was adapted from a questionnaire by Bales
and Couch that was designed to provide the value profile of the respondent.[2]
The questions used on the nursing student questionnaire were designed to
measure one particular value, that of individualism. The questions used required a Likert scale type of response. Note that the standard answer sheet
can accommodate both true-false responses (as in Section II) and Likert
items (as in Section III).

It is important to note at this point that the questionnaire was designed
using a variety of sources for the questions. Some of the questions were
original, while others were adapted from other studies or instruments. Furthermore, the type of response required for these questions varied. Part I
included both open-ended and closed-ended questions, Part II was made up
of true false questions, and Part III used a Likert scale.

While it is not necessary to mix one's questions in this manner, it is
often the necessary result when you use several different sources and measures in your questionnaire. It is not uncommon to find questionnaires that
contain all Likert scale questions or those with a mixture as in this study. One
important part of constructing an instrument is organization. The questionnaire sections serve an important function. The subject can respond with
ease, and therefore, accuracy. The distinct demarcation between sections,
plus the addition of various instructions to respondents, results in a coherent,
simplified design. Each section has a distinct focus and fairly unified answering system. This results in added ease in filling in the responses, as well as
scoring results.

Now, note some of the general characteristics of this questionnaire.
The instructions are quite clear and they are included for each separate part.
They are designed to be sufficiently specific to cover all questions a subject

Figure 19.2   Sample Standard Answer Sheet

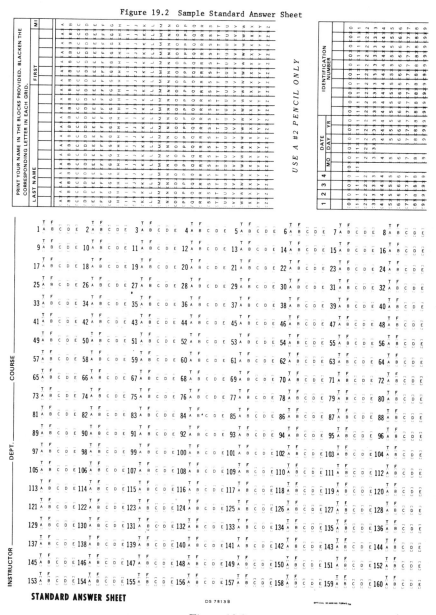

Figure 19.2.

may have about how to proceed. Second, the questionnaire can be completed quickly and easily. It is important not to have a form that is so long that it discourages the respondent. Third, the questions are worded in such a way that misunderstandings and misinterpretations can be avoided. Fourth, the visual layout of the instrument is set up in an orderly and organized fashion to minimize errors of respondents.

Once the questions to be used on the questionnaire were selected, some thought had to be given to how the data would be processed since this would affect the layout of the questionnaire. In this study, a variety of methods will be used to process the data. In particular,

Questions	Type	Method for Processing Data
Part I Questions 1–4	Closed-ended biographical	Computer library program for tallying the frequency of responses.
Part I Questions 5–10	Open-ended biographical	Manual summarization and categorization.
Part I Question 11	Closed-ended biographical	Manual tallying.
Part II Questions 1–27	True-false, ego strength scale	Total score determined for each respondent by scoring with answer key. Computer library program used to obtain descriptive statistics on total scores for entire group. (Need to find mean score and the resulting distribution for the whole group.)
Part III Questions 1–10	Likert scale value profile	Total score determined for each respondent by scoring with answer key. This scoring process involves the handling of five possible scores for each item as opposed to two in the true-false. Computer library program used to obtain descriptive statistics on total scores for entire group. (Need to find mean score and the resulting distribution for the whole group.)

The final step in the process was to distribute the questionnaires to the nursing students involved in the study. They would also be involved, as individuals, in analyzing the data and presenting the results about the entire group. In this particular case, the questionnaires were given to 74 undergraduate nursing students enrolled in an introductory research course.

DATA ANALYSIS

After the questionnaires have been returned, the student must begin the process of tallying, summarizing, and analyzing the data. In this section, we will examine how this is done for several of the questions.

To summarize the results of the first four questions in Part I (the closed-ended biographical questions), the computer program discussed in Section 16.3 was used. As you may recall, this program was a library program in the computer system.

In brief, this program requires the user to first type in the coded responses to each of the first four questions on all the 74 questionnaires. Then, when the program is run, a summary is printed that indicates, for *each* question, the frequency of *each* response. Thus, the program would list, for question 1, the percentage of respondents who were RN students. Figure 19.3 depicts the computer output that resulted from the processing of the questionnaires used in this study.

Note that the data had been entered prior to the "running" of this program. This step basically entailed typing in the response circled by each subject directly from the questionnaire. For a review of how this was done, refer back to Section 16.3. As you can see from Figure 19.3, 90.5 percent of the respondents were basic students and 9.5 percent were RN students. How many of the respondents decided to become nurses while they were in the last years of high school? How many had decided before they were 12 years old?

```
              COMPUTER OUTPUT AS A RESULT OF
              PROCESSING THE QUESTIONNAIRES

DO YOU NEED INSTRUCTIONS ABOUT THIS PROGRAM?

?  NO

HOW MANY QUESTIONNAIRES DO YOU HAVE?   74

HOW MANY QUESTIONS ON EACH QUESTIONNAIRE?   4


NO. ZEROS ONES TWOS THRS FOURS FIVES SIXES SVENS EGHTS NINES
 1    0.0  90.5  9.5  0.0   0.0   0.0
 2    0.0  18.9 37.8 39.2   4.1   0.0
 3    0.0  40.5 56.8  0.0   2.7   0.0
 4    0.0  14.9 36.6 10.8  29.7   8.1

NOTE:  ALL TABLE FIGURES ARE PERCENTAGES

READY
```

Figure 19.3

As you can see, this is a very useful technique for summarizing the data. In addition to these questions, all of the questions in Part II and Part III could have been similarly processed. Certainly, the same information can be tallied manually by setting up tally sheets for each question and counting up the number of marks under each heading. Although use of a pocket calculator would decrease the time spent if the researcher was doing everything by hand, this method is far more time-consuming than using the computer for processing.

For example, consider question 11 in Part I. One way to obtain the results is to prepare tally sheets and tabulate the data by hand. Figure 19.4 illustrates a tally sheet. Each questionnaire is reviewed and a tally mark is placed next to the appropriate response to question 11. When all questionnaires have been reviewed, the number of tally marks is totaled for each response and the percentages are then calculated by dividing each response total by the total number of respondents. Table 19.1 summarizes these results.

Open-ended questions are much more difficult to analyze because of the variety of responses that are usually obtained. The great advantage in utilizing this type of question lies in the richness of in-depth information that can be gathered in response to this unstructured query. Figure 19.5 lists each of the responses the subjects wrote in for question 5 of Part I. It is clear that while there are a variety of statements that were recorded for these questions, many of them are quite similar. For example, the responses to question 5 (What was your primary motivation for choosing nursing as a profession?) include helping sick people regain health, working with and helping people, to help people, I enjoy helping people, and working to help others. These responses could be combined in one category called "desire to help people." In much the same way, other responses could be combined into categories. It is the job of the person who is analyzing such open-ended questions to try and establish meaningful categories as a way of reducing the large volume of

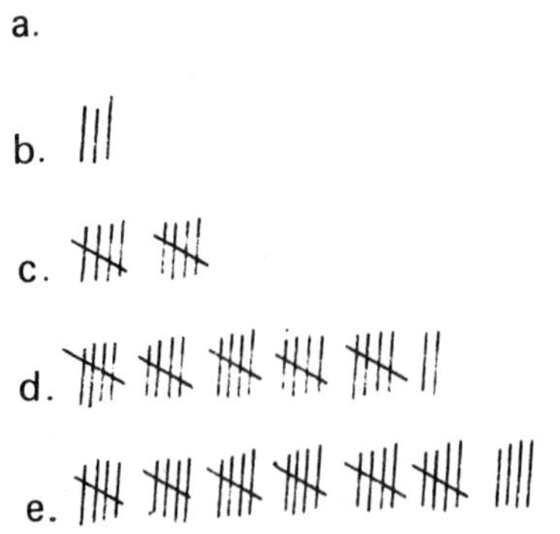

Figure 19.4. Tally sheets for tabulating data by hand.

Table 19.1
Percentage of Responses to Each Part
of Question 11 in Part I

Answer Choice	Number of People Responding	Percentage of Total Respondents
A	0	0.0
B	3	4.0
C	10	13.5
D	27	36.5
E	34	46.0

responses to a more manageable set. The categories that were finally selected for question 5 are listed in Figure 19.6. Students worked in small groups during this task to ensure consensus about category labels. Note that these labels are a concise description of the group's primary motivations for choosing nursing as a profession. A rough gauge of the relative weight of each category is indicated by the frequency of items that have been placed within it. It should be noted that various individuals could set up categories that differ in some minor way. However, the important general themes of the responses should appear in the results despite the minor variations.

Inspection of the responses should point to a common problem that is encountered in this type of data: numerous responses contain multiple themes. The categorizers in this instance decided to split the response into separate categories as appropriate. Thus, one subject's compound response could be subdivided and listed separately in two lists. One example of a compound response is "interest in medical field and desire to help others."

Part II contained the true-false questions that were part of the Thomas-Zander Ego Strength Scales. This section of each questionnaire had to be "scored." A respondent's score was equal to the number of true responses that were made. This score could be obtained manually or by a computer program. In our example, the standard answer sheets shown in Figure 19.2 were used. These types of computer-related programs require that the answers be recorded using a #2 pencil. Most of us have had ample opportunity to fill out these forms in a variety of situations ranging from course evaluations to entrance examinations. These forms are then machine processed and scored. Most educational institutions have a "testing service" that provides the means for scoring results in this form. You may have heard of the optical scanning machine used for this purpose. The scores for Part II for the 74 nursing students in this study are listed in Table 19.2.

The instructions given with the answer key for the Thomas-Zander Ego Strength Scales indicate that a high score represents high ego strength. The

Open Ended Biographical Responses

5. What was your primary motivation for choosing nursing as a profession?

Book on Florence Nightingale.

Working in nursing home.

Field I can learn well and do something worthwhile for people and myself.

Desire to know what is wrong physically with people who are not functioning normally.

Interested in medical profession, to help and work with people.

Love to deal with and help people.

Work as a nurse's aide.

Enjoy helping people.

Help me become a more unique individual.

A nurse is a high-rated professional.

Helping sick people regain health.   2

Enjoyed science subjects, know a young woman who was a nurse.

Next best thing to being a doctor.

Inner feeling to help.

To help people.   10

Interest in science, working with people, interesting (non-desk) occupation.

Interest in science and people.

Help people who are hurt.

Get involved with people and care for them.

Working to help others.

Its various applications to the professional world (teaching, health education, research, etc.).

For me, most rewarding in terms of a professional health science career. I'm aspiring to be a physical therapist.

Like to work with people, feel like I'm helping someone. Medicine fascinates me.

Profession in which I can incorporate medicine, psychology and philosophy.

Need to give.

Death of grandmother.

I like people.

What I wanted for a lifelong career.

Fascination for medicine.

Caring and help for others.

To have a profession which entails responsibility, integrity, interests.

Interaction with people and money.

Desire to help others, personal achievement.

Interesting, challenging, improvement, people.

Death of my mother.

Chance for professional advancement.

Many opportunities and facets of the career.

Fulfilling experience of helping others and helping myself grow.

(Continued)

Figure 19.5.

Wanted to work in health field.
Working with and helping people.
Help people and relate to them as people, not objects.
Enjoy people and feel that ill people are treated as objects—wish to change this in my role as a nurse.
Working with and helping people.
Life-long desire.
To help people.   5
Interest in medical field and desire to help others.
Helping people in something I enjoy.
Couldn't think of anything else at the time—I wanted a person-oriented career.
Liked working with sick people and helping them.

Figure 19.5. (cont.)

scores in Table 19.2 are listed by individual respondent. It would, however, be useful to have an ego strength profile for the entire group.

To summarize these individual ego strength scores, a computer library program was needed to provide the descriptive statistics that would represent the group standing. COSAP is the name of one of the statistical programs at many universities that can be used for obtaining descriptive statistics.

Categories constructed in Analysis of Question 5 on Part I of the Questionnaire

5. What was your primary motivation for choosing Nursing as a profession?

To help, care for, and work with others	(42)
General interest in a health science career	(12)
Academically related interests	(8)
Personal gratification and achievement	(8)
Humanistic aspects of the profession	(6)
Opportunities for professional advancement	(3)
Personal contact through work or acquaintances	(3)
Status of the profession	(3)
Death of a relative	(2)
Through literature	(1)
Monetary reasons	(1)
Couldn't think of an alternative	(1)

Figure 19.6.

Table 19.2
Ego Strength Scores

1.	12	26.	17	51.	17
2.	12	27.	16	52.	20
3.	19	28.	23	53.	17
4.	16	29.	12	54.	15
5.	21	30.	16	55.	12
6.	21	31.	21	56.	15
7.	17	32.	19	57.	10
8.	12	33.	12	58.	15
9.	14	34.	20	59.	21
10.	17	35.	14	60.	20
11.	12	36.	11	61.	13
12.	15	37.	23	62.	13
13.	19	38.	24	63.	18
14.	13	39.	17	64.	15
15.	18	40.	21	65.	18
16.	15	41.	16	66.	21
17.	18	42.	17	67.	19
18.	17	43.	8	68.	17
19.	14	44.	2	69.	20
20.	20	45.	2	70.	15
21.	18	46.	14	71.	14
22.	16	47.	17	72.	19
23.	17	48.	21	73.	9
24.	15	49.	23	74.	15
25.	19	50.	17		

When the COSAP program was run, the student was asked to type in the data. The data consisted of the 74 scores listed in Table 19.2 which were then typed into the computer at a computer terminal. The students had a choice of selecting any of the programs listed in Figure 19.7 for use with the data they had entered. The program that was initially selected for use was called EL (for *EL*ementary statistics). This program computes the mean, standard deviation, standard error maximum, minimum, and range (highest and lowest scores) of your data. In addition, a program called HI was used to display the data in the form of a histogram. Figure 19.8 illustrates the interactive nature of the COSAP package and the composite group results obtained for the ego strength scores. Note that the display of the data in the form of a histogram is a very good way to get an overall "picture" of how the group scored. The information supplied by the authors indicated that the possible scores on the test could range from a low of 0 (very low ego strength) to a high score of 27 (very high ego strength.) Thus, the theoretical midpoint between low and high amounts of ego strength is 13.5 (the range of a possible 27 points divided by 2). Theoretically, scores falling between 13.5 and 27 indicate high ego strength as is evidenced in this group of nursing students with a mean of 16.2. This can be visualized in Figure 19.8.

List of Some of the Programs for Student Use in the COSAP Computer Program

EL	Elementary statistics	HI	Produce histograms of data
RE	Regression analysis	CO	Correlation analysis
CH	Change data values	CT	Crosstabulations
TT	Statistical t-test		

Figure 19.7

```
WHICH UTILITY OR ANALYSIS ('FINISH' IF NO MORE)? EL

THIS PROGRAM COMPUTES ELEMENTARY STATISTICS.

VARIABLE    MEAN      STD. DEV   STD.ERROR   MAXIMUM   MINIMUM    RANGE
SCORES      16.189     4.180      0.486       24.00     2.00      22.00

WHICH UTILITY OR ANALYSIS ('FINISH' IF NO MORE)? HI

THIS PROGRAM PRINTS OUT A HISTOGRAM.

WHAT IS THE NAME OF THE VARIABLE? SCORES

TYPE A PRINT CHARACTER FOR THE HISTOGRAM   *? E

SPECIFY THE NUMBER OF INTERVALS. MAXIMUM IS 10 *? 8

FREQUENCY    2    0    3    8   17   22   18    4
--------+----+----+----+----+----+----+----+----+----+----
   22                                 E
   21                                 E
   20                                 E
   19                                 E
   18                                 E    E
   17                            E    E    E
   16                            E    E    E
   15                            E    E    E
   14                            E    E    E
   13                            E    E    E
   12                            E    E    E
   11                            E    E    E
   10                            E    E    E
    9                            E    E    E
    8                       E    E    E    E
    7                       E    E    E    E
    6                       E    E    E    E
    5                       E    E    E    E
    4                       E    E    E    E    E
    3             E         E    E    E    E    E
    2        E    E         E    E    E    E    E
    1        E    E         E    E    E    E    E
--------+----+----+----+----+----+----+----+----+----+----
      2 4.750   10.250    15.750    21.250
```

PRESENTING THE RESULTS

Once all of the appropriate data have been tallied, summarized, and analyzed, it is necessary to integrate the results into a unified set of statements about the subjects. The researcher should prepare some conclusions relating to the purpose of the study, which in this case was to describe a group of nursing students on the basis of selected personal and professional characteristics.

The scores on the value profile scale were handled in a similar fashion. The 74 scores were entered into the computer for use with the same computer program for descriptive statistics. The results from the EL program and the histogram displaying the scores can be visualized in Figures 19.9 and 19.10. Note that the mean or average score of the nursing students is 27.07.

The directions indicated that the range of possible scores on the profile could extend from a low score of 10 (indicating extreme amounts of value on individuality) to a high score of 50 (indicating a value on conformity). Since the theoretical midpoint is 30, it can easily be noted in Figure 19.11 that the nursing students' mean score of 27.07 placed them in the individualistic zone. This pictorial representation of the results serves to indicate that the students tend to be closer to a neutral standing rather than being strong individualists.

Although the actual results section should present numbers to describe the groups and to substantiate points, the majority of the section should be presented in a narrative format. The results should be clearly noncontroversial (the group of nursing students obtained a mean score of 16.2 indicating a high amount of ego strength), but the interpretations can vary according to the viewpoint of the author. There is no one correct way to combine infor-

```
            THE RESULTS OF THE EL PROGRAM FOR THE
            74 SCORES ON THE VALUE PROFILE SCALE

VALUE PROFILE = INDIVIDUALISM

WHICH UTILITY OR ANALYSIS ('FINISH' IF NOT MORE)? EL

THIS PROGRAM COMPUTES ELEMENTARY STATISTICS.

VARIABLE   MEAN   STD. DEV   STD. ERROR   MAXIMUM   MINIMUM   RANGE
TOTAL     37.068   6.403      0.744        40.00     10.00    30.00
```

Figure 19.9.

```
VALUE PROFILE = INDIVIDUALISM

WHICH UTILITY OR ANALYSIS ('FINISH' IF NO MORE)? HI

THIS PROGRAM PRINTS OUT A HISTOGRAM.

WHAT IS THE NAME OF THE VARIABLE? TOTAL

TYPE A PRINT CHARACTER FOR THE HISTOGRAM  *? I

SPECIFY THE NUMBER OF INTERVALS. MAXIMUM IS 10 *? 8

FREQUENCY    2    5    7   10   15   19   14    2
--------+----+----+----+----+----+----+----+----+----+----+---
  19                               I
  18                               I
  17                               I
  16                               I
  15                          I    I
  14                          I    I    I
  13                          I    I    I
  12                          I    I    I
  11                          I    I    I
  10                     I    I    I    I
   9                     I    I    I    I
   8                     I    I    I    I
   7                I    I    I    I    I
   6                I    I    I    I    I
   5           I    I    I    I    I    I
   4           I    I    I    I    I    I
   3           I    I    I    I    I    I
   2      I    I    I    I    I    I    I    I
   1      I    I    I    I    I    I    I    I
--------+----+----+----+----+----+----+----+----+----+----+---
       13.750     21.250     28.750     36.250
            17.500     25.000     32.500     40.000
```

DO YOU WISH ANOTHER HISTOGRAM? NO

POSSIBLE RANGE OF SCORES 10-50

10 = INDIVIDUALISTS   50 = CONFORMISTS

Figure 19.10. Results from running the histogram program for the 74 scores on the Value Profile Scale.

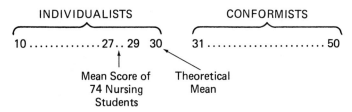

Figure 19.11. Visualizing results of the individualism score on the value profile.

mation in the section of a report dealing with the study results. The section should be clear, concise, and organized. Appropriate tables and figures should be included to emphasize important points.

Two actual student presentations have been reproduced in Commentaries 19.1 and 19.2. It is interesting to note the different approaches taken by each student to construct a report on the findings from the same data set.

Commentary 19.1
Report by Student Group A

The purpose of this study was to describe a group of nursing students on the basis of selected personal and professional characteristics. A questionnaire consisting of three parts—the coded and open-ended biographical data, the ego strength scale, and the value profile on individualism—was administered to 74 nursing students of whom 90.7 percent were basic students and 9.3 percent were RNs returning for their degrees.

Of the students questioned, 77 percent responded that they had decided to enter nursing when they were between 13 and 18 years of age. More than half (56.8 percent) responded that nursing was interesting and that they would continue in it as long as it fit into other aspects of their lives. Another 40.5 percent regarded nursing as their primary career. On the following question 36.5 percent of the subjects responded that marriage and children would interfere with their nursing. This seems to contradict the previous responses of 56.8 percent and 40.5 percent with nursing as a career. It does not seem that the nursing students are as committed as they had previously stated. These results can be visualized in Figure 1.

In the open-ended biographical data section, some of the responses received were very interesting. The least appealing aspects of nursing for the subjects (61.1 percent) were the stereotypic ideas, such as boredom, routine, menial work, competition. What a person/ nurse gets out of nursing is entirely up to her. Other less than appealing aspects were death, suffering, pain, and blood. These accounted for 23.6 percent of all responses. Nursing involves all of these aspects. This would appear to be a large percentage of people who have chosen nursing as their profession. The most appealing aspect about nursing was the idea of helping and caring for the sick. This response was given by 63.8 percent of the nursing students.

Two other questions concerned (1) what the nursing students

would be doing immediately following their baccalaureate program, and (2) what they would have achieved five years after their graduation. Many responded to the first question by saying that they would be staff nurses (57.9 percent). While in five years following graduation 78.09 percent were hoping to have the graduate degrees of MS, MA, or PhD. The most prevalent responses to these open-ended biographical questions could be classified under the headings of educational advancement and the giving of direct patient care.

Part II of the questionnaire measured personal characteristics. This was the ego strength scale. The subjects of the nursing class responding to this test scored higher than average. Because the mean found was 16.189 and the theoretical mean was 13.5 with a possible range of 27, these nurses could be considered to be self-confident and self-directed.

Part III of the questionnaire also measured personal characteristics. The value profile is based on the amount of individualism the subject has. The result of this test was very surprising. In the ego strength test, as you will recall, the nursing students scored very high in self-confidence and self-direction. The mean of the value profile

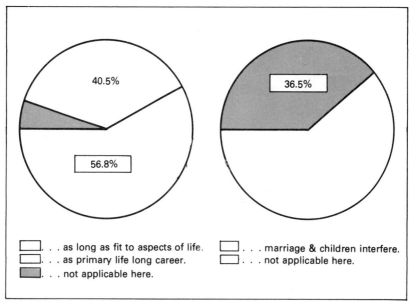

Commentary Fig. 1. Sample table from report by Student Group A.

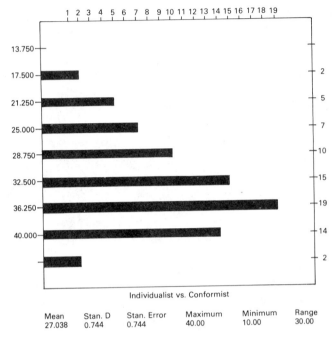

Commentary Fig. 2. Individualist vs. Conformist.

was found to be 27.038. The theoretical mean of this test was 30. This group of subjects barely scored as individualists, keeping in mind that a low score represents individualism while a high score represents a conformist. But when they were put on a graph (refer to figure above), the graph revealed that they were actually more centered in the conformist area. Being a conformist tends to contradict the high self-confident and self-directed scores of the previous ego strength test.

Summarizing these results as nursing implications, according to the percentages and means with graphs, these students are:

1. Not as committed to their profession as they should be because they responded that marriage and children would interfere when there are many shifts, hours, and part-time jobs nurses could reorganize themselves into.
2. The least appealing aspects are those of stereotyping, where these subjects could be more positive and get more out of nursing.
3. The appealing aspects of nursing were more idealistic than realistic. Nursing is more than just helping people to get well.

4. This group is very conforming to the traditional and stereotyped nursing. Nursing needs more positive attitudes to be recognized and expand from servant to individual patient care.

5. The conflicting note of this whole questionnaire is the ego strength scale. These subjects scored as self-confident, but the other questions break down this aspect. Nursing needs more self-confident workers, individualists who will take the initiative on their own and make decisions.

This questionnaire reveals that the nursing students of this study are not going to change the nursing profession, which was rather surprising to the researcher. It was felt before doing this questionnaire that this group was more positive about nursing. Even with all the research and theory taught during the subjects' education, it seems these nurses are going to follow previous patterns of marriage/family and staff nursing. There just does not seem to be enough of a trend toward change and improvement going on.

Courtesy of E. Broderick '80

Commentary 19.2
Report by Student Group B

This questionnaire describes a group of 74 sophomore (and RN) students now attending a baccalaurate School of Nursing on the basis of selected professional and personal characteristics. The majority of subjects were basic students while the remainder (9.5 percent) were RN students.

The first part of the questionnaire deals with professional characteristics. Many subjects decided on a career in nursing while still in their early teens: 37.9 percent decided to become nurses when they were between ages 13 and 15. While more subjects (39.2 percent) decided to become nurses while in their last years of high school. To the question "How important is nursing to you?" more than half of the students (56.8 percent) answered that they would continue in nursing as long as it fit into other aspects of their lives. The remaining 40.5 percent regarded nursing as their lifelong professional career. Surprisingly no one saw nursing "only as a way of earning a living." To the next question, "What do you think might interfere with or disrupt your nursing plans?", most subjects (36.5 percent) felt that marriage and/or children would disrupt their nursing career; while 29.7 percent felt that nothing would interfere with their career plans as far as they could see. These two questions showed that these subjects tended to be more traditionally oriented than modern in their views of nursing as a profession.

The majority of the subjects held humanistic ideas about nursing. Most chose nursing as a profession in order to help people. Helping and working with people was also the most appealing thing about the nursing profession to the majority of subjects. Therefore, the least appealing thing would logically be seeing people hurt, suffering, and dying; this in fact turned out to be the response of the subjects questioned. Other unappealing aspects about nursing were the working hours, the lack of independence—especially having to follow doctors orders—and the menial, routine tasks. These other unappealing aspects were probably reasons why 42.1 percent of the subjects planned on working for a Master's degree in some aspect of nursing within five years of their graduation. And even though half of the subjects planned on being staff nurses immediately after graduation, over 82 percent planned on continuing their education in some form.

Parts II and III of the questionnaire asked about the personal characteristics of the subjects. Part II consisted of an ego strength scale (from *Measures of Social Psychological Attitudes* by Robinson). The 27 true-false items asked were keyed for high scores, meaning that the higher the score the higher the level of self-confidence a person has and the more "self-directing" and able to "control and discharge tension he is." The mean score for this test was 16.189. This tells us that since the highest possible score was 27 and the theoretical average is 13.5, the majority of people scored high on the ego strength scale. No one scored the highest possible score of 27, the highest score received was 24, and 21.61 percent of the subjects scored 20 or over. Over half of the students (56.75 percent) scored between 13.5 and 19 on the scale. So most of the nursing students questioned did see themselves as self-directing, self-confident, and able to control tension.

Part III consisted of ten statements of general attitudes and values held in society. Subjects determined how much they agreed or disagreed with each statement. These questions tested the subjects' individualism. According to these statements, an individualist is a person who believes that to be superior a person must try to control his own life and avoid dependence on persons or things. He must be a nonconformist. The highest possible score a subject could get was 50, the lowest was 10; the theoretical mean was 30. A low score showed individualist, and above 30 showed that a person was a conformist. The mean score for the subjects tested were individualistic but not to a very great degree.

The nursing students tested were in general self-confident, slightly individualistic, self-directed persons, whose career aspirations were rather high in planning to achieve a high level of education and in helping and working with people, but to whom nursing was not a lifelong commitment. However this questionnaire failed to ask in which aspects nursing would be second in a subjects' life. A large number of subjects (40.5 percent) did see nursing as their "primary, lifelong professional career," but most of the subjects in the study were women and no consideration was made for the fact that many of them planned to have children. In that case it can be seen how nursing would no longer be primary, but more equivalent to other aspects of the subjects' lives.

There are significant implications of this study to nursing as a profession. First, the subjects' main motivation for choosing nursing as a profession was the same as the one they found most appealing in nursing: to help and work with people. This can only lead to better patient care and more concern and dedication to the patient. Second, the high level of self-confidence and self-direction, along with the fact that most subjects planned to continue their education beyond the baccalaureate program, points toward an increase in the professionalism of nursing. This will aid nursing in its quality of patient care and as a profession and a science in itself.

Courtesy of D. Schneller '80.

SKILLS DEVELOPED IN THE DATA ANALYSIS STUDY

At the end of the study, the nursing students were asked what skills or valuable experiences they felt were developed as a result of carrying out their data analysis project. The following is a list of the most frequently made responses.

1. The ability to use the computer to analyze data.
2. The ability to use descriptive statistics.
3. The ability to use figures and tables to illustrate a point about the data.
4. The ability to convert nominal data to categories.
5. The ability to use standardized scales that have been designed to measure factors such as ego strength and value dimensions.

6. The ability to create a multifaceted questionnaire with a variety of different types of questions.
7. The ability to tally some data manually.
8. The ability to score a questionnaire.
9. The ability to examine specific variables in depth (*e.g.*, selected personal and professional characteristics).
10. The ability to summarize information so that it can be communicated most effectively.
11. The ability to discern important points or issues from a mass of information.
12. The ability to blend tables and figures with a narrative description.
13. The ability to write up results in an organized, coherent, and concise manner.
14. The recognition that data can be interpreted and presented in different ways by different people.
15. An awareness of the creative and innovative ways in which data can be displayed.

In addition, many of the nursing students commented on their fascination with the topic itself. They found that working on a study that described something of keen personal interest was very rewarding. They found it interesting to see how the total group of 74 students averaged in contrast to their own personal score on the instrument.

ADDITIONAL ANALYSES THAT MIGHT HAVE BEEN PERFORMED

Whenever a research project or paper is completed, it is often worthwhile to reflect on what additional studies or analyses might be carried out with the data. Since those data have already been collected, additional research can be conducted with somewhat less effort.

For example, the following questions may be worth investigation:

1. How do basic students compare with RN students with respect to personal and professional characteristics?
2. Are there any characteristics that described all members of the group? None?
3. How would this group of nursing students compare on the ego strength and value profile dimensions with a group of non-nursing students? (Additional data would be necessary to satisfactorily answer this question.)

4. Is there a relationship between the respondents' stated degree of confidence in making the right decision in selecting nursing, and their ego strength score?

Some of the students were interested in reworking the data to see if they could answer some of the additional questions they wished to pose. The questionnaires were sorted several different times according to the responses given to some of the questions in Section I of the instrument. (The example shows some of the results of subdividing questions 1, 2, and 11.) The number of subjects in some of the newly constituted groups are very small, but it should be kept in mind that this represents the actual number of subjects and that the process was enacted to try to find interesting areas for further study. The average scores on the ego strength and individualism scores for each subgroup appear in Table 19.3.

The researcher might search for areas that might be fruitful topics of further study by noting the mean scores that are the most different from the actual group of theoretical mean. In inspecting this table, you may note that the groups which stand out in this regard each have fewer than ten subjects (groups 1, 2, and 9.) Although this small trend may be interesting, it is far too small to provide a basis for any conclusions.

The researcher may wish to do an "item analysis" for a subgroup on a group of selected questions. Figure 19.12 provides a graphic item analysis for

---

RN Student's Responses (n = 7)

Question 2.	a. /	3. a. ///	4. a. //	10. Goals	11. a.
	b. //	b. ///	b. //	Nurse-midwife	b. /
	c. ///	c.	c. /	Masters Degree in Child Health	c. /
	d.	d. /	d. /	MS Degree	d. ///
				MS in Maternal Child Health	e. //
				Good job and Continue School	
				Nurse Practitioner in Pediatrics with MS Degree	

Figure 19.12. An example of an item analysis.

Table 19.3
Ego Strength and Individualism Mean Scores for Newly Constituted Subgroups

Group	Ego Strength Mean Score (Total Group Mean Score = 16.189) Theoretical Mean Score = 13.5) Above 16.189 = high ego strength Below 18.189 = low ego strength	Individualism Mean Score (Total Group Mean Score = 27.07 Theoretical Mean Score = 30.00) Above 27.07 = conformist Below 27.07 = individualistic
1. RN students (n = 7)	17	20.57
2. Very low confidence 40–60% (n = 3)	11.67	23.67
3. Mod. low confidence 60–80% (n = 10)	16.8	30.8
4. Mod. high confidence 80–90% (n = 26)	16	26.96
5. High confidence 90–100% (n = 34)	16.79	26.21
6. Very early decision under 12 (n = 14)	15.36	26.71
7. Early decision 13–15 years (n = 28)	16.75	27.64
8. Routine decision 16–18 years (n = 29)	16.62	26.28
9. Late decision – over 19 (n = 3)	15	31

the small group of RN students on questions 2, 3, 4, 10, and 11. We can check back with the original questionnaire (Figure 19.1) and see how this group of subjects selected response items for the designated questions.

Again, it may be interesting to note that all of the seven RN students selected further education beyond the baccalaureate program as a goal. Although this is a surprising finding for a group that is not yet halfway through a baccalaureate program, it is still too small a number to produce a great amount of speculation. This could lead to a future study of the career-related academic aspirations of RN students.

An additional procedure was performed to determine whether the amount of confidence about the decision to choose nursing as a career related in any significant way to the ego strength scores of the subjects. To answer this question, the subjects were sorted into two groups in light of their answer to question 11. Subjects indicating a confidence level below 80 percent (n = 14) were placed in a subgroup labeled LOW CONFIDENCE. The HI CONFIDENCE group scoring above 80 percent consisted of 60 subjects. A t-test was performed to see if the mean scores of the two subgroups were significantly different from each other. The information in Figure 19.13 shows the results. The mean scores of the two groups do not appear to be very different (15.6 versus 16.5), yet we require a t-test to determine if there is a significant difference. A t-value of −.708776 resulted from the calculation. Please note the message at the bottom of the computer printout in Figure 19.13. It indicates the time it took for the computer to execute the calculations involved in the t-test for the 74 numbers. Note that it took less than a single second! Bet you can't do it that fast by hand. This t-value, when compared to

---

An Example of a t-Test

WHAT PROGRAM DO YOU WISH TO USE?   t-test
WHAT ARE THE NAMES OF THE TWO VARIABLES FROM YOUR DATA
? LOWCONFIDENCE
? HICONFIDENCE

VARIABLE	MEAN	VARIANCE
LOWCONFIDENCE	15.6154	21.9231
HICONFIDENCE	16.45	13.3703

STUDENT'S T .... −.708776
DEGREES OF FREEDOM...... 71
TIME   0.1 SECONDS

Figure 19.13.

the table of t-values in Appendix C is not greater than the appropriate number in the table, and is therefore *not* significant. This leads us to the conclusion that there is no real difference between the high and low confidence groups with regard to ego strength. Suppose the authors had originally set up a study to test the following hypothesis:

> H: Subjects with a high degree of confidence about their career choice will demonstrate significantly higher levels of ego strength than subjects with a low degree of confidence.

What would have been the decision regarding action on the hypothesis? It would have been *rejected* in this instance.

What other types of questions could you think up about these data on personal and professional characteristics of nursing students? What areas need to be studied in more depth? What changes would you make if you set out to repeat the study?

This small exercise has provided a few examples of the way research is intertwined with both the use of measurement techniques (both words and numbers) and computer applications.

REFERENCES

1. Thomas-Zander Ego Strength Scales (Thomas and Zander 1960). In Robinson and Shaver: Measures of Social Psychological Attitudes. Survey Research Center, Institute for Social Research, 1973.

2. Value Profile (Bales and Couch 1969). In Robinson and Shaver: Measures of Social Psychological Attitudes. Survey Research Center, Institute for Social Research, 1973.

CHAPTER

20

Getting Actively Involved in Research

THE INFORMATION EXPLOSION

Computers are being installed in hospitals to assist with various functions, such as keeping track of the patient census or transmitting messages to various work areas like the pharmacy and dietary department. Some hospitals even use computers to store the vital patient-related information in place of the traditional handwritten chart. Other clinical facilities keep daily tabs on nursing care "variables" by computer and use the retrievable information as the basis for planning in-service programs for staff. Nurses are being asked to assist in research projects in varying capacities, from assuming the role of subject to that of principal research investigator, including the myriad steps in between. While nursing students are encountering more research-related courses in their basic educational programs, they are looking more frequently to their role models in clinical facilities for guidance. This assistance is requested most often for help in identifying meaningful nursing problems, as well as for support in conducting small-scale studies.

Modern health care literature is bombarding nurses (as well as the general public) with all kinds of statistics, computations, tables, graphs, and figures that relate directly to the work they are doing. Procedures, such as nursing assessments and nursing audits call for the organization, extraction, and condensation of large masses of data. The move toward increased utilization of research-related techniques has already begun. The nursing students who have had the opportunity to develop and practice these types of skills are enthusiastic about the long-range impact these abilities will have on their professional careers. You can take a few steps to make this process easier for you:

ORGANIZING YOUR EFFORTS

Start a Research File

Start at the outset to develop the habit of recording information from the research articles you read. Get a special notebook or a set of index cards to preserve the key information from your articles. It may be easier in the beginning to make Xerox copies of your articles since you may want to read them over more than once. After you become skilled in reading these studies, you will be able to efficiently summarize the important points on your file cards and conserve time and energy. Your diligence in the beginning will "pay off" at a later time. Always jot down the complete bibliographical information (author, title, publisher, date of publication, etc.) so that you can relocate the article if needed or quote it in a paper you might write at a later time.

Organize Research Articles into Sections

Each research study can be broken down into several distinct sections. They often seem less formidable if approached from this viewpoint. The broad areas are as follows.

The Abstract

Most studies begin with an abstract, which is a brief summary of the entire study from start to finish. Abstracts are very helpful for those who are unfamiliar with the key points of research studies. Make sure to reread the abstract after going through the entire study to get a better handle on the important points.

The Introductory Material

The researchers will explain the main problem they were studying in this section. The purpose of the investigation will be spelled out in detail. This section usually contains a summary of the published literature on the topic, as well as statements about the theoretical knowledge to which it relates.

The Means of Conducting the Study

This section informs the reader about the actual steps that were followed in carrying out the study. Specific items are covered, such as the instrument used to collect information, the number and kind of subjects used, and the way in which they were selected.

The Results of the Study

The research findings are set forth in detail in the final narrative section of the study report. The author will report some of the results in terms of numbers or statistical formulations to let the reader see the basis for the statements he is making. The very end of this section usually contains suggestions for promising avenues of further research.

The References

The final section of a research study lists the main references utilized by the author in the course of the investigation. The quality of these references gives you a clue about the substance of the basis of the study. It is also an often overlooked source of related bibliographical references on the topic area.

USE YOUR RESOURCES

There are many, many resources available to help you stay active in research and, in fact, make it easier for you to do so. Certainly, hospital and university libraries provide a large service in this regard. Not only are they likely to have material relevant to your own area of interest, but through a borrowing system called "interlibrary loan," they can lend materials to libraries that are in need of additional reference sources. A list of some of the major medical libraries appears below.

1. New England Region (Conn., Me., Mass., N.H., R.I., Vt.)
    Francis A. Countway Library of Medicine
    10 Shattuck St., Boston, Me. 02115
2. New York and Northern New Jersey Region (New York and the 11 northern counties of New Jersey)
    New York Academy of Medicine Library
    2 East 103 St., New York, N.Y. 10029
3. Mideastern Region (Pa., Del., and the ten southern counties of New Jersey)
    Library of the College of Physicians
    19 South 22 St., Philadelphia, Pa. 19103
4. Mid-Atlantic Region (Va., W.Va., Md., D.C., N.C.)
    National Library of Medicine
    8600 Rockville Pike, Bethesda, Md. 20014
5. East Central Region (Ky., Mich., Ohio)
    Wayne State University Medical Library
    4325 Brush St., Detroit, Mich. 48201
6. Southeastern Region (Ala., Fla., Ga., Miss., S.C., Tenn., Puerto Rico)
    A. W. Calhoun Medical Library
    Emory University, Atlanta, Ga. 30322
7. Midwest Region (Ill., Ind., Iowa, Minn., N.D., Wis.)
    John Crerar Library
    35 West 33 St., Chicago, Ill. 60616
8. Midcontinental Region (Colo., Kans., Mo., Neb., S.D., Utah, Wyo.)
    University of Nebraska Medical Center
    42nd St. & Dewey Ave., Omaha, Neb. 68105
9. South Central Region (Ark., La., N.M., Okla., Tex.)
    University of Texas Southwestern Medical School at Dallas
    5323 Harry Hines Blvd., Dallas, Tex. 75235
10. Pacific Northwest Region (Alaska, Idaho, Mont., Oreg., Wash.)
    University of Washington
    Health Sciences Library
    Seattle, Wash. 98105
11. Pacific Southwest Region (Ariz., Calif., Hawaii, Nev.)
    Center for the Health Sciences
    University of California
    Los Angeles, Calif. 90024

In addition, many of these libraries have computer literature search services (as described in Chapter 5) which allow the user to obtain a computer-produced listing of articles and book titles in a particular area of interest.

Certainly, professional journals provide the best resource for the nurse who wishes to stay active in research. Keeping "current" will contribute a great deal to both personal and professional growth. Appendix G contains a listing of some of the health-related journals that may be of interest to you.

EVALUATING A RESEARCH REPORT

As a professional nurse, you will be required to critically evaluate research reports in journals related to your particular field of interest. In addition, it will be necessary for you to stay informed about what is being reported in the literature. To do this, you must be able to distinguish between good and bad research. Simply because a study is published does not mean that it is necessarily a good one.

Most of what you have learned in the earlier chapters of this book will help you critically evaluate a research report. With this in mind, the following steps can be used as an aide to your evaluation.

1. Read the report in its entirety.
2. Is the statement of the problem clear and concise?
3. Are the variables to be used in the study defined?
4. Is there a review of the literature on the subject?
5. Are the references that are cited relevant to the topic of the report?
6. Are the sources that are cited reasonably current?
7. Is there a clear statement about which hypotheses are to be tested?
8. Do the hypotheses describe an expected relationship between two variables?
9. Are the hypotheses testable?
10. Does the report describe the characteristics of the population that is being studied?
11. Is the method for selecting the sample truly random?
12. Is the method for selecting the sample described?
13. Is the sample that was finally selected representative of the population?
14. Is the sample size sufficient for the analysis that is to be done?
15. Is the data-gathering instrument described adequately?
16. Was the particular instrument that was used well designed?
17. Does the instrument measure what it claims to measure?
18. If there are scoring procedures to be followed when the questionnaire is processed, are they adequately described?
19. Was the instrument pretested?
20. How were the data processed?

21. If a computer was used, are the specific techniques and programs that were used clearly specified?
22. What statistical procedures were used to summarize and analyze the data?
23. Were the statistical techniques appropriate?
24. Should additional statistical tests have been made?
25. Are the statistical tests of significance that are used adequately explained?
26. Are the results statistically significant? (At what level?)
27. Are the tables and graphs that present the data accurate, complete, and well organized?
28. Are the results clearly presented?
29. Are the results related to the original hypotheses that were stated?
30. Are the results generalized? If so, is it justifiable?
31. Are the implications of any findings discussed?
32. Are recommendations for future research indicated?
33. Is a bibliography included?
34. Reread the abstract. Does it correctly describe the research study?
35. On reflection, does it appear that any variables were left out of the study?
36. Can the study be easily replicated by other researchers?
37. How can the findings be applied to nursing practice?

While this list may seem somewhat exhaustive, you will find that after using it to evaluate several research reports you will become quite good at critiquing these reports. It is important to recognize that one does not casually read a research article. It is sometimes necessary to reread it several times. Yet this is a critical dimension of one's professional growth.

It is often helpful to have a framework for gathering information from a published study as you first read it. Figure 20.1 is an example of a set of guidelines that has been used for this purpose by nursing students. The Research Reading Guidelines form in Figure 20.1 was completed by a student for the study presented in Chapter 4 of this text. Note that the reference identification section provides a place to note all the important information which would be needed to relocate the article or to list it in a bibliography at a later date without having to spend the time to look it up in the library once again. The last section helps the reader to begin the process of objectively "stepping back" from the article to gain a perspective from which it can be meaningfully evaluated.

After some practice with a form similar to the one pictured in Figure 20.1 the researchers often switch to notes on index cards for easy storage for later use. Whatever system works best for you, summarize the major findings as soon as you finish reading the study and list related resources on the card.

1. Reference Identification (In format for listing in Bibliography):

2. List the *sources* you used to locate the article:

3. Introductory Material:
   A. Research Problem (in your own words):

   B. Purpose of the study:

   C. Summarize the relevant points of the literature cited:

4. *Methodology:*
   A. Overall plan or design of the study (in your own words):

   B. Describe the following:
      1. Subjects:

      2. Variables (or factors) being studied:

      3. Instrument:

      4. Procedures (what was done to the subjects):

Figure 20.1.
Research Reading Guidelines.

437

5. *Results*

A. Summarize the main results:

B. Any additional interesting features:

6. *Demonstrate* one way you could use material from this article in a formal paper (an example of either a direct quote or an example of paraphrasing):

A. Example:

B. Footnote Format:

7. *Evaluation*

A. Your comprehension level of article

_____ fairly easy to understand

_____ some difficulty

_____ very complicated

B. Overall value of the study to the field

_____ very worthwhile

_____ average

_____ questional contribution

Figure 20.1 (cont.)

This takes but a few minutes and gives you an instant topical file of research that is related to your professional area.

The following references may be helpful to you in gathering more information on evaluating or critiquing research reports:

Downs, F. S. and Newman, M.: Elements of a research critique. In A Source Book of Nursing Research, Philadelphia, F. A. Davis, 1977, pp. xi–xvi.

Fleming, J. W. and Hayter, J.: Reading research reports critically. Nursing Outlook 22 (March 1974): 172–175.

Heidgerken, L. E.: Evaluation of reported research in nursing. In H. H.

Werley (ed.): Report on Nursing Research Conference, 24 February–7 March 1959. Washington D.C., Walter Reed Army Institute of Research, 1961, pp. 116–147.

Kariel, P. E.: A suggested approach to the reading of research. Tomorrow's Nurse 2 (October–November 1961): pp. 8–10.

Leininger, M. M.: The research critique: nature, function, and art. In M. V. Batey (ed.): Communicating Nursing Research: The Research Critique, Volume 1. Boulder, Colo., Western Interstate Commission for Higher Education, 1968, pp. 20–32. (Also in Nursing Research 17 [September–October 1968]: 444–459.

National League for Nursing, Research and Studies Service. Search or research? criteria for a research report. Nursing Outlook 12 (August 1964): p. 60.

Pitel, M.: Critique as an interaction process. In Second Nursing Research Conference, Phoenix, Arizona, February 28 March 1–2, 1966. New York, American Nurses' Association, n.d., pp. 1–8.

The research critique. (Editorial) Nursing Research 15 (Summer 1966): p. 195.

WRITING A RESEARCH REPORT

Whether it is an integral part of your research course or a part of your professional activities, you will at some time write a research report of your own. While the previous chapters have dealt with the various technical and methodological aspects of performing research, there has been no formal discussion of the format of the final report. This chapter presents factors to be considered in writing your results.

1. Make sure you have a copy of a writing style manual. As was noted in Chapter 5, there are several of these available. The most important criterion is to be consistent. These manuals are particularly helpful when preparing the technical aspects of papers such as bibliographies, appendices, tables, and figures.

2. Write clearly. This is certainly the most important part of the entire process. If you cannot communicate well, even significant results will go unnoticed. Simple language is often the key to clarity.

3. Before your study begins, prepare an outline of the research report. In particular, it is helpful to sketch what tables and graphs are likely to be used. In this way, as you proceed through your research, you can keep your data and findings appropriately organized. Some researchers find it helpful to keep a file folder for each section and subsection of the report. As the research study progresses, information and/or author's notes can be filed in the appropriate folder. This greatly facilitates the later preparation of the report.

4. The writing style should facilitate an objective and factual presentation. (Remember to avoid subjective statements, personal pronouns, and emotional phrasing.)
5. Take the time to ensure that words are spelled correctly, that the grammar is correct, and that the correct punctuation was used. These factors greatly color the reader's perception of the validity of the report.
6. When the final copy has been typed, read it through twice to ensure that there are no typographical errors. Once again, this is not too much to expect of a professional report. Proofread carefully.
7. The research report itself should contain most of the sections outlined in Appendix A. Of course, the specific sections used sometimes vary from one study to another. Each of the items in this outline has been discussed elsewhere in the text.
8. Be prepared to make two to three revisions of your report.
9. If the study is to be published in a journal, it will have to be shorter than the report that is prepared using the outline in Appendix A.
    (a) First, carefully read the journals in your professional area and select two or three that may be appropriate publications for your report. Note the organization, format and length of their published studies. (You should submit your work to only one journal at a time, however.)
    (b) Look on the editorial page to obtain information on the specifications for submitting a manuscript to this journal, or contact the journal directly for a copy of their author's guide on format, style, and length.
    (c) Prepare an abstract of 100 words or less that describes your research study. By reviewing other abstracts, you can get a pretty good idea of what summary information needs to be included.

The motivation for doing a research report may have been that it is an academic requirement, a necessary ingredient for professional success, a part of your job responsibilities, or simply a topic that you are very interested in learning more about. Whatever the reason, you should always strive to make your report of publishable quality and seek to share your results with those in your professional community.

The best way to reinforce your new research activities is to utilize some aspect of your newly acquired information as soon as possible. It would be best to aim for a two-pronged use. One method would be the mention of some aspect of one of the studies you read while conversing with colleagues. Another method would entail using some aspect of the research in your professional practice. This could include activities that range from the organization and collection of patient data to the application of study results in your nursing care.

APPENDIX A
Format of a Typical Nursing Research Paper

A. *Front Matter*
  I. *Title Page*
   Title of Study
   Authors' Names
   Course Title
   Instructor's Name
   Date
  II. *Table of Contents* (indicate page numbers for each listing)
   Divide content for each chapter into headings and subheadings
   Back Notes
   Bibliography
   Appendices
B. *Sections of the Paper*
   The Research Problem
    Chapter I: *The Introduction to the Problem*
         Presentation of the Problem
         Need to Investigate the Problem
         Personal Interest
         Purpose of the Study
         Scope of the Study
    Chapter II: *Review of the Literature*
         (Divide into subheadings as necessary)
    Chapter III: *Theoretical Framework*
         (Divide into subheadings as necessary)
   Methodology
    Chapter IV: *Research Orientation and Expectations*
         Research Approach and Design, with Rationale
         Statement of Purpose
         Definition of Variables in Statement of Purpose
         Operational Definitions
         Criterion Measure Defined
         Method of Sampling, with Rationale
         Population, Study Group, and Setting
         Extraneous Variables Defined, with Rationale
    Chapter V: *Data Collection*
         Method and Technique Selected, with Rationale
         Description of Instrument, with Rationale for
           Developed Items

Pretest and Resultant Changes
Method of Processing Data
Data Analysis Plan

Results

Chapter VI: *Analysis of Results*
Analysis of Data (include tables, graphs, etc.)
Interpretation of Results
Relationship of Extraneous Variables to Results
Relationship of Results to the Problem and
    Theoretical Framework
Implications for Nursing

Chapter VII: *Discussion*
Summary
Conclusions
Limitations of the Study
Recommendations for Further Study

C. *Back Matter*
   I.   Back Notes
   II. Bibliography
   III. Appendices
        Copy of Instrument
        Tally Sheets
        Correspondence

APPENDIX B

Table of Areas under the Normal Curve

$\dfrac{X - \mu}{\sigma}$ (1)	Area under the curve between μ and X (2)	Ordinate (Y) of the curve at X (3)	$\dfrac{X - \mu}{\sigma}$ (1)	Area under the curve between μ and X (2)	Ordinate (Y) of the curve at X (3)
.00	.00000	.39894	.40	.15542	.36827
.01	.00399	.39892	.41	.15910	.36678
.02	.00798	.39886	.42	.16276	.36526
.03	.01197	.39876	.43	.16640	.36371
.04	.01595	.39862	.44	.17003	.36213
.05	.01994	.39844	.45	.17364	.36053
.06	.02392	.39822	.46	.17724	.35889
.07	.02790	.39797	.47	.18082	.35723
.08	.03188	.39767	.48	.18439	.35553
.09	.03586	.39733	.49	.18793	.35381
.10	.03983	.39695	.50	.19146	.35207
.11	.04380	.39654	.51	.19497	.35029
.12	.04776	.39608	.52	.19847	.34849
.13	.05172	.39559	.53	.20194	.34667
.14	.05567	.39505	.54	.20540	.34482
.15	.05962	.39448	.55	.20884	.34294
.16	.06356	.39387	.56	.21226	.34105
.17	.06749	.39322	.57	.21566	.33912
.18	.07142	.39253	.58	.21904	.33718
.19	.07535	.39181	.59	.22240	.33521
.20	.07926	.39104	.60	.22575	.33322
.21	.08317	.39024	.61	.22907	.33121
.22	.08706	.38940	.62	.23237	.32918
.23	.09095	.38853	.63	.23565	.32713
.24	.09483	.38762	.64	.23891	.32506
.25	.09871	.38667	.65	.24215	.32297
.26	.10257	.38568	.66	.24537	.32086
.27	.10642	.38466	.67	.24857	.31874
.28	.11026	.38361	.68	.25175	.31659
.29	.11409	.38251	.69	.25490	.31443
.30	.11791	.38139	.70	.25804	.31225
.31	.12172	.38023	.71	.26115	.31006
.32	.12552	.37903	.72	.26424	.30785
.33	.12930	.37780	.73	.26730	.30563
.34	.13307	.37654	.74	.27035	.30339
.35	.13683	.37524	.75	.27337	.30114
.36	.14058	.37391	.76	.27637	.29887
.37	.14431	.37255	.77	.27935	.29659
.38	.14803	.37115	.78	.28230	.29431
.39	.15173	.36973	.79	.28524	.29200

Appendix B (cont.)

$\dfrac{X - \mu}{\sigma}$ (1)	Area under the curve between μ and X (2)	Ordinate (Y) of the curve at X (3)	$\dfrac{X - \mu}{\sigma}$ (1)	Area under the curve between μ and X (2)	Ordinate (Y) of the curve at X (3)
.80	.28814	.28969	1.20	.38493	.19419
.81	.29103	.28737	1.21	.38686	.19186
.82	.29389	.28504	1.22	.38877	.18954
.83	.29673	.28269	1.23	.39065	.18724
.84	.29955	.28034	1.24	.39251	.18494
.85	.30234	.27798	1.25	.39435	.18265
.86	.30511	.27562	1.26	.39617	.18037
.87	.30785	.27324	1.27	.39796	.17810
.88	.31057	.27086	1.28	.39973	.17585
.89	.31327	.27849	1.29	.40147	.17360
.90	.31594	.26609	1.30	.40320	.17137
.91	.31859	.26369	1.31	.40490	.16915
.92	.32121	.26129	1.32	.40658	.16694
.93	.32381	.25888	1.33	.40824	.16474
.94	.32639	.25647	1.34	.40988	.16256
.95	.32894	.25406	1.35	.41149	.16038
.96	.33147	.25164	1.36	.41309	.15822
.97	.33398	.24923	1.37	.41466	.15608
.98	.33646	.24681	1.38	.41621	.15395
.99	.33891	.24439	1.39	.41774	.15183
1.00	.34134	.24197	1.40	.41924	.14973
1.01	.34375	.23955	1.41	.42073	.14764
1.02	.34614	.23713	1.42	.42220	.14556
1.03	.34850	.23471	1.43	.42364	.14350
1.04	.35083	.23230	1.44	.42507	.14146
1.05	.35314	.22988	1.45	.42647	.13943
1.06	.35543	.22747	1.46	.42786	.13742
1.07	.35769	.22506	1.47	.42922	.13542
1.08	.35993	.22265	1.48	.43056	.13344
1.09	.36214	.22025	1.49	.43189	.13147
1.10	.36433	.21785	1.50	.43319	.12952
1.11	.36650	.21546	1.51	.43448	.12758
1.12	.36864	.21307	1.52	.43574	.12566
1.13	.37076	.21069	1.53	.43699	.12376
1.14	.37286	.20831	1.54	.43822	.12188
1.15	.37493	.20594	1.55	.43943	.12001
1.16	.37698	.20357	1.56	.44062	.11816
1.17	.37900	.20121	1.57	.44179	.11632
1.18	.38100	.19886	1.58	.44295	.11450
1.19	.38298	.19652	1.59	.44408	.11270

Appendix B (cont.)

$\dfrac{X - \mu}{\sigma}$ (1)	Area under the curve between μ and X (2)	Ordinate (Y) of the curve at X (3)	$\dfrac{X - \mu}{\sigma}$ (1)	Area under the curve between μ and X (2)	Ordinate (Y) of the curve at X (3)
1.60	.44520	.11092	2.00	.47725	.05399
1.61	.44630	.10915	2.01	.47778	.05292
1.62	.44738	.10741	2.02	.47831	.05186
1.63	.44845	.10567	2.03	.47882	.05082
1.64	.44950	.10396	2.04	.47932	.04980
1.65	.45053	.10226	2.05	.47982	.04879
1.66	.45154	.10059	2.06	.48030	.04780
1.67	.45254	.09893	2.07	.48077	.04682
1.68	.45352	.09728	2.08	.48124	.04586
1.69	.45449	.09566	2.09	.48169	.04491
1.70	.45543	.09405	2.10	.48214	.04398
1.71	.45637	.09246	2.11	.48257	.04307
1.72	.45728	.09089	2.12	.48300	.04217
1.73	.45818	.08933	2.13	.48341	.04128
1.74	.45907	.08780	2.14	.48382	.04041
1.75	.45994	.08628	2.15	.48422	.03955
1.76	.46080	.08478	2.16	.48461	.03871
1.77	.46164	.08329	2.17	.48500	.03788
1.78	.46246	.08183	2.18	.48537	.03706
1.79	.46327	.08038	2.19	.48574	.03626
1.80	.46407	.07895	2.20	.48610	.03547
1.81	.46485	.07754	2.21	.48645	.03470
1.82	.46562	.07614	2.22	.48679	.03394
1.83	.46638	.07477	2.23	.48713	.03319
1.84	.46712	.07341	2.24	.48745	.03246
1.85	.46784	.07206	2.25	.48778	.03174
1.86	.46856	.07074	2.26	.48809	.03103
1.87	.46926	.06943	2.27	.48840	.03034
1.88	.46995	.06814	2.28	.48870	.02965
1.89	.47062	.06687	2.29	.48899	.02898
1.90	.47128	.06562	2.30	.48928	.02833
1.91	.47193	.06438	2.31	.48956	.02768
1.92	.47257	.06316	2.32	.48983	.02705
1.93	.47320	.06195	2.33	.49010	.02643
1.94	.47381	.06077	2.34	.49036	.02582
1.95	.47441	.05959	2.35	.49064	.02522
1.96	.47500	.05844	2.36	.49086	.02463
1.97	.47558	.05730	2.37	.49111	.02406
1.98	.47615	.05618	2.38	.49134	.02349
1.99	.47670	.05508	2.39	.49158	.02294

Appendix B (cont.)

$\dfrac{X - \mu}{\sigma}$ (1)	Area under the curve between μ and X (2)	Ordinate (Y) of the curve at X (3)	$\dfrac{X - \mu}{\sigma}$ (1)	Area under the curve between μ and X (2)	Ordinate (Y) of the curve at X (3)
2.40	.49180	.02239	2.80	.49744	.00792
2.41	.49202	.02186	2.81	.49752	.00770
2.42	.49224	.02134	2.82	.49760	.00748
2.43	.49245	.02083	2.83	.49767	.00727
2.44	.49266	.02033	2.84	.49774	.00707
2.45	.49286	.01984	2.85	.49781	.00687
2.46	.49305	.01936	2.86	.49788	.00668
2.47	.49324	.01889	2.87	.49795	.00649
2.48	.49343	.01842	2.88	.49801	.00631
2.49	.49361	.01797	2.89	.49807	.00613
2.50	.49379	.01753	2.90	.49813	.00595
2.51	.49396	.01709	2.91	.49819	.00578
2.52	.49413	.01667	2.92	.49825	.00562
2.53	.49430	.01625	2.93	.49831	.00545
2.54	.49446	.01585	2.94	.49836	.00530
2.55	.49461	.01545	2.95	.49841	.00514
2.56	.49477	.01506	2.96	.49846	.00499
2.57	.49492	.01468	2.97	.49851	.00485
2.58	.49506	.01431	2.98	.49856	.00471
2.59	.49520	.01394	2.99	.49861	.00457
2.60	.49534	.01358	3.00	.49865	.00443
2.61	.49547	.01323	3.01	.49869	.00430
2.62	.49560	.01289	3.02	.49874	.00417
2.63	.49573	.01256	3.03	.49878	.00405
2.64	.49585	.01223	3.04	.49882	.00393
2.65	.49598	.01191	3.05	.49886	.00381
2.66	.49609	.01160	3.06	.49889	.00370
2.67	.49621	.01130	3.07	.49893	.00358
2.68	.49632	.01100	3.08	.49897	.00348
2.69	.49643	.01071	3.09	.49900	.00337
2.70	.49653	.01042	3.10	.49903	.00327
2.71	.49664	.01014	3.11	.49906	.00317
2.72	.49674	.00987	3.12	.49910	.00307
2.73	.49683	.00961	3.13	.49913	.00298
2.74	.49693	.00935	3.14	.49916	.00288
2.75	.49702	.00909	3.15	.49918	.00279
2.76	.49711	.00885	3.16	.49921	.00271
2.77	.49720	.00861	3.17	.49924	.00262
2.78	.49728	.00837	3.18	.49926	.00254
2.79	.49736	.00814	3.19	.49929	.00246

Appendix B (cont.)

$\dfrac{X - \mu}{\sigma}$ (1)	Area under the curve between μ and X (2)	Ordinate (Y) of the curve at X (3)	$\dfrac{X - \mu}{\sigma}$ (1)	Area under the curve between μ and X (2)	Ordinate (Y) of the curve at X (3)
3.20	.49931	.00238	3.60	.49984	.00061
3.21	.49934	.00231	3.61	.49985	.00059
3.22	.49936	.00224	3.62	.49985	.00057
3.23	.49938	.00216	3.63	.49986	.00055
3.24	.49940	.00210	3.64	.49986	.00053
3.25	.49942	.00203	3.65	.49987	.00051
3.26	.49944	.00196	3.66	.49987	.00049
3.27	.49946	.00190	3.67	.49988	.00047
3.28	.49948	.00184	3.68	.49988	.00046
3.29	.49950	.00178	3.69	.49989	.00044
3.30	.49952	.00172	3.70	.49989	.00042
3.31	.49953	.00167	3.71	.49990	.00041
3.32	.49955	.00161	3.72	.49990	.00039
3.33	.49957	.00156	3.73	.49990	.00038
3.34	.49958	.00151	3.74	.49991	.00037
3.35	.49960	.00146	3.75	.49991	.00035
3.36	.49961	.00141	3.76	.49992	.00034
3.37	.49962	.00136	3.77	.49992	.00033
3.38	.49964	.00132	3.78	.49992	.00031
3.39	.49965	.00127	3.79	.49992	.00030
3.40	.49966	.00123	3.80	.49993	.00029
3.41	.49968	.00119	3.81	.49993	.00028
3.42	.49969	.00115	3.82	.49993	.00027
3.43	.49970	.00111	3.83	.49994	.00026
3.44	.49971	.00107	3.84	.49994	.00025
3.45	.49972	.00104	3.85	.49994	.00024
3.46	.49973	.00100	3.86	.49994	.00023
3.47	.49974	.00097	3.87	.49995	.00022
3.48	.49975	.00094	3.88	.49995	.00021
3.49	.49976	.00090	3.89	.49995	.00021
3.50	.49977	.00087	3.90	.49995	.00020
3.51	.49978	.00084	3.91	.49995	.00019
3.52	.49978	.00081	3.92	.49996	.00018
3.53	.49979	.00079	3.93	.49996	.00018
3.54	.49980	.00076	3.94	.49996	.00017
3.55	.49981	.00073	3.95	.49996	.00016
3.56	.49981	.00071	3.96	.49996	.00016
3.57	.49982	.00068	3.97	.49996	.00015
3.58	.49983	.00066	3.98	.49997	.00014
3.59	.49983	.00063	3.99	.49997	.00014

APPENDIX C
Table of the *T*-Distribution

Level of Significance

d.f.	0.9	0.8	0.7	0.6	0.5	0.4	0.3	0.2	0.1	0.05	0.02	0.01	0.001
1	.158	.325	.510	.727	1.000	1.376	1.963	3.078	6.314	12.706	31.821	63.657	636.619
2	.142	.289	.445	.617	.816	1.061	1.386	1.886	2.910	4.303	6.965	9.925	31.598
3	.137	.277	.424	.584	.765	.978	1.250	1.638	2.353	3.182	4.541	5.841	12.941
4	.134	.271	.414	.569	.741	.941	1.190	1.533	2.132	2.776	3.747	4.604	8.610
5	.132	.267	.408	.559	.727	.920	1.156	1.476	2.015	2.571	3.365	4.032	6.859
6	.131	.265	.404	.553	.718	.906	1.134	1.440	1.943	2.447	3.143	3.707	5.959
7	.130	.263	.402	.549	.711	.896	1.119	1.415	1.895	2.365	2.998	3.499	5.405
8	.130	.262	.399	.546	.706	.889	1.108	1.397	1.860	2.306	2.896	3.355	5.041
9	.129	.261	.398	.543	.703	.883	1.100	1.383	1.833	2.262	2.821	3.250	4.781
10	.129	.260	.397	.542	.700	.879	1.093	1.372	1.812	2.228	2.764	3.169	4.587
11	.129	.260	.396	.540	.697	.876	1.088	1.363	1.796	2.201	2.718	3.106	4.437
12	.128	.259	.395	.539	.695	.873	1.083	1.356	1.782	2.179	2.681	3.055	4.318
13	.128	.259	.394	.538	.694	.870	1.079	1.350	1.771	2.160	2.650	3.012	4.221
14	.128	.258	.393	.537	.692	.868	1.076	1.345	1.761	2.145	2.624	2.977	4.140
15	.128	.258	.393	.536	.691	.866	1.074	1.341	1.753	2.131	2.602	2.947	4.073

df													
16	4.015	2.921	2.583	2.120	1.746	1.337	1.071	.865	.690	.535	.392	.258	.128
17	3.965	2.898	2.567	2.110	1.740	1.333	1.069	.863	.689	.534	.392	.257	.128
18	3.922	2.878	2.552	2.101	1.734	1.330	1.067	.862	.688	.534	.392	.257	.127
19	3.883	2.861	2.539	2.093	1.729	1.328	1.066	.861	.688	.533	.391	.257	.127
20	3.850	2.845	2.528	2.086	1.725	1.325	1.064	.860	.687	.533	.391	.257	.127
21	3.819	2.831	2.518	2.080	1.721	1.323	1.063	.859	.686	.532	.391	.257	.127
22	3.792	2.819	2.508	2.074	1.717	1.321	1.061	.858	.686	.532	.390	.256	.127
23	3.767	2.807	2.500	2.069	1.714	1.319	1.060	.858	.685	.532	.390	.256	.127
24	3.745	2.797	2.492	2.064	1.711	1.318	1.059	.857	.685	.531	.390	.256	.127
25	3.725	2.787	2.485	2.060	1.708	1.316	1.058	.856	.684	.531	.390	.256	.127
26	3.707	2.779	2.479	2.056	1.706	1.315	1.058	.856	.684	.531	.390	.256	.127
27	3.690	2.771	2.473	2.052	1.703	1.314	1.057	.855	.684	.531	.389	.256	.127
28	3.674	2.763	2.467	2.048	1.701	1.313	1.056	.855	.683	.530	.389	.256	.127
29	3.659	2.756	2.462	2.045	1.699	1.311	1.055	.854	.683	.530	.389	.256	.127
30	3.646	2.750	2.457	2.042	1.697	1.310	1.055	.854	.683	.530	.389	.256	.127
40	3.551	2.704	2.423	2.021	1.684	1.303	1.050	.851	.681	.529	.388	.255	.126
60	3.460	2.660	2.390	2.000	1.671	1.296	1.046	.848	.679	.527	.387	.254	.126
120	3.373	2.617	2.358	1.980	1.658	1.289	1.041	.845	.677	.526	.386	.254	.126
∞	3.291	2.576	2.326	1.960	1.645	1.282	1.036	.842	.674	.524	.385	.253	.126

Table of Squares and Square Roots

n	n^2	$\sqrt{n}$	$\sqrt{10n}$	$1/n$	n	n^2	$\sqrt{n}$	$\sqrt{10n}$	$1/n$
1.00	1.0000	1.00000	3.16228	1.000000	1.50	2.2500	1.22474	3.87298	.666667
1.01	1.0201	1.00499	3.17805	.990099	1.51	2.2801	1.22882	3.88587	.662252
1.02	1.0404	1.00995	3.19374	.980392	1.52	2.3104	1.23288	3.89872	.657895
1.03	1.0609	1.01489	3.20936	.970874	1.53	2.3409	1.23693	3.91152	.653595
1.04	1.0816	1.01980	3.22490	.961538	1.54	2.3716	1.24097	3.92428	.649351
1.05	1.1025	1.02470	3.24037	.952381	1.55	2.4025	1.24499	3.93700	.645161
1.06	1.1236	1.02956	3.25576	.943396	1.56	2.4336	1.24900	3.94968	.641026
1.07	1.1449	1.03441	3.27109	.934579	1.57	2.4649	1.25300	3.96232	.636943
1.08	1.1664	1.03923	3.28634	.925926	1.58	2.4964	1.25698	3.97492	.632911
1.09	1.1881	1.04403	3.30151	.917431	1.59	2.5281	1.26095	3.98748	.628931
1.10	1.2100	1.04881	3.31662	.909091	1.60	2.5600	1.26491	4.00000	.625000
1.11	1.2321	1.05357	3.33167	.900901	1.61	2.5921	1.26886	4.01248	.621118
1.12	1.2544	1.05830	3.34664	.892857	1.62	2.6244	1.27279	4.02492	.617284
1.13	1.2769	1.06301	3.36155	.884956	1.63	2.6569	1.27671	4.03733	.613497
1.14	1.2996	1.06771	3.37639	.877193	1.64	2.6896	1.28062	4.04969	.609756
1.15	1.3225	1.07238	3.39116	.869565	1.65	2.7225	1.28452	4.06202	.606061
1.16	1.3456	1.07703	3.40588	.862069	1.66	2.7556	1.28841	4.07431	.602410
1.17	1.3689	1.08167	3.42053	.854701	1.67	2.7889	1.29228	4.08656	.598802
1.18	1.3924	1.08628	3.43511	.847458	1.68	2.8224	1.29615	4.09878	.595238
1.19	1.4161	1.09087	3.44964	.840336	1.69	2.8561	1.30000	4.11096	.591716
1.20	1.4400	1.09545	3.46410	.833333	1.70	2.8900	1.30384	4.12311	.588235
1.21	1.4641	1.10000	3.47851	.826446	1.71	2.9241	1.30767	4.13521	.584795
1.22	1.4884	1.10454	3.49285	.819672	1.72	2.9584	1.31149	4.14729	.581395
1.23	1.5129	1.10905	3.50714	.813008	1.73	2.9929	1.31529	4.15933	.578035
1.24	1.5376	1.11355	3.52136	.806452	1.74	3.0276	1.31909	4.17133	.574713
1.25	1.5625	1.11803	3.53553	.800000	1.75	3.0625	1.32288	4.18330	.571429
1.26	1.5876	1.12250	3.54965	.793651	1.76	3.0976	1.32665	4.19524	.568182
1.27	1.6129	1.12694	3.56371	.787402	1.77	3.1329	1.33041	4.20714	.564972
1.28	1.6384	1.13137	3.57771	.781250	1.78	3.1684	1.33417	4.21900	.561798
1.29	1.6641	1.13578	3.59166	.775194	1.79	3.2041	1.33791	4.23084	.558659
1.30	1.6900	1.14018	3.60555	.769231	1.80	3.2400	1.34164	4.24264	.555556
1.31	1.7161	1.14455	3.61939	.763359	1.81	3.2761	1.34536	4.25441	.552486
1.32	1.7424	1.14891	3.63318	.757576	1.82	3.3124	1.34907	4.26615	.549451
1.33	1.7689	1.15326	3.64692	.751880	1.83	3.3489	1.35277	4.27785	.546448
1.34	1.7956	1.15758	3.66060	.746269	1.84	3.3856	1.35647	4.28952	.543478
1.35	1.8225	1.16190	3.67423	.740741	1.85	3.4225	1.36015	4.30116	.540541
1.36	1.8496	1.16619	3.68782	.735294	1.86	3.4596	1.36382	4.31277	.537634
1.37	1.8769	1.17047	3.70135	.729927	1.87	3.4969	1.36748	4.32435	.534759
1.38	1.9044	1.17473	3.71484	.724638	1.88	3.5344	1.37113	4.33590	.531915
1.39	1.9321	1.17898	3.72827	.719424	1.89	3.5721	1.37477	4.34741	.529101
1.40	1.9600	1.18322	3.74166	.714286	1.90	3.6100	1.37840	4.35890	.526316
1.41	1.9881	1.18743	3.75500	.709220	1.91	3.6481	1.38203	4.37035	.523560
1.42	2.0164	1.19164	3.76829	.704225	1.92	3.6864	1.38564	4.38178	.520833
1.43	2.0449	1.19583	3.78153	.699301	1.93	3.7249	1.38924	4.39318	.518135
1.44	2.0736	1.20000	3.79473	.694444	1.94	3.7636	1.39284	4.40454	.515464
1.45	2.1025	1.20416	3.80789	.689655	1.95	3.8025	1.39642	4.41588	.512821
1.46	2.1316	1.20830	3.82099	.684932	1.96	3.8416	1.40000	4.42719	.510204
1.47	2.1609	1.21244	3.83406	.680272	1.97	3.8809	1.40357	4.43847	.507614
1.48	2.1904	1.21655	3.84708	.675676	1.98	3.9204	1.40712	4.44972	.505051
1.49	2.2201	1.22066	3.86005	.671141	1.99	3.9601	1.41067	4.46094	.502513
1.50	2.2500	1.22474	3.87298	.666667	2.00	4.0000	1.41421	4.47214	.500000
n	n^2	$\sqrt{n}$	$\sqrt{10n}$	$1/n$	n	n^2	$\sqrt{n}$	$\sqrt{10n}$	$1/n$

APPENDIX E
Table of Chi-Square (χ^2) Values

d.f.	0.99	0.98	0.95	0.90	0.80	0.70	0.50	0.30	0.20	0.10	0.05	0.02	0.01
1	0.000157	0.000628	0.00393	0.0158	0.0642	0.148	0.455	1.074	1.642	2.706	3.841	5.412	6.635
2	0.0201	0.0404	0.103	0.211	0.446	0.713	1.386	2.408	3.219	4.605	5.991	7.824	9.210
3	0.115	0.185	0.352	0.584	1.005	1.424	2.366	3.665	4.642	6.251	7.815	9.837	11.345
4	0.297	0.429	0.711	1.064	1.649	2.195	3.357	4.878	5.989	7.779	9.488	11.668	13.277
5	0.554	0.752	1.145	1.610	2.343	3.000	4.351	6.064	7.289	9.236	11.070	13.388	15.086
6	0.872	1.134	1.635	2.204	3.070	3.828	5.348	7.231	8.558	10.645	12.592	15.033	16.812
7	1.239	1.564	2.167	2.833	3.822	4.671	6.346	8.383	9.803	12.017	14.067	16.622	18.475
8	1.646	2.032	2.733	3.490	4.594	5.527	7.344	9.524	11.030	13.362	15.507	18.168	20.090
9	2.088	2.532	3.325	4.168	5.380	6.393	8.343	10.656	12.242	14.684	16.919	19.679	21.666
10	2.558	3.059	3.940	4.865	6.179	7.267	9.342	11.781	13.442	15.987	18.307	21.161	23.209
11	3.053	3.609	4.575	5.578	6.989	8.148	10.341	12.899	14.631	17.275	19.675	22.618	24.725
12	3.571	4.178	5.226	6.304	7.807	9.034	11.340	14.011	15.812	18.549	21.026	24.054	26.217
13	4.107	4.765	5.892	7.042	8.634	9.926	12.340	15.119	16.985	19.812	22.362	25.472	27.688
14	4.660	5.368	6.571	7.790	9.467	10.821	13.339	16.222	18.151	21.064	23.685	26.873	29.141
15	5.229	5.985	7.261	8.547	10.307	11.721	14.339	17.322	19.311	22.307	24.996	28.259	30.578
16	5.812	6.614	7.962	9.312	11.152	12.624	15.338	18.418	20.465	23.542	26.296	29.633	32.000
17	6.408	7.255	8.672	10.085	12.002	13.531	16.338	19.511	21.615	24.769	27.587	30.995	33.409
18	7.015	7.906	9.390	10.865	12.857	14.440	17.338	20.601	22.760	25.989	28.869	32.346	34.805
19	7.633	8.567	10.117	11.651	13.716	15.352	18.338	21.689	23.900	27.204	30.144	33.687	36.191
20	8.260	9.237	10.851	12.443	14.578	16.266	19.337	22.775	25.038	28.412	31.410	35.020	37.566
21	8.897	9.915	11.591	13.240	15.445	17.182	20.337	23.858	26.171	29.615	32.671	36.343	38.932
22	9.542	10.600	12.338	14.041	16.314	18.101	21.337	24.939	27.301	30.813	33.924	37.659	40.289
23	10.196	11.293	13.091	14.848	17.187	19.021	22.337	26.018	28.429	32.007	35.172	38.968	41.638
24	10.856	11.992	13.848	15.659	18.062	19.943	23.337	27.096	29.553	33.196	36.415	40.270	42.980
25	11.524	12.697	14.611	16.473	18.940	20.867	24.337	28.172	30.675	34.382	37.652	41.566	44.314
26	12.198	13.409	15.379	17.292	19.820	21.792	25.336	29.246	31.795	35.563	38.885	42.856	45.642
27	12.879	14.125	16.151	18.114	20.703	22.719	26.336	30.319	32.912	36.741	40.113	44.140	46.963
28	13.565	14.847	16.928	18.939	21.588	23.647	27.336	31.391	34.027	37.916	41.337	45.419	48.278
29	14.256	15.574	17.708	19.768	22.475	24.577	28.336	32.461	35.139	39.087	42.557	46.693	49.588
30	14.953	16.306	18.493	20.599	23.364	25.508	29.336	33.530	36.250	40.256	43.773	47.962	50.892

APPENDIX F
Basic Math Review

Most of us need an occasional review of some basic mathematics. Often through lack of use, we forget even some of the simple arithmetic operations. Since many of the errors that are commonly made in statistical analyses are not mistakes in statistics, but rather mistakes in simple arithmetic, we shall review a few of the basic rules.

WORKING WITH FRACTIONS

In the fraction ⅜, the numerator is 3 and the denominator is 8. Many of the operations with fractions involve the numerator or denominator, or both. The above fraction is a simple fraction. If the numerator is larger than the denominator (such as $5/3$) the fraction is called an improper fraction. Any number that has a whole number and a fraction (such as 5⅜) is called a mixed number.

You can convert a number from a mixed number to an improper fraction by the following method:

	Result
Convert 5⅜ to an improper fraction.	
1. Multiply the whole number by the denominator.	40
2. Add the numerator.	43
3. Place this result over the denominator.	$\frac{43}{8}$

You can convert an improper fraction to a mixed number by using the following technique:

Convert $43/8$ to a mixed number.	
1. Divide the numerator by the denominator and get the closest whole number.	5
2. Place the remainder over the denominator.	⅜
3. Combine these two as a mixed number.	5⅜

In the discussion that follows, it will be assumed that all mixed numbers have been converted to improper fractions. In practice, it is often easier to perform arithmetic with fractions if this is the case.

It is often necessary to reduce a fraction to its lowest terms. The rule to remember in this case is that if you divide both the numerator and the denominator by the same number, the value of the fraction doesn't change. This should be done until no more reductions are possible.

For example, reduce the fraction $^{84}/_{180}$.

1. Divide both terms by 2.	$^{42}/_{90}$
2. Divide both terms by 3.	$^{14}/_{30}$
3. Divide both terms by 2.	$^{7}/_{15}$

When two or more fractions are to be added, they must have the same denominator. If the denominators are the same, you merely add the numerators together and place this number over the "common denominator."

For example:

$$\frac{1}{8} + \frac{12}{8} + \frac{3}{8} = \frac{16}{8}$$

$$\frac{1}{3} + \frac{8}{3} + \frac{1}{3} = \frac{10}{3}$$

If the denominators are not the same, some arithmetic operations must be performed to get a common denominator. The easiest, though certainly not the most efficient, way of doing this is as follows:

Solve:

$$\frac{5}{3} + \frac{2}{7} + \frac{1}{2}$$

1. Multiply all of the denominators.

$$(3)\,(7)\,(2) = 42$$

2. Multiply each numerator by each of the *other* denominators (not including its own).

$$(5)\,(7)\,(2) = 70$$
$$(2)\,(3)(2) = 12$$
$$(1)\,(3)\,(7) = 21$$

3. Add the results from Step 2.   103
4. Place the answer from Step 3 over the answer from Step 1. $\frac{103}{42}$

5. Reduce to lowest terms. $\frac{103}{42}$

When two or more fractions are to be subtracted, they must also have the same denominator. The rules are the same as those for addition except that a subtraction is performed where appropriate. A few examples should clarify this.

a. $\dfrac{12}{11} - \dfrac{2}{11} + \dfrac{3}{11} - \dfrac{4}{11} = \dfrac{12 - 2 + 3 - 4}{11} = \dfrac{9}{11}$

b. $\dfrac{1}{4} + \dfrac{9}{5} - \dfrac{1}{2}$

Rule 1: (4) (5) (2) = 40
Rule 2: (1) (5) (2) = 10
$\qquad$ (9) (4) (2) = 72
$\qquad$ (−1) (4) (5) = −20
Rule 3: 10 + 72 − 20 = 62
Rule 4: $\dfrac{62}{40}$
Rule 5: $\dfrac{31}{20}$

Note: In the application of Rule 3, a subtraction was called for in the original problem.

To multiply fractions, you need only multiply all of the numerators to get the numerator of the answer. Then multiply all the denominators to get the denominator of the answer. For example:

a. $\dfrac{2}{5} \times \dfrac{3}{7} \times \dfrac{2}{4} \times \dfrac{1}{2} = \dfrac{12}{280}$

Reducing to lowest terms = $3/70$

$\dfrac{9}{2} \times 5 \times 2\dfrac{2}{3} \times \dfrac{9}{2} \times \dfrac{5}{1} \times \dfrac{8}{3} = \dfrac{360}{6} = 60$

In example b, the whole number 5 was made into a fraction $5/1$ and the mixed number $2^2/3$ was made into a fraction $8/3$.

The reciprocal of a fraction is a fraction with its numerator and denominator "switched." Thus, the reciprocal is very useful when dividing by fractions.

To divide a number by a fraction, you simply multiply that number by the reciprocal of that fraction. Thus,

a. $\dfrac{\frac{5}{1}}{\frac{1}{3}} = 5 \times \dfrac{3}{1} = 15$ $\qquad\qquad$ b. $\dfrac{\frac{1}{2}}{\frac{1}{4}} = \dfrac{1}{2} \times \dfrac{4}{1} = \dfrac{2}{1} = 2$

c. $\dfrac{2\frac{1}{8}}{3\frac{3}{4}} = \dfrac{17/8}{15/4} = \dfrac{17}{8} \times \dfrac{4}{15} = \dfrac{68}{120} = \dfrac{17}{30}$

Please note carefully all of the operations in example c.

Before moving on to other math topics, mastery of the material in this section should be determined by solving the following problems:

1. If 10 ounces of sugar are added to 25 ounces of water, what part of the finished solution is water?
2. Four out of every ten children visiting a health clinic were vaccinated against smallpox. What fraction of the group were vaccinated? If 420 children visited the clinic, how many were vaccinated?
3. A tablet contains 9 grains of a particular drug, if you want to give a patient 3 grains, what fraction of the tablet will you use?
4. Change the following improper fractions to mixed numbers.

    a. $\dfrac{75}{18}$ b. $\dfrac{649}{320}$ c. $\dfrac{94}{21}$

    d. $\dfrac{327}{7}$ e. $\dfrac{563}{280}$ f. $\dfrac{55}{11}$

5. Change the following mixed fractions to improper fractions:

    a. $2\dfrac{3}{17}$ b. $13\dfrac{4}{7}$ c. $132\dfrac{2}{3}$

    d. $23\dfrac{5}{9}$ e. $112\dfrac{13}{25}$ f. $95\dfrac{1}{2}$

6. A tablet of morphine contains ⅓ grain of the drug. If you used ¾ of a tablet, how much of the drug would be used?
7. If a patient receives 2⅔ tablets of Inderal and each tablet contains 1¼ grains, how much of the drug will she receive?
8. Perform the indicated arithmetic operations of the following fractions.

    a. $\dfrac{1}{50} \div \dfrac{3}{8}$ f. $3\dfrac{3}{5} \div 4\dfrac{1}{8}$

    b. $25\dfrac{2}{3} \times \dfrac{1}{8}$ g. $25\dfrac{1}{5} \times 6 + \dfrac{1}{3}$

    c. $250 \div 5\dfrac{3}{5}$ h. $28 \div 56$

    d. $\dfrac{1}{4} + \dfrac{1}{3} + \dfrac{5}{8}$ i. $7\dfrac{1}{8} + 5 + 2\dfrac{2}{3} - 1\dfrac{1}{2}$

    e. $2\dfrac{1}{2} - 3\dfrac{3}{4} + \dfrac{2}{3} + 4$ j. $3\dfrac{1}{3} - 4\dfrac{1}{3} + 6\dfrac{1}{8}$

WORKING WITH DECIMALS

A decimal is a fraction whose denominator is some power of 10 (i.e., 10, 100, 1,000, 10,000 etc.). Thus $^{45}/_{100}$ can be written as .45 instead of as a fraction. The first number after the decimal point is tenths, the second represents hundredths, and so on.

A decimal is formed by dividing the numerator of a fraction by its denominator and carrying the answer out to as many decimal positions as you wish. Thus, if we begin with the fraction $^8/_{15}$, its decimal equivalent would be:

$$
\begin{array}{r}
.533 \\
15 \overline{\smash{\big)}\ 8.000} \\
-7.5 \\
\hline
50 \\
-45 \\
\hline
50 \\
-45 \\
\hline
5
\end{array}
$$

Multiplying a decimal by a power of 10 is merely a matter of moving the decimal point. You move the decimal point one place to the right for each zero in the power of 10 you are multiplying by.

Therefore,

$$
\begin{aligned}
.533 \times 10 &= 5.33 \\
.533 \times 100 &= 53.3 \\
.533 \times 1,000 &= 533.
\end{aligned}
$$

If you are dividing by a power of 10, you move the decimal point one place to the *left* for each zero in the power of 10 you are dividing by. So:

$$
\frac{.533}{10} = .0533
$$

$$
\frac{.533}{100} = .00533
$$

$$
\frac{.533}{1,000} = .000533
$$

Adding and subtracting decimals is done in the same way as with whole numbers. Before the operation takes place, however, all decimal points are aligned. For example,

a. Add 11.7, 36.75 and 28.032

$$
\begin{array}{r}
11.700 \\
36.750 \\
+28.032 \\
\hline
76.482
\end{array}
$$

b. Subtract 8.39 from 16.965

$$
\begin{array}{r}
16.965 \\
-\ 8.390 \\
\hline
8.575
\end{array}
$$

When multiplying decimal, together, you multiply them just as if they were whole numbers. The number of decimal places you are supposed to have in your answer is equal to the sum of the number of decimal *places* you had in the original factors. Thus,

a.
$$\begin{array}{r} 3.8 \\ \times\ 9.1 \\ \hline .38 \\ 34.2 \\ \hline 34.58 \end{array}$$

b. $3.4 \times 8.6 \times 1.5$

$$\begin{array}{r} 3.4 \\ \times\ 8.6 \\ \hline 2.04 \\ 27.2 \\ \hline 29.24 \end{array} \qquad \begin{array}{r} 29.24 \\ \times\ 1.5 \\ \hline 14.620 \\ 29.24 \\ \hline 43.860 \end{array}$$

The rules for dividing one decimal by another are as follows:

Divide 36.30 by 1.5	Result
1. Move the decimal point in the divisor to the right until you have a whole number	15
2. Move the decimal point in the dividend the same number of positions to the right as you did in Step 1.	364.0
3. Proceed with the division	$\begin{array}{r} 24.2 \\ 15\overline{)363.00} \\ 30 \\ \hline 63 \\ 60 \\ \hline 30 \\ 30 \\ \hline 0 \end{array}$

Finally, it is sometimes necessary to convert from a decimal to a fraction.

For example, convert .612 to a fraction.	Result
1. The numerator of the fraction is found by moving the decimal point to the right until you have a whole number.	612
2. The denominator of the fraction is found by raising 10 to the same power as the number of places you had to move the decimal point to in Step 1.	$10^3 = 1,000$
3. Reduce the fraction to lowest terms	$\dfrac{612}{1,000} = \dfrac{153}{250}$

For practice in working with decimal, you should solve the following problems.

1. Express the following fractions as decimals.

   a. $\dfrac{3}{8}$

   b. $7\dfrac{11}{15}$

   c. $\dfrac{350}{10,000}$

   d. $4\dfrac{7}{8}$

   e. $172\dfrac{99}{150}$

2. Add the following decimals.
   a. $3.025 + 17 + 11.962$
   b. $1.005 + 1.030 + .0463$
   c. $.8 + .3 + .8 + .1$
   d. $340.6 + .8$
   e. $9.89 + .106 + 140.35$

3. A distraught male has taken 15 capsules of tuinal in a suicide attempt. If each capsule contains .025 grains of secobarbital sodium and amobarbital sodium, what is the total amount of the drug that was taken?

4. A particular patient needs to get 1½ grains of digitalis over a period of 24 hours. How many .2 gram tablets will be needed?

5. Convert the following decimals to fractions.
   a. 0.00328
   b. 0.65
   c. 0.541
   d. 0.1755
   e. 0.5
   f. 0.00601

6. Perform the indicated arithmetic operations for each of the following problems.
   a. $1896.32 \div 4.8$
   b. $908.6582 \div .00005$
   c. $4 \div 100.6$
   d. $5.520 \div 8.671$
   e. $1.625 - .0039$
   f. $7.6314 \times \text{⅛}$
   g. $37\text{¼} \div 0.5$
   h. $0.851 + 96.32 + 8.2 - .6$

i. 33.333 × 33.333
j. 972.652 ÷ 3.1

FINDING AND USING PERCENTS

Percent means "by the hundred." Thus, a percent is really a fraction with 100 as its denominator. For example 92 percent is the same as $^{92}/_{100}$. You can also represent this percent as the decimal .92 by using the rules for converting from fractions to decimals that was given earlier. Care must be taken when representing percents as decimals as can be seen in the example below:

$$.92 \text{ does not equal } .92\%$$

$$.92 = \frac{92}{100} \qquad\qquad .92\% = \frac{.92}{100}$$

To change decimal numbers into percents, move the decimal point two places to the right and add the percent sign at the end. For example:

a. .365 = 36.5%
b. 1.10 = 110%
c. 0.004 = .4%

To change fractions into percents,

1. Change the fraction into a decimal number.
2. Move the decimal point to the right two places and add the percent sign.

a.
$$\begin{array}{r} .25 \\ 1/4\overline{)\,1.00} \\ -.8 \quad = 25\% \\ \hline 20 \\ -\,20 \\ \hline 0 \end{array}$$

b.
$$\begin{array}{r} .375 \\ 3/8\overline{)\,3.000} \\ -2.4 \quad = 37.5\% \\ \hline 60 \\ -\,56 \\ \hline 0 \end{array}$$

It is useful to note that many percentage problems involve a very simple formula:

Formula 1: Percent = $\dfrac{\text{Part}}{\text{Whole}}$

This can also be written in two other forms:

Formula 2: Part = Whole × Percent

Formula 3: Whole = $\dfrac{\text{Part}}{\text{Percent}}$

(The percent is always in its decimal form.)

If any two of these quantities are known, the third can always be found. For example:

a.   Find 20% of 60.

$$Percent = .20$$
$$Part = ?$$
$$Whole = 60$$

Use Formula 2: Part = 60 × .20 = 12

b.   12 is what percent of 48?

$$Percent = ?$$
$$Part = 12$$
$$Whole = 48$$

Use Formula 1: Percent = 12/48 = 1/4 = .25 = .25%

c.   30 percent of what number is equal to 15?

$$Percent = .30$$
$$Part = 15$$
$$Whole = ?$$

Use Formula 3: Whole = 15/.30 = $\frac{15}{3/10}$ = 15 × 10/3 = $\frac{150}{3}$ = 50

Very often, it is necessary to find the percentage of an increase or a decrease. To do this, it is first necessary to find the amount of the increase or decrease and divide this amount by the "base" or starting number. For example:

A patient's weight increased from 205 pounds to 220 pounds. Find the percentage of increase.

$$Amount\ of\ increase = 15$$
$$Base\ number = 205$$
$$Percentage\ of\ increase = \frac{15}{205} = \frac{3}{41} = .73 = 7.3\%$$

The number of orders for Valium decreased from 75 to 25 in one day. Find the percentage of decrease in Valium orders.

$$Amount\ of\ decrease = 50$$
$$Base\ number = 75$$
$$Percentage\ of\ decrease = \frac{50}{75} = \frac{2}{3} = .667 = 66.7\%$$

The following problems deal with percents.

1.   A nurse earns $1,400 per month and spends $1,200. What percentage of her monthly salary does she save?

2.   About 3 percent of the nurses graduating from a certain university become involved in rape counseling. If there are 400 graduates, how many become rape counselors?

3.   Between December 1973 and December 1976, nursing salaries increased from $9,000 per year to $12,000 per year. What percentage is this?

4.   If a data collection effort reveals that 30 fathers were present during the

birth of their first child, and this represents 25 percent of those interviewed, how many fathers were interviewed?

5. A research report states that the number of nurses at a particular hospital has dropped from 155 to 120 in the past year. What is the percentage of decrease?

6. Solve the following:
   a. Find 60 percent of 450.
   b. 40 is what percent of 350?
   c. You send out 3,500 questionnaires as part of a research project. You got 1,250 returns. What was your response rate?

7. Change the following fractions into percents.
   a. $\dfrac{3}{8}$

   b. $\dfrac{60}{135}$

   c. $\dfrac{950}{2,100}$

   d. $\dfrac{8}{54}$

   e. $\dfrac{19}{20}$

SQUARE ROOTS

In statistical analysis, the student will find many instances in which a square root needs to be taken. Appendix D contains the square root for whole numbers from 1 to 1,000. The square root of a number is obtained by identifying a number that, when multiplied by itself equals the original number. Thus, the square root of 16 is 4 (since $4 \times 4 = 16$). The symbol $\sqrt{}$ (called the radical) is used to denote the square root of a number. The previous example would have been written as: $\sqrt{16} = 4$

Occasionally, you will need to know the square root of a number that is not a whole number (and thus is not contained in Appendix D). While detailed arithmetic techniques are available (as are desk calculators), it is often sufficient to approximate the answer through trial and error. For example, if you were looking for $\sqrt{1525}$ you might try the following:

$$35 \times 35 = 1,225 \text{ (too low)}$$
$$40 \times 40 = 1,600 \text{ (too high)}$$
$$39 \times 39 = 1,521 \text{ (close enough)}$$

Try the following problems:

1. Use the tables in Appendix D to find the following square roots.
    a. $\sqrt{35}$
    b. $\sqrt{952}$
    c. $\sqrt{300}$
    d. $\sqrt{175}$
    e. $\sqrt{18}$
2. Approximate the following square roots.
    a. $\sqrt{36.2}$
    b. $\sqrt{1.896}$
    c. $\sqrt{37,592}$
    d. $\sqrt{\dfrac{38}{5}}$

NEGATIVE NUMBERS

There are special rules for performing arithmetic with negative numbers.

Addition

To add numbers that all have a minus sign in front of them, you simply add the numbers and put a minus sign in front of the answer. For example:

$$(-6) + (-30) + (-5) = -41$$

When signs are mixed (i.e., some positive and some negative), you add all the positive numbers (put a plus sign in front of the result) and add all the negative numbers (and place a minus sign in front of that total). You are now left with two numbers, one positive and one negative. The final step is to take the difference between these two numbers (disregarding signs) and give the sign of the largest number to the answer. For example: Add the following-
    a. $-8 + 10.2 - 15.2 + 8 - 2.1 - 3 = +18.2 - 28.3 = -10.1$
    b. $+36.5 - 8.3 = +28.2$
    c. $-18.6 + 9 = -9.6$

Subtraction

When subtracting a negative number, change its sign, and proceed as you did in addition.

$$
\begin{array}{r} 42 \\ -(-5) \\ \hline 47 \end{array}
\qquad
\begin{array}{r} -17 \\ -(-3) \\ \hline -14 \end{array}
\qquad
\begin{array}{r} -3.6 \\ -(-8.9) \\ \hline +5.3 \end{array}
$$

Multiplication

Whenever you are multiplying a series of numbers together, the sign (plus or minus) of the answer is a function of how many negative signs were in the set of numbers. If there are an even number, the answer is positive. If there are an odd number of minus signs, the answer is negative.

a. $(-6) \times (-5) = +30$
b. $(-4) \times (+3) = -12$
c. $(-3) \times (-8) \times (-4) \times (-2) = +192$
d. $(-2) \times (+3) \times (-1) \times (-2) = -12$

Division

When a number is divided by a number with the same sign, the answer is always positive. When the signs are different, the answer is always negative.

a. $\dfrac{+18}{+13} = +6$

b. $\dfrac{-18}{+3} = -6$

c. $\dfrac{+18}{-3} = -6$

d. $\dfrac{-18}{-3} = +6$

You should test your knowledge of how to deal with negative numbers by solving the following problems.

1. $-90 + 96.1 - 8 - 5.6 + 32.5 - 121$
2. $^1/_4 + ^3/_8 - 5^2/_3 + 2^1/_4$
3. $62.5 - (-8)$

4. $3^3/_8 - (-1^1/_2)$
5. -6×-3.2
6. $-^1/_8 \times 1^1/_3$
7. $3^3/_5 \div -5^1/_4$
8. $18.6 - {}^5/_6 + 1^1/_4 - 1$
9. $-19.5 - 18.1 + 18.6 - 3.2$
10. $9^1/_2 - .005 + 1.5 - .75$

THE NUMBER ZERO

Sometimes, the number zero causes students difficulty. However, there really is nothing to it! There are two key rules to remember about the number zero.

1. Anything that is multiplied by zero is equal to zero. Examples:
   a. $56.3 \times 0 = 0$
   b. $(5) \times (^1/_8) \times (0) \times (35.6) = 0$
2. Division by zero is not a legitimate arithmetic operation and is not allowed.
3. Dividing zero by anything leaves you with zero. Thus,

$$0 \div {}^1/_4 = 0$$

At this point, you should be more confident in your ability to work with numbers.

APPENDIX G
Selected References in Research, Statistics, and Computers

Advances in Nursing Science. Aspen Systems Corporation, P. O. Box 335, Dover, New Jersey 07801.

International Journal of Nursing Studies. Pergamon Press, Maxwell House, Fariview Park, Elmsford, New York 10523.

Issues in Mental Health Nursing. McGraw-Hill Book Co., 1221 Avenue of the Americas, New York, New York 10020.

Journal of Advanced Nursing. Blackwell Scientific Publications Ltd., Osney Mead, Oxford, England.

Journal of Nursing Education. Charles B. Slack, Inc., 6900 Grove Road, Thorofare, New Jersey 08086.

Journal of Obstetric, Gynecologic and Neonatal Nursing. Medical Department, Harper & Row Publishers, 2350 Virginia Ave., Hagerstown, MD 21740.

Journal of Psychiatric Nursing and Mental Health Services. Charles B. Slack Inc., 6900 Grove Road, Thorofare, New Jersey 08086.

Nursing Administration Quarterly. Aspen Systems Corporation, 20010 Century Boulevard, Germantown, MD 20767.

Nursing Forum. Nursing Publications, Inc. Box 218, Hillsdale, New Jersey 07642.

Nursing Research. 10 Columbus Circle, New York, New York 10019.

Maternal-Child Nursing Journal. 3505 Fifth Avenue, Pittsburgh, PA 15213.

Research in Nursing & Health. John Wiley & Sons, Inc. Publishers, 605 Third Avenue, New York, NY 10016.

Western Journal of Nursing Research. Philips-Allen, Publishers, 1330 S. State College Blvd., Anaheim, CA 92806.

Research Reference Books

Abdellah, F. and Levine, E. *Better Patient Care Through Nursing Research*, (2nd ed.). New York: Macmillan Co., 1978.

Downs, N. and Newman, M. *A Source Book of Nursing Research*, (2nd ed.). Philadelphia: F. A. Davis Co., 1977.

Fox, D. *Fundamentals of Research in Nursing*, (2nd ed.). New York: Appleton Century Crofts, 1970.

Hardyck, C. & Petrinovich, L. *Understanding Research in the Social Sciences*. Philadelphia: W. B. Saunders Co., 1975.

Kerlinger, F. *Foundations of Behavioral Research*. New York: Holt, Rinehart & Winston, 1973.

Mayo, C. and La France, M. *Evaluating Research in Social Psychology*. Montery, Calif.: Brooks/Cole Publishing Co., 1977.

Notter, L. *Essentials of Nursing Research*, (2nd ed.). New York: Springer Publishing Co., 1978.

Polit, D. and Hungler, B. *Nursing Research*. Philadelphia: J. B. Lippincott Co., 1978.

Treece, E. & Treece, J. *Elements of Research in Nursing*, (2nd ed.). St. Louis: C. V. Mosby Co., 1977.

Verhonick, P. & Seaman, C. *Research Methods for Undergraduate Students in Nursing*. New York: Appleton-Century-Crofts, 1978.

Wandelt, M. *Guide for the Beginning Researcher*. New York: Appleton-Century-Crofts, 1970.

Selection of Periodicals That Contain Computer Information

Computerworld
Creative Computing
Datamation
Personal Computing
Physician's Microcomputer Report

Computer Reference Books

Awad, E.M. *Business Data Processing*. 5th ed. Englewood Cliffs, NJ: Prentice Hall, 1980

Collen, M.F. (ed) *Hospital Computer Systems*. New York: Wiley, 1974.

Hennenfeld, Julien. *Using BASIC*. Boston: Prindle, Weber & Schmidt, Inc. 1978

Mulcahy, Michael. *Conversational BASIC*. Boston: CBI Publishing Company. 1980

O'Brien, James A. *Computers in Business Management*. Illinois: Richard D. Irwin, Inc., 1979

Rothman, S. and C. Mossman. *Computers and Society*, 2nd ed. Chicago: Science Research Associates, 1976

Teague, R., and C. Erickson. *Computers and Society*. St. Paul, MN: West Publishing Co., 1974

Reference Books in Statistics

Arkin, Herbert. Statistical Methods. New York: Barnes and Noble, Inc., 1970

Arkin, Herbert. Tables for Statisticians. New York: Barnes and Noble, Inc., 1970

Hoel, Paul. Elementary Statistics. New York: John Wiley and Sons, Inc., 1976

Kilpatrick, James. Statistical Principles in Health Care Information. Baltimore: University Park Press, 1973

Moore, Richard. Introduction to the Use of Computer Packages for Statistical Analysis. New Jersey: Prentice Hall, Inc., 1978

Nie, Norman et al. SPSS Statistical Package for the Social Sciences. New York: McGraw-Hill, 1975

APPENDIX H
Examples of Research Studies Conducted by Nursing Students

Nurses' Perceptions of Their Roles and Responsibilities in Discharge Planning

Factors Influencing Nurses' Attitudes Toward Abortions

A Study of Nurses' Perceptions of Breast Feeding Problems

Hypertension: Knowledge and Attitudes of the Black Male College Student

Attitudes of Residents of a Suburban Community Toward Utilizing an Independent Nurse Practitioner as Their Primary Health Care Provider

Fears of the Primiparous Woman in the Process of Childbirth: A Comparison of Women Prepared in the Lamaze Method and Those Who Were Not

Factors Influencing the Decision for Home Delivery

Nurses' Perceptions of Their Role and Responsibilities in the Deinstitutionalization of Long-term Psychiatric Patients

A Study of the Acceptance of Change in a Patient Data-recording Procedure Involving a Selected Group of Nurses

A Study of the Needs, Reactions, and Problems of Expectant Fathers in the First, Second, and Third Trimesters of Pregnancy

Health Knowledge and Attitudes of the College Population Regarding Heart Disease and Its Prevention

A Study of Registered Nurses' Attitudes Toward Malpractice Insurance as a Means of Protection Against Liabilities

An Investigation of Patient Characteristics and Situational Factors Influencing Noncompliance in Keeping Appointments in a Venereal Disease Clinic

A Study of the Confidence Levels of Nursery Nurses in Caring for Newborns with Heart Defects

Crying Behavior of Children After Elective Surgery

Patients' Attitudes About Evaluating the Quality of Their Nursing Care

A Study of the Level of Sexual Knowledge of Adolescents Seeking Abortions in a Community Clinic

Health Needs and Concerns of Unwed Pregnant Adolescents

A Study of the Attitudes and Motivational Factors Which Influence the Practice of Breast Self-Examination in Female College Students

Attitudes of Doctors and Nurses Toward the Value and Utilization of Nurses' Notes

A Study of the Health Consumer—His Knowledge of His Medications, His Source of Information, and Implication for Nursing

A Study of Anxieties of Preoperative Children Exhibited in Play Therapy Sessions with Nursing Students

Nurses' Attitudes About Having Patients Evaluate Their Professional Work

The Nurses' Therapeutic Use of Touch as Related to the Age Factor of the Critically Ill Patient

A Study of the Health Care Needs of a Selected Population of Residents in an Urban Housing Project for the Elderly

Factors Influencing the Staff Nurses' Assessment of Possible Child Abuse

A Study of the Kindergarten Child's Knowledge and Recollections of His Recent Tonsillectomy and Adenoidectomy

A Study of Cardiac Patients' Knowledge About Their Prescribed Medications

The Development of the Role of the Pediatric Nurse Practitioner

A Study of the Anxieties of Mothers of Hospitalized Children

Medical Nurses' Attitudes Toward the Transexual Patient

Attitudes of Nurses Toward Euthanasia

Anxieties of Patients Participating in a Cardiac Rehabilitation Program

A Study of the Confidence Levels of Nurses in Handling Emergency Situations

A Study of Alcoholic Patients' Perceptions of the Role of the Nurse

Nurses' Knowledge About Occupational Health Information

A Study of Expectant Fathers' Attitudes About Participating in the Natural Childbirth Process

An Investigation of Nurses' Reactions and Participation in the Implementation of a New Bath Procedure

A Study of Nursing Students' Behavior and Motivation with Regard to Smoking Practices

Identification of the Importance Staff Nurses Place on Selected Personality Characteristics of Clinical Nursing Leaders

A Study of Nurses' Priorities in Teaching Health-related Information to Hospitalized Patients Recovering from a Cerebral Vascular Accident

Health Teaching Needs of Pregnant Diabetics

Clinical Nurses' Perceptions of the Nursing Profession

Nurses' Attitudes Toward Caring for Dying Patients: A Comparative Study of Nurses Working in an Oncology Unit and Nurses Working in Routine Medical-Surgical Units

Patients' Perceptions of Their Needs for Nursing Care After Undergoing Surgical Procedures Resulting in Drastic Changes in Body Image

APPENDIX I
Answers to Selected Problems in the Text

Chapter 10

1. Directions
    The demographic section
    Research questions
    The answering system.
2. *Mutually exclusive*: if one answer to a particular question is chosen, then another cannot be.
    Collectively exhaustive: all possible choices have been provided as answers to a particular question.
3. Many, often, unusually, fairly, occasionally, etc.
4. Personal interview
    Telephone survey
    Mailing questionnaires
    Small groups
5. How representative a sample is desired?
    How expensive is the data-gathering effort?
    What response rate is desired?

Chapter 11

1.

	Treatment A	Treatment B
Mean	$51^8/_9$	$52^1/_9$
Median	52	49
Mode	40	45

2. Mean $8.47
    Median $8.00
    Mode $8.00
    Range $5
    Standard Deviation 1.345

APPENDIX F

Problems with fractions:

1. 5/7
2. 2/5 168 children
3. 1/3
4. (a) 4 1/6 (b) 2 9/320 (c) 4 10/21 (d) 46 5/7 (e) 2 3/280 (f) 5
5. (a) 37/17 (b) 95/7 (c) 398/3 (d) 212/9 (e) 2,813/25 (f) 191/2

6. 1/4 grain
7. 3 1/3 grains
8. (a) 4/75
    (b) 77/24
    (c) 625/14
    (d) 29/24
    (d) 3 3/4
    (f) 144/165
    (g) 451/3
    (y) 1/2
    (i) 13 1/4
    (j) 5 1/8

Problems with decimals:

1. (a) .375
    (b) 7.733
    (c) .035
    (d) 4.875
    (e) 172.66
2. (a) 31.987
    (b) 2.0813
    (c) 2.0
    (d) 341.4
    (e) 150.346
3. .375 grains
4. 7.5 tablets
5. (a) 328/100,000 or 41/12,500
    (b) 65/100 or 13/20
    (c) 541/1,000
    (d) 1,755/10,000 or 351/2,000
    (d) 1/2
    (f) 601/100,000
6. (a) 395.066
    (b) 18,173,164
    (c) .03976
    (d) .6366
    (e) 1.6211
    (f) .9539
    (g) 298
    (h) 104.0051
    (i) 1,111.0888
    (j) 313.7587

Finding and using percents:

1. 14.29% is saved
2. 12 graduates
3. 33.33% increase
4. 120
5. 22.58%
6. (a)   270
    (b)   11.42%
    (c)   35.71%
7. (a)   37.5%
    (b)   44.44%
    (c)   79.166%
    (d)   14.8%
    (e)   95%

Square roots:

1. (a)   5.916
    (b)   30.854
    (c)   17.3205
    (d)   13.228
    (e)   4.242
2. (a)   6.015
    (b)   1.38
    (c)   193
    (d)   2.75

Negative numbers:

1.   −96
2.   −2 2/3
3.   73
4.   4 7/8
5.   19.2
6.   −1/6
7.   −.6857
8.   18.0167
9.   −22.2
10. 10.245

Index

Note: Page numbers in *italics* indicate figures; pages numbers followed by t indicate tables.

Abstract(s)
  definition of, 40
  of health science periodicals, *79, 80*
Alphanumeric data, 339
American Nurses' Association
  Commission on Nursing Research,
    human rights guidelines of,
    153–154
    priorities set by, 24–25
    research recommendations of,
    18–20
  commitment to research and, 22
American Statistics Index (ASI), 82
Analysis
  of collected data, 394–395, 396t–397t,
    398–399. *See also* Data, col-
    lected, analysis of
  of population sample, 256–259
  research method and, 109
Anesthesiologist, computer training of,
    315
Annotations, of article content, 76
Area of interest, in normal curve, 248–
    256

Artifacts, in research, 164
ASI, 82
Assembly language, of computer, 339
Attitude(s)
  of nurses, toward contraceptives,
    111–112
    toward dying patients, 52–62
    toward patients' "sick roles," 26–27
Attitude scales, 179, 181, *179, 180*
Audiovisual materials, indexes of, 80

Baccalaureate programs, research
    courses in, 16, 17, 18, 19
Bar graph, 287–288, *287–289*
BASIC, computer language, 346
Beehive Medical Electronic computer
    system, 299–300
Behavioral changes, in research, 33–34
Bibliographic data. *See* Data, biblio-
    graphic
Bibliography
  of computer information, 466–467
  of nursing research, 81